Comprehensive Gynecology and Obstetrics

Series Editors
Ikuo Konishi, National Kyoto Medical Center, Kyoto, Kyoto, Japan

Hidetaka Katabuchi, Department of Obstetrics and Gynecology
Kumamoto University, Kumamoto, Kumamoto, Japan

This series presents the current and future perspectives of medical science in gynecology and obstetrics. The authors fully describe the current understanding of a disease including clinical features, imaging, pathology, and molecular biology, and also include the historical aspects and theories for exploring the etiology of the disease. Also, recent developments in diagnostic strategy, medical treatment, surgery, radiotherapy, prevention, and better health-care methods are clearly shown. Thus, each volume in the series focuses on the scientific basis for the pathogenesis of a disease and provides clinical applications that make it possible to offer personalized treatment for each patient. Over the past 20 years, physicians have been working to develop a standard treatment and publish clinical guidelines for a disease based on epidemiological evidence, mainly through the use of randomized clinical trials and meta-analyses. Recently, however, comprehensive genomic and genetic analyses have revealed the differences and variations in biological characteristics even among patients with the same diagnosis and have been focusing on personalized therapy. Now all physicians and patients are entering a new world of "precision medicine" through the use of genomic evidence. We are confident that readers will greatly benefit from the contents of the series with its purview of the exciting and promising future of gynecology and obstetrics.

Daisuke Aoki
Editor

Recent Topics on Prevention, Diagnosis, and Clinical Management of Cervical Cancer

Springer

Editor
Daisuke Aoki
Akasaka Sanno Medical Center
International University of Health and Welfare Graduate School
Tokyo, Japan

ISSN 2364-1932 ISSN 2364-219X (electronic)
Comprehensive Gynecology and Obstetrics

ISBN 978-981-99-9398-7 ISBN 978-981-99-9396-3 (eBook)
https://doi.org/10.1007/978-981-99-9396-3

This Springer imprint is published by the registered company Springer Nature Singapore Pte Ltd.
The registered company address is: 152 Beach Road, #21-01/04 Gateway East, Singapore 189721, Singapore

Paper in this product is recyclable.

Contents

Part I

Pathogenesis and Epidemiology of Cervical Cancer

Recent Topics of Human Papillomavirus and Cervical Cancer

1

Iwao Kukimoto

Abstract

Human papillomavirus (HPV) infection is the leading cause of cervical cancer, resulting in a significant global disease burden. HPV consists of a large family of small DNA viruses; with a limited protein-coding capacity due to its ~8000-bp genome, HPV relies heavily on host cell proteins to support the viral life cycle, both productive and persistent phases of infection. Although the viral oncoproteins E6 and E7 (targeting TP53 and RB1, respectively) play critical roles in cervical carcinogenesis, accumulation of somatic mutations in the host genome is required for cancer progression. With regard to this latter point, APOBEC3 cytosine deaminases, which are upregulated by E6/E7, are a major mutagenic source of the HPV-related cancer genome. Moreover, deep sequencing of HPV genomes has shown high levels of variability in the viral genomic sequences in clinical specimens, and elucidated evolutionary pressures on the HPV genome. Cellular mechanisms hijacked by HPV include the intracellular transport pathways for infectious cell entry, DNA damage responses and homologous recombination repair for viral genome replication, and double-strand DNA break repair for viral integration into the host genome. These novel insights pave the way for the development of promising anti-HPV therapeutics to treat and eliminate HPV-infected lesions.

Keywords
Human papillomavirus · Cervical cancer · APOBEC3 · Replication · Integration

I. Kukimoto (✉)
Pathogen Genomics Center, National Institute of Infectious Diseases, Tokyo, Japan
e-mail: ikuki@niid.go.jp

D. Aoki (ed.), *Recent Topics on Prevention, Diagnosis, and Clinical Management of Cervical Cancer*, Comprehensive Gynecology and Obstetrics,
https://doi.org/10.1007/978-981-99-9396-3_1

1.1 Introduction

Viral infections are generally classified as either acute or persistent. The former can efficiently produce large numbers of viral progeny in a short period of time, whereas the latter allows the virus to persist or survive in the host with limited virus production for an extended period of time. Among the viruses that establish persistent infections, papillomaviruses are unique in that they target epithelial cells of the skin or mucosa and are involved in the development of a variety of diseases, from benign warts to malignant tumors, of which cervical cancer is the most representative. Disease manifestations are closely related to the viral life cycle, which is strictly regulated by the epithelial differentiation program. Since the identification of human papillomavirus (HPV) as the causative agent of cervical cancer in 1983 [1], the elucidation of viral oncogenic mechanisms has had a major impact on human tumor biology. Of particular note were the findings that the tumor suppressor proteins TP53 and RB1 are inactivated by the viral oncoproteins E6 and E7, respectively. This chapter describes recent progress in basic research focused on HPV and the mechanisms by which it drives carcinogenesis.

1.2 HPV and Cervical Cancer

Papillomaviruses (*Papillomaviridae*) are a family of small DNA viruses that are able to infect the skin and mucosa of vertebrates. The host range of the *Papillomaviridae* family is highly species specific, and papillomaviruses are named after their hosts, such as human papillomavirus (HPV). HPV has a circular double-stranded DNA genome of approximately 8000 bp, encapsulated in a non-enveloped capsid of 50–55 nm diameter. During a long history of virus-host co-evolution, HPV has acquired high levels of genetic heterogenicity. To date, more than 400 distinct genotypes have been identified based on a > 10% difference in the *L1* capsid gene sequence, and are phylogenetically classified into five genera: Alpha-, Beta-, Gamma-, Mu-, and Nu-papillomaviruses [2].

HPVs infect epithelial basal cells in either cutaneous or mucosal tissues, and around 40 genotypes of Alpha-papillomaviruses are recognized as mucosa-tropic genotypes. Mucosal HPVs are considered to be sexually transmitted, and at least 15 types (HPV16, 18, 31, 33, 35, 39, 45, 51, 52, 56, 58, 59, 68, 73, and 82) are causatively associated with the development of human malignancies, including cervical, vaginal, vulvar, anal, penile, and head-and-neck cancers, thus called "high-risk" HPVs (Fig. 1.1) [3]. Almost all cervical cancer cases are attributable to infections with high-risk HPVs. HPV16 is the most frequently detected type in cervical cancer, followed by HPV18, and the two types account for about 70% of cervical cancer cases worldwide [4]. It is estimated that high-risk HPV infection is responsible for at least 90% of anal cancers and 40% of vaginal, vulvar, and penile cancers [5]. Among mucosal HPVs, HPV6 and 11 cause condyloma acuminatum, a condition of the male and female reproductive organs, and are called "low-risk" HPVs.

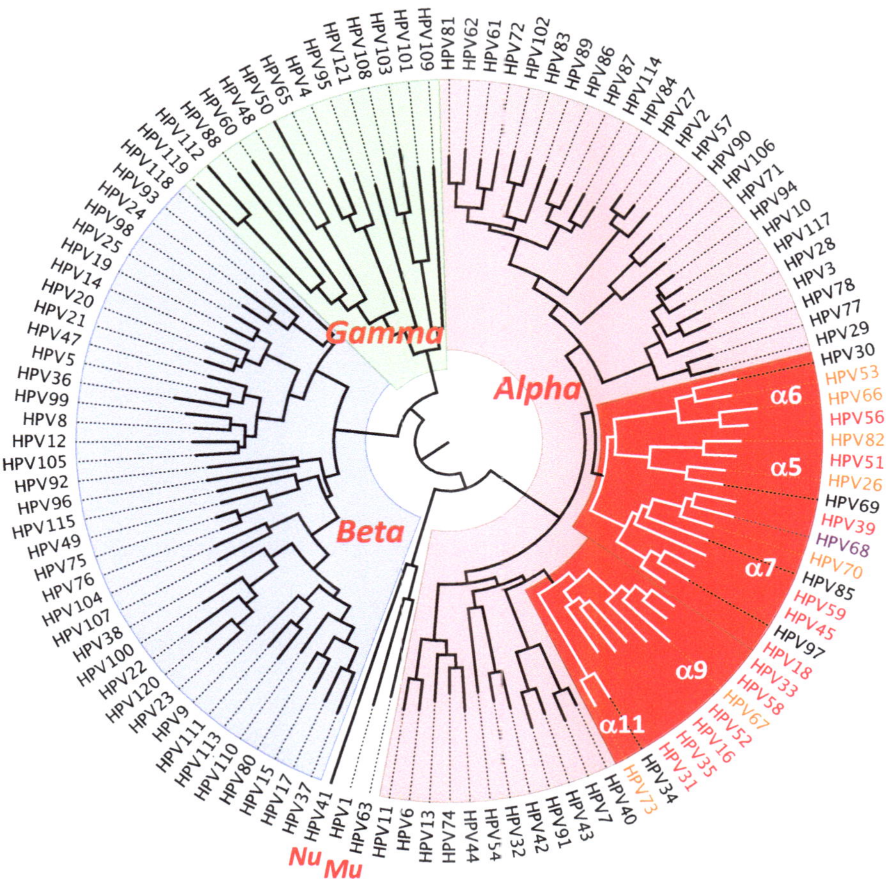

Fig. 1.1 Phylogenetic tree of 116 human papillomavirus types inferred from the nucleotide sequence of *L1*. The tree was constructed using the maximum likelihood method in RAxML-NG v.1.0.2. The clades of Alpha-, Beta-, Gamma-papillomaviruses are shown in pink (including red), blue, and green area. The high-risk types classified as carcinogenic (Group 1), probably carcinogenic (Group 2A), and possibly carcinogenic (Group 2B) are highlighted in red, purple, and orange fonts, respectively

Mucosal HPVs infect the basal cells of the genital epidermis through micro lesions and establish a state where the viral genome is maintained as a nuclear episome [6]. When the infected basal cells divide, the viral genomes also replicate and are distributed to the daughter cells, leading to persistent infection in epithelial stem cells. When the infected basal cells begin epidermal differentiation, vegetative virus replication occurs in the suprabasal layers of the epithelia, followed by production of the capsids for generating progeny virions. The transformation zone of the cervix (the border between the squamous and columnar epithelium) is a site of rapid cell proliferation and thought to be more susceptible to HPV infection. If productive

HPV infection occurs in cervical stratified epithelia, low-grade lesions called cervical intraepithelial neoplasia grade 1 (CIN1) occur, but most CIN1 lesions are cleared spontaneously by the host's immune responses. However, if HPV infection persists in the transformation zone, precancerous lesions called CIN2 are generated, and if not appropriately treated, CIN2 can further progress into CIN3, a direct precursor of invasive cervical cancer.

Most sexually active individuals become infected with high-risk HPV at some point in their lives, but only a small proportion of them become chronically infected and even fewer of these develop cancer [5]. HPV-infected cells are transformed and immortalized by the viral oncoproteins E6 and E7, but have not yet acquired malignant phenotypes such as invasive or metastatic potentials. It is generally accepted that the HPV carcinogenic process takes more than 10 years of viral persistent infection; during this period, additional mutations and/or chromosomal abnormalities accumulate in the host genome, which is prerequisite for generating invasive cervical cancer.

1.3 Cervical Cancer and APOBEC3 Cytosine Deaminase

Among various intrinsic and extrinsic factors that are responsible for introducing somatic mutations into the cancer genome, the apolipoprotein B mRNA editing catalytic polypeptide-like 3 (APOBEC3) enzymes are primary contributors to the generation of multiple types of human cancer, including breast, bladder, cervical, and head-and-neck cancers [7]. The APOBEC3 enzymes enable the innate immune response by deaminating cytosine bases in viral genomes and retroelements to restrict infection and limit retrotransposition [8]. In humans, the APOBEC3 family consists of seven members (A3A, B, C, D, F, G, and H), which are evolutionally amplified and clustered on chromosome 22. The APOBEC3 proteins convert cytosine to uracil by deamination in single-stranded DNA, resulting in C-to-T base substitutions after proper replication across a uracil base, or C-to-G base substitutions possibly caused by error-prone DNA polymerase activity at an abasic site. APOBEC3-mediated cytosine deamination preferentially occurs at motifs involving a thymine immediately 5′ to the target cytosine, referred to as the "TCW" motif, where W corresponds to an A or T [9]. Such target preference is clearly observed in single base substitution (SBS) signatures 2 and 13 from Catalogue Of Somatic Mutations In Cancer (COSMIC). These two signatures were extracted from cancer genome sequences by the negative matrix factorization method and experimentally defined for their etiologies. The high prevalence of SBS2 and SBS13 across multiple cancer genomes suggests that deamination by APOBEC3 enzymes is a frequent source of somatic mutation in human tumors [10].

Comprehensive cancer genomics studies have revealed that APOBEC3-associated mutations are responsible for many mutations of genes in HPV-associated carcinogenesis pathways, including common *PIK3CA* point mutations [11]. In HPV-positive head-and-neck and cervical cancers, mutations in *PIK3CA* are almost exclusively detected as E542K (c.1624G > A) and E545K (c.1633G > A) corresponding to a C-to-T base substitution at a TCW motif, indicative of APOBEC3-induced mutagenesis [12]. In contrast, these mutations are less frequent in HPV-negative head-and-neck cancers, suggesting that APOBEC3 activity is the major source of *PIK3CA* mutations in HPV-driven carcinogenesis. An enrichment of APOBEC3 mutations was also found in other cancer-related genes, such as *EP300*, *FBXW7*, and *PTEN* [11]. The high prevalence of APOBEC3 mutations in these cancer genomes likely reflects upregulation of APOBEC3 activity in HPV-driven cancers. Indeed, E6 induces A3B gene expression via the TEAD4 transcription factor [13, 14], and E7 stabilizes the A3A protein by inhibiting its ubiquitination-dependent proteasomal degradation [15]. A3B was originally deemed a major source of the C-to-T/G mutations that accumulate in the genomes of various human cancers. This was because A3B expression is elevated in cancer specimens and there is prominent localization of the protein in the nuclei of tumor cells [16]. However, more recent studies indicate a predominant role for A3A in cancer mutagenesis [17–19].

1.4 HPV Genomics and Evolution

HPV genome sequences are relatively stable compared to those of RNA viruses because HPV replication relies fully on host cell high-fidelity DNA polymerases. Within individual genotypes, however, HPV exhibits another level of genetic complexity, called intra-type variation, which gives rise to variants with less than 10% differences in their complete viral genome sequence [20]. In this context, 1.0–10% and 0.5–1.0% nucleotide differences are phylogenetically classified as variant lineages and sublineages, respectively. Recent large-scale genomics studies of HPV16 and HPV31 clinical isolates revealed thousands of slightly different viral genome sequences among cervical specimens [21, 22]. Such high levels of minor genetic variation are most likely the result of the long evolutionary history of virus-host interaction.

Recent advances in next-generation sequencing technologies have led to a detailed understanding of viral genetic diversity within and between infected individuals [21, 23–25]. HPV genomes within individual clinical specimens harbor a large number of minor genetic variants, the so-called within-host genomic variability. In the HPV16 genome, for example, C-to-T base substitutions predominate in these variants, clearly implicating cellular APOBEC3 cytosine deaminases in their generation (Fig. 1.2). Such a particular mutation pattern is more frequently detected in normal or low-grade specimens of the cervix [23, 26], suggesting that single-stranded DNA exposed during viral genome replication is a major target for APOBEC3-mediated deamination. However, APOBEC3 editing of the HPV genome is much less frequent than that observed with retroviruses such as human immunodeficiency virus type 1 (HIV-1), making HPV elimination by APOBEC3 highly incidental. Other prominent within-host mutations detected in HPV genomes are C-to-A and T-to-C base substitutions. The potential source of C-to-A mutations is reactive oxygen species (ROS) generated within the cell, since the most common

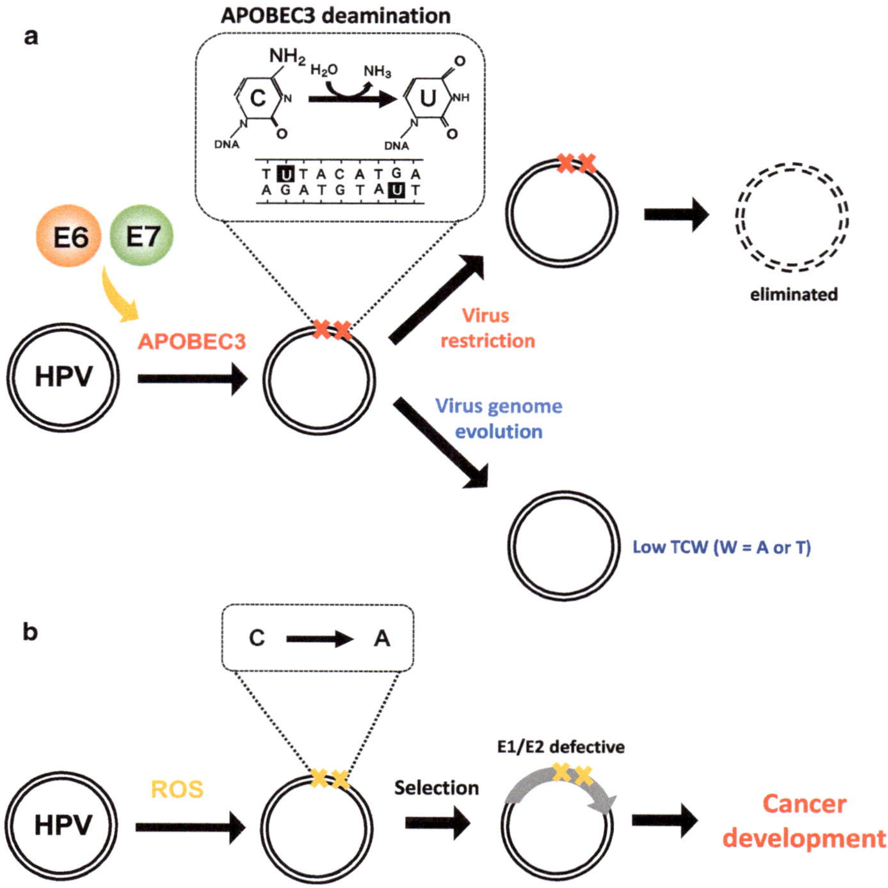

Fig. 1.2 Mechanisms of HPV genome mutagenesis. (**a**) APOBEC3, upregulated by E6/E7, is involved in editing the HPV genome in low-grade cervical lesions, and contributes to the evolution of the HPV genome. (**b**) Non-APOBEC3 mutagenesis, such as C-to-A mutations caused by reactive oxygen species (ROS), can disrupt the functions of *E1/E2*, leading to the development of cervical cancer via upregulation of *E6/E7*

type of genomic damage caused by ROS is G-to-T transversion [27]. T-to-C mutations, on the other hand, can be introduced during translesion DNA synthesis with host cell error-prone DNA polymerases, such as DNA polymerase eta, which is known to preferentially cause A-to-G transition when copying undamaged DNA [28]. Notably, E6 increases cellular ROS levels when expressed in HPV-negative cervical cancer cells [29], while E7 activates the translesion synthesis pathway in human foreskin keratinocytes [30].

Specific nucleotide variants in the HPV16 genome are enriched to relatively high levels in some malignant and precancerous samples [23, 31]. These intra-host, high-frequency mutations tend to be non-APOBEC3 mutations and are more frequently detected in viral *E1* and *E2* genes compared to other viral genomic regions [32]. *E1* encodes for a DNA helicase required for the initiation and progression of viral genome replication, whereas *E2* encodes for a DNA-binding protein that recruits the E1 helicase to the viral genome and also represses transcription of the viral promoter driving *E6*/*E7* expression. Interestingly, some of intra-host, high-frequency *E1*/*E2* mutations are mostly non-synonymous nucleotide substitutions and affect their abilities to support viral replication and transcription [32]. These observations suggest that such E1/E2 variants are positively selected for during cervical cancer progression, and that dysfunction of E1/E2 may contribute to tumorigenesis. By contrast, non-synonymous mutations in *E7* gene sequences are not found in frank cervical cancer, suggesting they are not tolerated, whereas those in low-grade cervical lesions have substantial numbers of non-synonymous substitutions. This suggests that the conservation of E7 amino acid sequences is critical for full-blown viral carcinogenesis [21].

In cervical cancer and precancerous lesions, the HPV genome is often integrated into the host genome, and is no longer able to produce progeny viruses [33]. Even without viral integration, cervical cancer/precancerous lesions containing circular HPV genomes do not generally support virion production because of the lack of epithelial differentiation in the malignant lesions. Thus, intra-host mutations in the viral genome found in malignant and premalignant specimens are not expected to contribute to viral genome evolution. On the other hand, low-grade cervical lesions like CIN1 can produce a large number of virions consisting of a cloud of variant genomes, which would be placed under evolutionary selection based on viral transmissibility and fitness costs to the host. In this regard, HPV genome sequences show characteristic dinucleotide patterns; TC and CG dinucleotides are significantly less frequent than would be expected by chance. TC depletion is likely a result of APOBEC3 editing of the viral genome during a long period of virus-host interplay [34]. In contrast, CG dinucleotides are a specific motif recognized by toll-like receptor 9 (TLR9), and might have been evolutionally reduced to avoid endosomal detection of the viral genome by TLR9 [35].

Given the antiviral activity of APOBEC3 proteins, some viruses have unique accessory proteins that effectively inhibit APOBEC3 activity [8]. Viral infectivity factor protein of HIV-1 targets A3G for proteasomal degradation [36]. Ribonucleotide reductase large subunits of Epstein–Barr virus, Kaposi's sarcoma-associated herpesvirus, and herpes simplex virus-1 directly bind, repress, and relocalize A3A and A3B to protect lytic phase viral DNA replication intermediates from APOBEC3-catalyzed deamination [37]. In sharp contrast, HPV does not encode such viral proteins that counteract APOBEC3 activity, but instead increases APOBEC3 expression via the E6 and E7 oncoproteins. The underlying reason for this may be that RB1 plays a pivotal role in the epigenetic silencing of retrotransposons embedded in the host genome [38]. Since RB1 silences retrotransposons by associating with the E2F1 transcription factor complex, the degradation of RB1 by the HPV E7 protein is predicted to cause transcription of retrotransposons such as those of the long-interspersed element-1 family. Expression of these retrotransposons would have a negative impact on the survival of HPV-infected cells because the expressed retroelements are recognized as neoantigens and targeted by adaptive immune responses. Thus, HPV-dependent increases in APOBEC3 levels and subsequent silencing of reactivated retrotransposons facilitates viral persistence in host cells.

1.5 HPV Cell Entry

HPV utilizes intracellular vesicle trafficking for infectious cell entry, thereby evading the cytoplasmic DNA sensors that trigger the innate immune response [39]. Initial attachment of HPV virions to the cell is mediated by binding of the major capsid L1 protein to heparan sulfate proteoglycan on the cell surface or within the extracellular matrix. To date, no specific entry receptor has been identified that explains the tissue specificity of HPV infection, but virions are internalized by endocytosis after proteolytic modifications of the capsid, such as cleavage of the minor capsid L2 protein by the extracellular protease furin [40]. Once internalized, virions traffic through the endosomal compartments, where L2 insertion and protrusion from the vesicular membrane is facilitated by a cell-penetrating peptide (CPP) sequence close to its C-terminus [41]. Gamma-secretase and its adaptor protein p120-catenin promote insertion of L2 into the endosome membrane [42, 43]. Membrane spanning of L2 into the cytoplasm enables the recruitment of sorting nexins, such as SNX17 and SNX27, and the trimetric retromer complex composed of Vps26, Vps29, and Vps35, to the cytosolic region of L2 [44]. These steps are critical for the retrograde trafficking of L2/viral DNA complexes from the endosome to the *trans*-Golgi network (TGN).

Recent studies employing a genetic screen with a library of short randomized hydrophobic peptides have unveiled the detailed mechanisms that underlie the retrograde transport of the L2/viral DNA complex (Fig. 1.3) [45]. The interaction of L2 with the retromer complex recruits a Rab7 GTPase-activating protein, TBC1D5, to stimulate hydrolysis of Rab7-GTP at the endosome membrane, which induces retromer disassembly from L2, thereby delivering the virus to the retrograde pathway for transport to the TGN [46]. Of note, HPV trafficking requires cycling of Rab7 between GTP- and GDP-bound forms, whereas only the GTP-bound form is required for trafficking of cellular retromer cargos, such as cation independent mannose 6-phosphate receptor and divalent metal transporter 1-II.

Intriguingly, short synthetic peptides with the retromer-binding site and CPP sequence of L2 block retromer recruitment to incoming HPV virions and inhibit viral exit from the endosome, resulting in clearance of the viral components from the cell [47]. These results strongly suggest that the retrograde transport of HPV via retromer may be a potential target for antiviral agents.

Nuclear entry of the L2/viral DNA complex requires host cell progression into mitosis and nuclear envelope breakdown [39]. Upon G2/M transition, the vesicles containing L2/viral DNA are dispersed from Golgi stacks, and L2, which penetrates the vesicle, interacts with mitotic spindle motor proteins and transports viral DNA to the pericentriolar space in prometaphase, eventually reaching the metaphase chromosomes. The viral chromosome binding is mediated by a central

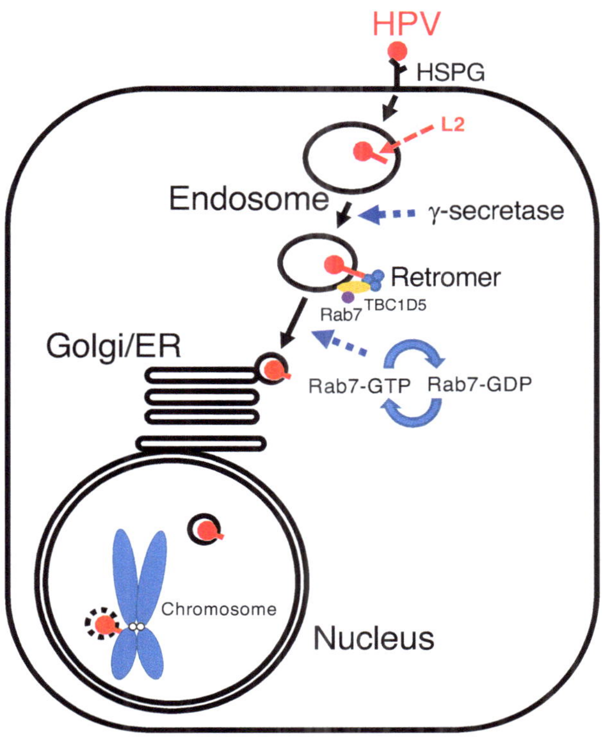

Fig. 1.3 Mechanisms of HPV cell entry. HPV virions attached to heparan sulfate proteoglycan (HSPG) on the cell surface are internalized by endocytosis, and trafficked through the endosome to the Golgi apparatus in the retrograde transport pathway. Gamma-secretase is required for protrusion of the L2 capsid protein into the endosome membrane, and the trimetric retromer complex enables the transport of the L2/viral DNA complex to the *trans*-Golgi network coupled with cycling of the Rab7 GTPase states. The L2/viral DNA complex finally reaches the metaphase chromosome during mitosis to establish infection

chromosome-binding region in L2, enabling L2-dependent chromosomal tethering of the vesicular L2/viral DNA complex during mitosis. Finally, incoming viral DNA is localized at nuclear sub-compartments, PML bodies, which are important sites that are utilized for successful infection. However, the mechanism by which this particular localization contributes to viral replication/transcription remains elusive.

1.6 HPV Replication and the Host DNA Damage Response

Activation of DNA damage response (DDR) pathways is necessary for HPV replication and differentiation-dependent amplification (Fig. 1.4) [48]. Human cells have high-fidelity DDR mechanisms to ensure the integrity of the host genome. Two major signaling pathways are engaged in DDR; one is the ataxia-telangiectasis

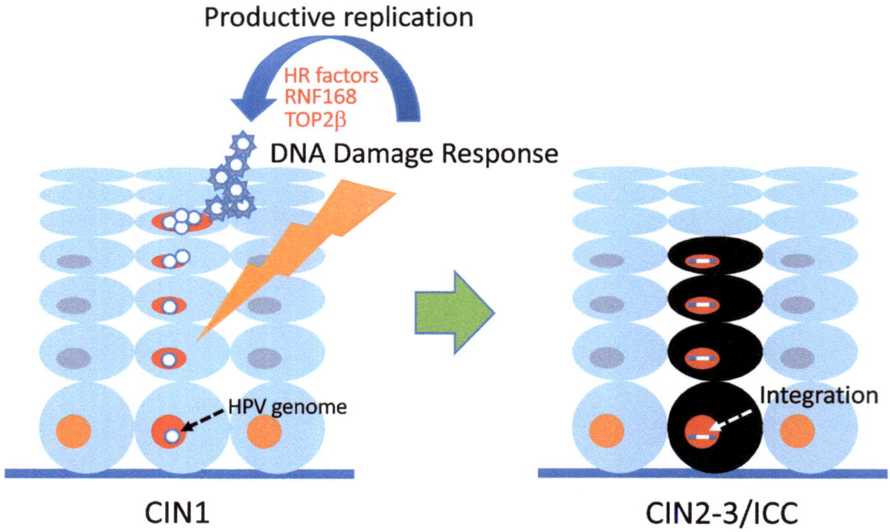

Fig. 1.4 HPV genome replication and integration in cervical lesions. In low-grade cervical lesions (CIN1), productive replication of the HPV genome requires DNA damage responses induced by viral proteins and utilizes host homologous recombination (HR) repair factors, such as RAD51 and BRCA1, E3 ubiquitin ligase RNF168, and topoisomerase 2β (TOP2β). In high-grade lesions (CIN2–3) and invasive cervical cancer (ICC), the viral genome is often integrated into the host genome losing the potential for virion production, which drives malignant transformation of infected cells

mutated kinase (ATM) pathway and the other is the ataxia-telangiectasis and RAD3-related kinase (ATR) pathway. The former is activated after DNA double-strand breaks (DSBs) and induces high-fidelity homologous recombination (HR) repair, whereas the latter is responsible for resolving DNA single-stranded breaks that occur during replication stress and fork stalling. These DDR pathways are constitutively activated by viral proteins during HPV infection, leading to the recruitment of DDR proteins to HPV episomes, and are utilized for vegetative viral replication [49]. Proteins of the DSB signaling and repair pathways, such as ATM and its substrate H2AX (γ-H2AX), the MRE11-RAD50-NBS1 complex, p53-binding protein 1 (53BP1), the breast cancer susceptibility gene 1 (BRCA1), the replication protein A, and RAD51, accumulate in nuclear structures called viral replication centers [50–52]. In particular, RAD51 and BRCA1 are absolutely necessary for HPV productive replication [53]. While HPV infection leads to constantly activated DDR, this could also impair the host genome integrity. The preferential recruitment of DDR proteins to HPV genomes can create a shortage of repair proteins and thereby lead to host genomic instability. Although E6 and E7 enhance the ability of HR proteins to form repair foci, both oncoproteins suppress HR-dependent repair by mislocalizing RAD51 from DSBs in the host genome toward the viral episomes [54]. Besides productive replication, siRNAs knockdown against the ATM and ATR pathways significantly reduced viral episomes [55], suggesting that these pathways also play a role in the maintenance of HPV episomes in infected basal cells.

A recent study has revealed a novel link between E7 from high-risk HPVs and host DSB repair [56]. E7 directly binds to RNF168, an E3 ubiquitin ligase required for proper DNA repair following DSBs, without affecting its enzymatic activity. Expression of E7 reduces the accumulation of RNF168 and its substrates at DSBs, thereby promoting HR repair, consistent with the observation that inhibition of RNF168 leads to increased repair by HR [57]. Notably, RNF168 knockdown also impairs viral genome amplification in differentiated keratinocytes, suggesting that E7 supports productive viral replication by utilizing RNF168 to increase the availability of HR factors. As RNF168 is a limiting factor during DSB repair and promotes efficient DNA replication by stabilizing replication forks in S phase [58], E7 may redirect this ubiquitin ligase to viral replication centers to facilitate the replication of its own genome. Importantly, HPV-positive cancer cells express high levels of RNF168, and accumulate high numbers of 53BP1 nuclear bodies, a marker of genomic instability induced by replication stress [56]. Given that RNF168 is essential for proper DNA repair, the hijacking of RNF168 functions by E7 suggests a novel mechanism by which HPV infection causes genomic instability and promote cancer progression.

Topoisomerase (TOP) 2β is a type II topoisomerase that induces DSBs at topologically associated domains to relieve torsional stress arising during replication and transcription. Interestingly, levels of TOP2 β are upregulated in cells containing high-risk HPV genomes, and TOP2β knockdown with short hairpin RNAs reduces DNA breaks in the cell and blocks HPV genome replication [59]. As episomal HPV genomes accumulate fewer DSBs than the host genome due to preferential recruitment of HR effector proteins to the viral genome [60], efficient HPV genome replication may require high levels of DNA breaks that are transiently induced by TOP2β and rapidly repaired by HR factors.

Another viral protein important for persistent infection is the truncated E2 protein, E8^E2, which regulates viral transcription and replication to maintain HPV persistence [61]. E8^E2 is a fusion protein of a short E8 peptide with the hinge and DNA-binding domain of E2. E8^E2 competes with full-length E2 for binding to the E2-binding sites in the viral genome and can suppress E2-dependent replication and transcriptional regulation. E8^E2 can also form heterodimers with full-length E2 proteins and inhibit E2's functions. In addition, the E8 portion of E8^E2 recruits the host nuclear co-repressor complex, NCOR/SMRT, to the HPV genome [62]. If E8^E2 is deleted, the HPV genome spontaneously enters the productive phase of its life cycle, inducing cellular DDR and inhibiting cell proliferation [63]. Thus, by suppressing the production phase, E8^E2 maintains a reservoir of viral genomes in basal cells, which is essential for persistent infection.

1.7 Novel Targets of E6/E7

As mentioned above, E6 and E7 play critical roles in driving viral carcinogenesis [64, 65]. E7 binds to and promotes the degradation of RB1, releasing the E2F transcription factors, thereby promoting S phase entry and DNA replication. High-risk E6 binds to the cellular ubiquitin ligase E6AP to form a complex that targets TP53 for proteasomal degradation, thereby blocking the apoptotic signaling that would otherwise be activated by E7. The inactivation of these tumor suppressor proteins is a major contributor to the carcinogenic potential of these oncoproteins; however, other functions of E6 and E7 are also essential for the viral life cycle and pathogenesis. Affinity purification and mass spectrometry have enabled a comprehensive survey of the cellular proteins that bind E6/E7 from alpha- and beta-HPVs [66].

The E6 proteins of the beta genus, such as HPV5 and HPV8, bind specifically to MAML1, a co-activator and effector of Notch-induced transcription [67, 68]. MAML1 forms a transcriptional activation complex that modulates expression of Notch target genes in conjunction with EP300 and CREBBP histone acetyltransferases, the RBPJ transcription factor and the intracellular domain of the Notch receptor. The association of beta-HPV E6 proteins with MAML1 inhibits Notch signaling, thereby delaying keratinocyte differentiation. Given the tumor suppressive role of the Notch pathway in skin epithelial cells, these findings implicate MAML1 in beta-HPV-driven cutaneous carcinogenesis. Interestingly, the E6-MAML1 interaction occurs via the LXXLL motif in MAML1, and the E6-E6AP interaction is also mediated via the same LXXLL motif in E6AP, suggesting that different binding partners of E6 have arisen during the evolution of alpha- and beta-HPVs, which may define their tissue tropisms for mucosal and cutaneous epithelia, respectively.

The non-receptor tyrosine phosphatase PTPN14 associates with E7 proteins from alpha- and beta-HPVs, but only high-risk HPV E7 proteins promote the proteasome-mediated degradation of PTPN14 [69, 70]. E7 binds to the C-terminal phosphatase domain of PTPN14, and the degradation of PTPN14 requires a complex formation between E7 and the ubiquitin ligase UBR4. The E7-mediated PTPN14 degradation represses keratinocyte differentiation, and PTPN14 degradation contributes to E6/E7-mediated immortalization of primary keratinocytes [71]. It has been long proposed that high-risk HPV E7 proteins exhibit transforming activity independent of RB1 inactivation, and analyses of HPV16 E7 variants revealed that E7-dependent inactivation of PTPN14 correlates with its RB1-independent activity and is thus likely an important contributor to viral oncogenesis.

E7-mediated PTPN14 degradation also enables HPV persistent infection in squamous epithelia [72]. PTPN14 interacts with YAP1, a transcriptional cofactor downstream of the Hippo signaling pathway. Here, PTPN14 functions as a tumor suppressor and blocks proliferation by promoting cytoplasmic translocation of YAP1 in a cell density-dependent manner; this does not require PTPN14 phosphatase activity. PTPN14 degradation by E7 relieves cytoplasmic retention of YAP1 and induces YAP1 nuclear translocation and YAP1-dependent transcriptional programs that extend the lifespan of primary keratinocytes, thereby contributing to the maintenance of basal cell identity. This E7 activity is critical for HPV persistence because YAP1 activation causes HPV-infected cells to be retained in the basal layer of stratified epithelia.

1.8 HPV Integration

Another important step in HPV-associated tumorigenesis is the integration of viral DNA into the host genome (Fig. 1.4) [33]. All high-risk HPVs have shown evidence of integration in cervical cancer at varying frequencies. For example, HPV integration is observed in nearly all HPV18-positive tumors, whereas 76% of HPV16-positive tumors show viral integration, indicating that viral genome integration is required for HPV18-associated tumorigenesis, but is not necessarily required for HPV16-driven malignant transformation [11]. The most common breakpoints in the viral genome are located within the *E1* and *E2* genes, and these integration events can trigger upregulation of *E6* and *E7,* because the E1/E2 proteins negatively regulate the viral LCR that drives *E6/E7* transcription [73]. In addition, *E1/E2* disruption downstream of the *E6/E7* genes may increase the stability of E6/E7 mRNAs expressed from the viral-host fusion transcripts, which likely leads to higher levels of viral oncogene expression [74].

Within the host genome, HPV integration tends to be observed in transcriptionally active regions of open chromatin rather than transcriptionally inactive heterochromatic regions, and also at or near common fragile sites [75]. Cellular genes that are frequently disrupted or amplified with HPV integration include the well-known oncogenes, *TP63* and *MYC* [75], and the tumor suppressor gene, *RAD51* [76]. Dysregulation of these genes via viral integration may confer cancer-promoting properties. Recently, a comprehensive analysis of large datasets from cervical and head-and-neck cancers revealed that integration breakpoints at HPV insertion sites were enriched in both FANCD2-associated fragile sites and enhancer-rich regions, and frequently showed adjacent focal DNA amplification [77]. The recurrent integration sites were also rich in super-enhancers, which may induce expression of cell-lineage genes. It has, therefore, been proposed that episomal HPV genomes associated with transcriptional regulatory hubs can be accidentally integrated into these regions, thereby promoting viral oncogene expression and driving carcinogenesis.

Unlike retroviruses, which encode viral integrases to allow their genomes to be actively incorporated into the host genome, HPV does not have such enzymes. Thus, HPV integration requires DNA DSBs to occur accidentally in the genomes of both host and virus, and cellular DNA repair mechanisms to recombine the host and viral DNAs. Notably, the host DNA repair pathways are dysregulated by E6 and E7, contributing to viral DNA integration. Two models are proposed for HPV integration [78]. One is a microhomology-mediated DNA repair model, in which host DNA repair mechanisms are involved in facilitating integration at regions of microhomology between the host and viral genomes near the integration site [79]. In this model, viral integration is the result of repairing DNA DSBs via microhomology-mediated DNA repair pathways. Indeed, HPV16 E7 alters DNA DSB repair pathways by promoting error-prone, microhomology-mediated end-joining [80]. The other is the "looping" model, in which the HPV genome first integrates to form a bridge between human DNA at two sites with DSBs. Then, the region containing HPV DNA forms a transient loop structure that is subsequently amplified during DNA replication, which explains the generation of various types of virus-host integrant concatemers at integration sites [81].

Recently, long-read sequencing technology has provided a more comprehensive view of large-range HPV-host integration events in cervical cancer. Employing the Nanopore sequencing platform, multiple clonal integration events, inter-chromosomal translocations, and extrachromosomal circular (ECC) virus-human hybrid structures were clearly demonstrated [82]. Of note, contrary to previous studies of HPV integration, a type of integration that lacks the *E6/E7* region was detected at high frequency, suggesting that cervical cancer can also be driven by E6/E7-independent mechanisms. Moreover, virus-human ECC DNA, which can replicate autonomously and lead to amplification of host oncogenes captured in ECC DNA, was also more prevalent than previously thought, suggesting that HPV-human ECC DNA plays an important role in driving cervical carcinogenesis [82].

1.9 Future Directions

Recent advances in basic HPV research have led to a deeper understanding of the mechanisms underlying the viral life cycle and carcinogenesis, but there are still unanswered questions. Differences in carcinogenicity between mucosal and cutaneous HPVs or between high-risk HPVs should be examined using relevant experimental systems, including three-dimensional tissue models, patient-derived xenografts in mice, and patient-derived tumor organoids [83]. It will also be important to investigate whether inhibiting APOBEC3 mutagenesis may limit tumor heterogeneity, metastasis and drug resistance in HPV-related cancer [84]. The replication of the HPV genome, both in the productive and persistent phases, requires host DDR factors, but the exact molecular mechanisms controlling these processes are not yet understood. By elucidating viral replication, it is thus hoped that new antiviral molecules can be developed to suppress the propagation of HPV in infected individuals and eliminate viral infection. As the history of successful HPV vaccine development demonstrates, basic research on HPV will continue to provide valuable insights into the underlying biological processes and contribute to realization of clinical applications for treatment of HPV-associated diseases.

References

1. Durst M, Gissmann L, Ikenberg H, Zur Hausen H. A papillomavirus DNA from a cervical carcinoma and its prevalence in cancer biopsy samples from different geographic regions. Proc Natl Acad Sci USA. 1983;80(12):3812–5.

2. McBride AA. Human papillomaviruses: diversity, infection and host interactions. Nat Rev Microbiol. 2021;20:95.
3. Munoz N, Bosch FX, de Sanjose S, Herrero R, Castellsague X, Shah KV, Snijders PJ, Meijer CJ, International Agency for Research on Cancer Multicenter Cervical Cancer Study G. Epidemiologic classification of human papillomavirus types associated with cervical cancer. N Engl J Med. 2003;348(6):518–27.
4. de Sanjose S, Quint WG, Alemany L, Geraets DT, Klaustermeier JE, Lloveras B, Tous S, Felix A, Bravo LE, Shin HR, et al. Human papillomavirus genotype attribution in invasive cervical cancer: a retrospective cross-sectional worldwide study. Lancet Oncol. 2010;11(11):1048–56.
5. Schiffman M, Doorbar J, Wentzensen N, de Sanjose S, Fakhry C, Monk BJ, Stanley MA, Franceschi S. Carcinogenic human papillomavirus infection. Nat Rev Dis Primers. 2016;2:16086.
6. Della Fera AN, Warburton A, Coursey TL, Khurana S, McBride AA. Persistent human papillomavirus infection. Viruses. 2021;13(2):321.
7. Alexandrov LB, Nik-Zainal S, Wedge DC, Aparicio SA, Behjati S, Biankin AV, Bignell GR, Bolli N, Borg A, Borresen-Dale AL, et al. Signatures of mutational processes in human cancer. Nature. 2013;500(7463):415–21.
8. Harris RS, Dudley JP. APOBECs and virus restriction. Virology. 2015;479-480:131–45.
9. Roberts SA, Lawrence MS, Klimczak LJ, Grimm SA, Fargo D, Stojanov P, Kiezun A, Kryukov GV, Carter SL, Saksena G, et al. An APOBEC cytidine deaminase mutagenesis pattern is widespread in human cancers. Nat Genet. 2013;45(9):970–6.
10. Burns MB, Temiz NA, Harris RS. Evidence for APOBEC3B mutagenesis in multiple human cancers. Nat Genet. 2013;45(9):977–83.
11. Cancer Genome Atlas Research N, Albert Einstein College of M, Analytical Biological S, Barretos Cancer H, Baylor College of M, Beckman Research Institute of City of H, Buck Institute for Research on A, Canada's Michael Smith Genome Sciences C, Harvard Medical S, Helen FGCC, et al. Integrated genomic and molecular characterization of cervical cancer. Nature. 2017;543(7645):378–84.
12. Henderson S, Chakravarthy A, Su X, Boshoff C, Fenton TR. APOBEC-mediated cytosine deamination links PIK3CA helical domain mutations to human papillomavirus-driven tumor development. Cell Rep. 2014;7(6):1833–41.
13. Vieira VC, Leonard B, White EA, Starrett GJ, Temiz NA, Lorenz LD, Lee D, Soares MA, Lambert PF, Howley PM, et al. Human papillomavirus E6 triggers upregulation of the antiviral and cancer genomic DNA deaminase APOBEC3B. MBio. 2014;5(6):e02234.
14. Mori S, Takeuchi T, Ishii Y, Yugawa T, Kiyono T, Nishina H, Kukimoto I. Human papillomavirus 16 E6 upregulates APOBEC3B via the TEAD transcription factor. J Virol. 2017;91(6):e02413.
15. Warren CJ, Xu T, Guo K, Griffin LM, Westrich JA, Lee D, Lambert PF, Santiago ML, Pyeon D. APOBEC3A functions as a restriction factor of human papillomavirus. J Virol. 2015;89(1):688–702.
16. Burns MB, Lackey L, Carpenter MA, Rathore A, Land AM, Leonard B, Refsland EW, Kotandeniya D, Tretyakova N, Nikas JB, et al. APOBEC3B is an enzymatic source of mutation in breast cancer. Nature. 2013;494(7437):366–70.
17. Chan K, Roberts SA, Klimczak LJ, Sterling JF, Saini N, Malc EP, Kim J, Kwiatkowski DJ, Fargo DC, Mieczkowski PA, et al. An APOBEC3A hypermutation signature is distinguishable from the signature of background mutagenesis by APOBEC3B in human cancers. Nat Genet. 2015;47(9):1067–72.
18. Law EK, Levin-Klein R, Jarvis MC, Kim H, Argyris PP, Carpenter MA, Starrett GJ, Temiz NA, Larson LK, Durfee C, et al. APOBEC3A catalyzes mutation and drives carcinogenesis in vivo. J Exp Med. 2020;217(12):e20200261.
19. Petljak M, Dananberg A, Chu K, Bergstrom EN, Striepen J, von Morgen P, Chen Y, Shah H, Sale JE, Alexandrov LB, et al. Mechanisms of APOBEC3 mutagenesis in human cancer cells. Nature. 2022;607(7920):799–807.
20. Burk RD, Harari A, Chen Z. Human papillomavirus genome variants. Virology. 2013;445(1–2):232–43.

21. Mirabello L, Yeager M, Yu K, Clifford GM, Xiao Y, Zhu B, Cullen M, Boland JF, Wentzensen N, Nelson CW, et al. HPV16 E7 genetic conservation is critical to carcinogenesis. Cell. 2017;170(6):1164–1174.e1166.
22. Pinheiro M, Harari A, Schiffman M, Clifford GM, Chen Z, Yeager M, Cullen M, Boland JF, Raine-Bennett T, Steinberg M, et al. Phylogenomic analysis of human papillomavirus type 31 and cervical carcinogenesis: a study of 2093 viral genomes. Viruses. 2021;13(10):1948.
23. Hirose Y, Onuki M, Tenjimbayashi Y, Mori S, Ishii Y, Takeuchi T, Tasaka N, Satoh T, Morisada T, Iwata T, et al. Within-host variations of human papillomavirus reveal APOBEC signature mutagenesis in the viral genome. J Virol. 2018;92(12):e00017.
24. Dube Mandishora RS, Gjotterud KS, Lagstrom S, Stray-Pedersen B, Duri K, Chin'ombe N, Nygard M, Christiansen IK, Ambur OH, Chirenje MZ, et al. Intra-host sequence variability in human papillomavirus. Papillomavirus Res. 2018;5:180–91.
25. Lagstrom S, van der Weele P, Rounge TB, Christiansen IK, King AJ, Ambur OH. HPV16 whole genome minority variants in persistent infections from young Dutch women. J Clin Virol. 2019;119:24–30.
26. Zhu B, Xiao Y, Yeager M, Clifford G, Wentzensen N, Cullen M, Boland JF, Bass S, Steinberg MK, Raine-Bennett T, et al. Mutations in the HPV16 genome induced by APOBEC3 are associated with viral clearance. Nat Commun. 2020;11(1):886.
27. Kuchino Y, Mori F, Kasai H, Inoue H, Iwai S, Miura K, Ohtsuka E, Nishimura S. Misreading of DNA templates containing 8-hydroxydeoxyguanosine at the modified base and at adjacent residues. Nature. 1987;327(6117):77–9.
28. Matsuda T, Bebenek K, Masutani C, Hanaoka F, Kunkel TA. Low fidelity DNA synthesis by human DNA polymerase-eta. Nature. 2000;404(6781):1011–3.
29. Cruz-Gregorio A, Manzo-Merino J, Gonzalez-Garcia MC, Pedraza-Chaverri J, Medina-Campos ON, Valverde M, Rojas E, Rodriguez-Sastre MA, Garcia-Cuellar CM, Lizano M. Human papillomavirus types 16 and 18 early-expressed proteins differentially modulate the cellular redox state and DNA damage. Int J Biol Sci. 2018;14(1):21–35.
30. Wendel SO, Stoltz A, Xu X, Snow JA, Wallace N. HPV 16 E7 alters translesion synthesis signaling. Virol J. 2022;19(1):165.
31. van der Weele P, King AJ, Meijer C, Steenbergen RDM. HPV16 variant analysis in primary and recurrent CIN2/3 lesions demonstrates presence of the same consensus variant. Papillomavirus Res. 2019;7:168–72.
32. Hirose Y, Yamaguchi-Naka M, Onuki M, Tenjimbayashi Y, Tasaka N, Satoh T, Tanaka K, Iwata T, Sekizawa A, Matsumoto K, et al. High levels of within-host variations of human papillomavirus 16 E1/E2 genes in invasive cervical cancer. Front Microbiol. 2020;11:596334.
33. McBride AA, Warburton A. The role of integration in oncogenic progression of HPV-associated cancers. PLoS Pathog. 2017;13(4):e1006211.
34. Warren CJ, Van Doorslaer K, Pandey A, Espinosa JM, Pyeon D. Role of the host restriction factor APOBEC3 on papillomavirus evolution. Virus Evol. 2015;1(1):vev015.
35. King KM, Rajadhyaksha EV, Tobey IG, Van Doorslaer K. Synonymous nucleotide changes drive papillomavirus evolution. Tumour Virus Res. 2022;14:200248.
36. Simon V, Bloch N, Landau NR. Intrinsic host restrictions to HIV-1 and mechanisms of viral escape. Nat Immunol. 2015;16(6):546–53.
37. Cheng AZ, Moraes SN, Shaban NM, Fanunza E, Bierle CJ, Southern PJ, Bresnahan WA, Rice SA, Harris RS. APOBECs and herpesviruses. Viruses. 2021;13(3):390.
38. Wallace NA, Munger K. The curious case of APOBEC3 activation by cancer-associated human papillomaviruses. PLoS Pathog. 2018;14(1):e1006717.
39. Ozbun MA, Campos SK. The long and winding road: human papillomavirus entry and subcellular trafficking. Curr Opin Virol. 2021;50:76–86.
40. Richards RM, Lowy DR, Schiller JT, Day PM. Cleavage of the papillomavirus minor capsid protein, L2, at a furin consensus site is necessary for infection. Proc Natl Acad Sci U S A. 2006;103(5):1522–7.

41. Zhang P, Monteiro da Silva G, Deatherage C, Burd C, DiMaio D. Cell-penetrating peptide mediates intracellular membrane passage of human papillomavirus L2 protein to trigger retrograde trafficking. Cell. 2018;174(6):1465–1476.e1413.
42. Inoue T, Zhang P, Zhang W, Goodner-Bingham K, Dupzyk A, DiMaio D, Tsai B. Gamma-secretase promotes membrane insertion of the human papillomavirus L2 capsid protein during virus infection. J Cell Biol. 2018;217(10):3545–59.
43. Harwood MC, Dupzyk AJ, Inoue T, DiMaio D, Tsai B. p120 catenin recruits HPV to gamma-secretase to promote virus infection. PLoS Pathog. 2020;16(10):e1008946.
44. Xie J, Zhang P, Crite M, DiMaio D. Papillomaviruses Go Retro. Pathogens. 2020;9(4):267.
45. Xie J, Zhang P, Crite M, Lindsay CV, DiMaio D. Retromer stabilizes transient membrane insertion of L2 capsid protein during retrograde entry of human papillomavirus. Sci Adv. 2021;7(27):eabh4276.
46. Xie J, Heim EN, Crite M, DiMaio D. TBC1D5-catalyzed cycling of Rab7 is required for Retromer-mediated human papillomavirus trafficking during virus entry. Cell Rep. 2020;31(10):107750.
47. Zhang P, Moreno R, Lambert PF, DiMaio D. Cell-penetrating peptide inhibits retromer-mediated human papillomavirus trafficking during virus entry. Proc Natl Acad Sci U S A. 2020;117(11):6121–8.
48. Anacker DC, Moody CA. Modulation of the DNA damage response during the life cycle of human papillomaviruses. Virus Res. 2017;231:41–9.
49. Spriggs CC, Laimins LA. Human papillomavirus and the DNA damage response: exploiting host repair pathways for viral replication. Viruses. 2017;9(8):232.
50. Moody CA, Laimins LA. Human papillomaviruses activate the ATM DNA damage pathway for viral genome amplification upon differentiation. PLoS Pathog. 2009;5(10):e1000605.
51. Gillespie KA, Mehta KP, Laimins LA, Moody CA. Human papillomaviruses recruit cellular DNA repair and homologous recombination factors to viral replication centers. J Virol. 2012;86(17):9520–6.
52. Anacker DC, Gautam D, Gillespie KA, Chappell WH, Moody CA. Productive replication of human papillomavirus 31 requires DNA repair factor Nbs1. J Virol. 2014;88(15):8528–44.
53. Chappell WH, Gautam D, Ok ST, Johnson BA, Anacker DC, Moody CA. Homologous recombination repair factors Rad51 and BRCA1 are necessary for productive replication of human papillomavirus 31. J Virol. 2015;90(5):2639–52.
54. Wallace NA, Khanal S, Robinson KL, Wendel SO, Messer JJ, Galloway DA. High-risk Alphapapillomavirus oncogenes impair the homologous recombination pathway. J Virol. 2017;91(20):e01084.
55. Edwards TG, Helmus MJ, Koeller K, Bashkin JK, Fisher C. Human papillomavirus episome stability is reduced by aphidicolin and controlled by DNA damage response pathways. J Virol. 2013;87(7):3979–89.
56. Sitz J, Blanchet SA, Gameiro SF, Biquand E, Morgan TM, Galloy M, Dessapt J, Lavoie EG, Blondeau A, Smith BC, et al. Human papillomavirus E7 oncoprotein targets RNF168 to hijack the host DNA damage response. Proc Natl Acad Sci U S A. 2019;116(39):19552–62.
57. Hustedt N, Durocher D. The control of DNA repair by the cell cycle. Nat Cell Biol. 2016;19(1):1–9.
58. Schmid JA, Berti M, Walser F, Raso MC, Schmid F, Krietsch J, Stoy H, Zwicky K, Ursich S, Freire R, et al. Histone ubiquitination by the DNA damage response is required for efficient DNA replication in unperturbed S phase. Mol Cell. 2018;71(6):897–910.e898.
59. Kaminski P, Hong S, Kono T, Hoover P, Laimins L. Topoisomerase 2beta induces DNA breaks to regulate human papillomavirus replication. MBio. 2021;12(1):e00005.
60. Mehta K, Laimins L. Human papillomaviruses preferentially recruit DNA repair factors to viral genomes for rapid repair and amplification. MBio. 2018;9(1):e00064.
61. Kuehner F, Stubenrauch F. Functions of papillomavirus E8;E2 proteins in tissue culture and in vivo. Viruses. 2022;14(5):953.

62. Dreer M, Fertey J, van de Poel S, Straub E, Madlung J, Macek B, Iftner T, Stubenrauch F. Interaction of NCOR/SMRT repressor complexes with papillomavirus E8;E2C proteins inhibits viral replication. PLoS Pathog. 2016;12(4):e1005556.
63. Straub E, Dreer M, Fertey J, Iftner T, Stubenrauch F. The viral E8;E2C repressor limits productive replication of human papillomavirus 16. J Virol. 2014;88(2):937–47.
64. Vande Pol SB, Klingelhutz AJ. Papillomavirus E6 oncoproteins. Virology. 2013;445(1–2):115–37.
65. Roman A, Munger K. The papillomavirus E7 proteins. Virology. 2013;445(1–2):138–68.
66. White EA, Howley PM. Proteomic approaches to the study of papillomavirus-host interactions. Virology. 2013;435(1):57–69.
67. Brimer N, Lyons C, Wallberg AE, Vande Pol SB. Cutaneous papillomavirus E6 oncoproteins associate with MAML1 to repress transactivation and NOTCH signaling. Oncogene. 2012;31(43):4639–46.
68. Tan MJ, White EA, Sowa ME, Harper JW, Aster JC, Howley PM. Cutaneous beta-human papillomavirus E6 proteins bind mastermind-like coactivators and repress notch signaling. Proc Natl Acad Sci U S A. 2012;109(23):E1473–80.
69. White EA, Munger K, Howley PM. High-risk human papillomavirus E7 proteins target PTPN14 for degradation. MBio. 2016;7(5):e01530.
70. Szalmas A, Tomaic V, Basukala O, Massimi P, Mittal S, Konya J, Banks L. The PTPN14 tumor suppressor is a degradation target of human papillomavirus E7. J Virol. 2017;91(7):e00057.
71. Hatterschide J, Bohidar AE, Grace M, Nulton TJ, Kim HW, Windle B, Morgan IM, Munger K, White EA. PTPN14 degradation by high-risk human papillomavirus E7 limits keratinocyte differentiation and contributes to HPV-mediated oncogenesis. Proc Natl Acad Sci U S A. 2019;116(14):7033–42.
72. Hatterschide J, Castagnino P, Kim HW, Sperry SM, Montone KT, Basu D, White EA. YAP1 activation by human papillomavirus E7 promotes basal cell identity in squamous epithelia. elife. 2022;11:11.
73. Romanczuk H, Howley PM. Disruption of either the E1 or the E2 regulatory gene of human papillomavirus type 16 increases viral immortalization capacity. Proc Natl Acad Sci U S A. 1992;89(7):3159–63.
74. Jeon S, Lambert PF. Integration of human papillomavirus type 16 DNA into the human genome leads to increased stability of E6 and E7 mRNAs: implications for cervical carcinogenesis. Proc Natl Acad Sci U S A. 1995;92(5):1654–8.
75. Bodelon C, Untereiner ME, Machiela MJ, Vinokurova S, Wentzensen N. Genomic characterization of viral integration sites in HPV-related cancers. Int J Cancer. 2016;139(9):2001–11.
76. Parfenov M, Pedamallu CS, Gehlenborg N, Freeman SS, Danilova L, Bristow CA, Lee S, Hadjipanayis AG, Ivanova EV, Wilkerson MD, et al. Characterization of HPV and host genome interactions in primary head and neck cancers. Proc Natl Acad Sci U S A. 2014;111(43):15544–9.
77. Warburton A, Markowitz TE, Katz JP, Pipas JM, McBride AA. Recurrent integration of human papillomavirus genomes at transcriptional regulatory hubs. NPJ Genom Med. 2021;6(1):101.
78. Porter VL, Marra MA. The drivers, mechanisms, and consequences of genome instability in HPV-driven cancers. Cancers (Basel). 2022;14(19):4623.
79. Hu Z, Zhu D, Wang W, Li W, Jia W, Zeng X, Ding W, Yu L, Wang X, Wang L, et al. Genome-wide profiling of HPV integration in cervical cancer identifies clustered genomic hot spots and a potential microhomology-mediated integration mechanism. Nat Genet. 2015;47(2):158–63.
80. Leeman JE, Li Y, Bell A, Hussain SS, Majumdar R, Rong-Mullins X, Blecua P, Damerla R, Narang H, Ravindran PT, et al. Human papillomavirus 16 promotes microhomology-mediated end-joining. Proc Natl Acad Sci U S A. 2019;116(43):21573–9.
81. Akagi K, Li J, Broutian TR, Padilla-Nash H, Xiao W, Jiang B, Rocco JW, Teknos TN, Kumar B, Wangsa D, et al. Genome-wide analysis of HPV integration in human cancers reveals recurrent, focal genomic instability. Genome Res. 2014;24(2):185–99.

82. Zhou L, Qiu Q, Zhou Q, Li J, Yu M, Li K, Xu L, Ke X, Xu H, Lu B, et al. Long-read sequencing unveils high-resolution HPV integration and its oncogenic progression in cervical cancer. Nat Commun. 2022;13(1):2563.
83. Lohmussaar K, Oka R, Espejo Valle-Inclan J, Smits MHH, Wardak H, Korving J, Begthel H, Proost N, van de Ven M, Kranenburg OW, et al. Patient-derived organoids model cervical tissue dynamics and viral oncogenesis in cervical cancer. Cell Stem Cell. 2021;28(8):1380–1396.e1386.
84. Swanton C, McGranahan N, Starrett GJ, Harris RS. APOBEC enzymes: mutagenic fuel for cancer evolution and heterogeneity. Cancer Discov. 2015;5(7):704–12.

Recent Epidemiologic Trends in Cervical Cancer

2

Satoyo Hosono

Abstract

Understanding the recent global pattern and trends in cervical cancer burden could enable us to prevent and control this condition.

First, we reviewed cervical cancer incidence and mortality according to the human development index (HDI) and geographical region. More than 80% of cancer cases and deaths occurred in areas with a lower or middle level of development. In addition, a remarkable geographic contrast in cervical cancer burden was observed. The highest incidence and mortality were observed in Eastern, Southern and Middle Africa, due to a lack of awareness of disease symptoms, limited access to appropriate prevention and medical services, and the concomitant human immunodeficiency virus (HIV) epidemic in this region.

Next, we reviewed sexual behavior, immunodeficiency disorders owing to HIV infection, history of sexually transmitted infection, tobacco smoking, endogenous and exogenous hormonal factors as risk factors associated with acquiring human papillomavirus (HPV) infection, and impaired immune response to HPV infection and progression of cervical intraepithelial neoplasia (CIN). Although HPV is a main etiological factor in cervical carcinogenesis, the noteworthy geographic contrast might also be attributable to exposure to these risk factors and inequalities in access to the healthcare system.

Eliminating cervical cancer requires—in addition to HPV vaccination, screening and treatment—consideration of lifestyle modification, including tobacco control, sexual education, and HIV control.

S. Hosono (✉)
Division of Cancer Screening Assessment and Management, Institute for Cancer Control, National Cancer Center, Tokyo, Japan
e-mail: shosono@ncc.go.jp

D. Aoki (ed.), *Recent Topics on Prevention, Diagnosis, and Clinical Management of Cervical Cancer*, Comprehensive Gynecology and Obstetrics,
https://doi.org/10.1007/978-981-99-9396-3_2

Keywords

Descriptive epidemiology · Human development index · Tobacco smoking · Sex hormonal factor · Human immunodeficiency virus

2.1 Introduction

Worldwide in 2008, an estimated 530,000 women developed cervical cancer and 275,000 women died of it, making it the third- and fourth-most common cause of female cancer incidence and mortality, respectively [1]. The knowledge that persistent human papillomavirus (HPV) infection is the major cause of cervical cancer spread widely in the 2000s. In particular, HPV type 16 and 18 are responsible for 71% of cervical cancers globally [2]. In consequence, prophylactic vaccines to prevent HPV infection and HPV assays were developed from the 2000s to 2010s. Despite recent advances in prophylactic HPV vaccines, and in screening, diagnosis and treatment, however, the number of cervical cancer cases and deaths continues to increase. In 2020, 604,000 cases and 342,000 deaths from cervical cancer were estimated worldwide, with about 88% of cases occurring in low-income and middle-income countries [3]. The increasing trend might be attributed to other environmental risk factors or inequality of access to healthcare systems, in addition to global aging and growing population.

In this chapter, we describe the current global pattern and trend in cervical cancer incidence and mortality. In particularly, we focus on risk factors related to HPV infection, such as high-risk sexual behavior [4, 5], human immunodeficiency virus (HIV) infection [6, 7], infection with other sexually transmitted diseases [8, 9], tobacco smoking [10], and endogenous and exogenous hormonal factors [11, 12].

2.2 Worldwide Estimate of Incidence and Mortality of Cervical Cancer

Table 2.1 illustrates the estimated number of incident cases and deaths of cervical cancer (ICD-10 code C53), the age-standardized incidence rate (ASIR) and age-standardized mortality rate (ASMR) using the world standard population in 2020, including the cumulative incidence and mortality rate. In addition, comparisons across the 4-tier Human Development Index (HDI, very high, high, middle, and low) defined by the United Nations Development Programme [13] and 21 predefined world regions [14] were conducted. These data were extracted from the Global Cancer Observatory (GLOBOCAN) database by the International Agency for Research on Cancer (IARC) [3].

In 2020, approximately 604,000 cases and 342,000 deaths from cervical cancer were estimated worldwide. All-age ASIR and ASMR was 13.3 and 7.3 per 100,000, respectively (Table 2.1). Among female malignancies, cervical cancer is the

Table 2.1 Estimated cervical cancer incidence and mortality in 2020 and human papillomavirus prevalence by HDI tier and subcontinent

	Number of cases	ASIR (/10[5] women)	CIR (%)	Rank (all ages)	Number of deaths	ASMR (/10[5] women)	CMR	Rank (all ages)	HPV prevalence (%) (95% CI) (ref. [16])
World	604,127	13.3	1.8	4	341,831	7.3	1.2	6	11.7 (11.6–11.7)
HDI level									
Very high	98,675	9.1	1.1		42,920	3.1	0.56		
High	240,400	12.7	1.7		129,444	6.5	1.2		
Medium	182,866	16.5	2.7		113,149	10.4	2		
Low	81,922	27.2	4.1		56,167	19.8	3.4		
World region									
Eastern Africa	54,560	40.1	5.7		36,497	28.6	4.6		33.6 (30.2–37.1)
Middle Africa	15,646	31.6	5		10,572	22.7	4.1		
Northern Africa	6971	6.3	1.1		4033	3.7	0.78		9.2 (7.3–11.3)
Southern Africa	12,333	36.4	5.7		6867	20.6	3.6		17.4 (15.9–18.9)
Western Africa	27,806	22.9	3.8		18,776	16.6	3.2		19.6 (18.5–20.8)
Caribbean	3857	13.7	2.3		2495	8.2	1.8		35.4 (29.0–42.2)
Central America	13,848	13.8	2.2		6866	6.8	1.4		13.0 (12.6–13.5)
Northern America	14,971	6.1	0.72		6343	2.1	0.36		4.7 (4.6–4.7)
South America	41,734	15.4	2.3		22,221	7.8	1.5		15.3 (14.7–15.8)
Eastern Asia	129,567	10.8	1.3		66,435	4.9	0.82		10.7 (10.4–10.9)
South-Central Asia	148,128	15.3	2.6		91,985	9.6	1.9		7.1 (6.7–7.4)
South-eastern Asia	68,623	17.8	2.7		38,530	10	2		14.0 (13.0–15.0)
Western Asia	5402	4.1	0.69		2951	2.3	0.49		1.7 (1.1–2.5)
Central and Eastern Europe	32,348	14.5	1.7		15,854	6.1	0.92		21.4 (20.1–22.7)
Northern Europe	6666	10.4	1.1		2134	2.2	0.42		10.0 (9.8–10.2)
Southern Europe	9053	7.7	0.93		3705	2.3	0.42		8.8 (8.5–9.0)

(continued)

Table 2.1 (continued)

	Number of cases	ASIR (/10^5 women)	CIR (%)	Rank (all ages)	Number of deaths	ASMR (/10^5 women)	CMR	Rank (all ages)	HPV prevalence (%) (95% CI) (ref. [16])
Western Europe	10,102	7	0.88		4296	2	0.41		9.0 (8.8–9.2)
Australia and New Zealand	1094	5.6	0.63		409	1.6	0.32		
Melanesia	1330	28.3	4.2		818	18.6	3.6		
Micronesia	53	18.7	2.8		24	8.2	2.1		
Polynesia	35	9.7	1.2		19	5.3	0.68		

ASIR age-standardized incidence rate, *CIR* cumulative incidence rate, *ASMR* age-standardized mortality rate, *CMR* cumulative moratlity rate, *HPV* human papillomavirus, *95% CI* 95% confidence interval, *HDI* human development index

fourth- and third-most common by incidence and mortality. Lifetime cumulative incidence rate (CIR) and mortality rate (CMR) in that year were 1.8% and 1.2%, meaning that one in 55.6 women developed cervical cancer in their lifetime and one in 83.3 women died from it (Table 2.1). The distribution of cervical cancer varies widely, according to HDI and world region.

2.2.1 Cervical Cancer Incidence and Mortality by the 4-Tier HDI

HDI is a summary measure of average achievement in key dimensions of human development: a health dimension measured by life expectancy at birth, an education dimension by mean of years of schooling for adults and expected years of schooling for children of school entry age, and a standard of living dimension by gross national income per capita. The HDI is a geometric mean of normalized indices for each of the three dimensions [13], and can therefore indicate the average socioeconomic development of each country. Here, the pattern of cervical cancer incidence and mortality was compared between the four HDI tiers (very high, high, middle, and low). Countries in the low and middle HDI tiers are located mainly in Eastern Africa, Middle Africa, Southern Africa, and Southern Asia.

As given in Table 2.1, the distribution of cervical cancer varies widely according to HDI tier. Approximately 19.5% of all cervical cancer cases and 14.4% of cervical cancer deaths occurred in the very high HDI category, while the rest of the global burden falls in areas with lower and middle levels of development. ASIR and ASMR increase with decreasing HDI tier, from 9.1 and 3.1 per 100,000 in countries in the very high HDI tier to 27.2 and 19.8 per 100,000 in countries in the low HDI tier, respectively. Lin et al. also reported a significant inverse correlation between HDI and cervical cancer incidence and mortality [15]. In addition, CIR and CMR also increased with decreasing HDI tier, from 1.1% and 0.56% in countries in the very high tier to 4.1% and 3.4% in those in the low tier, respectively.

2.2.2 Cervical Cancer Incidence and Mortality by Geographical Region

GLOBOCAN provides cervical cancer incidence data across 21 subcontinents, as given in Table 2.1. The different distribution in incidence and mortality are more evident when the focus is on subcontinents. African countries are grouped in five subcontinents: Eastern, Middle, Northern, Southern, and Western Africa. The highest incidence and mortality were observed in the East African subcontinent (40.1 and 28.6 per 100,000), followed in order by the Southern (36.4 and 20.6) and Middle African subcontinents (31.6 and 22.7; all respectively). Sub-Saharan Africa had among the highest HPV infection prevalence [16]. The high incidence and mortality of cervical cancer in sub-Saharan Africa is not unexpected, given the high rates of HPV and HIV infection, as well as the aging, population growth, lack of awareness of disease symptoms, and limited access to appropriate prevention and medical services in this region. Conversely, the incidence of cervical cancer is relatively low in the mainly Muslim countries of Northern Africa. These populations are considered to have more conservative sexual behavior, and the prevalence of HPV is accordingly low [17]. In the Caribbean, South America and Asia, the ASIR and ASMR of cervical cancer were relatively high. There are many low to high HDI countries in these regions, and cervical cancer screening programs are lacking or insufficient [18]. Non-existent or insufficient screening programs and limited access to adequate medical care have led to a majority cases being detected in the advanced stages of disease, and mortality in these regions is consequently higher.

2.2.3 Time Trends in Cervical Cancer Incidence and Mortality

Here, we focus on recent trends in cervical cancer worldwide, and the impact of screening together with other factors that influence cervical cancer risk. The eight selected countries are in the high or very high HDI tier (Table 2.2). Figure 2.1 shows the temporal trends in cervical cancer incidence and mortality from 1999 to 2018 among these eight countries, using the most recent data from GLOBOCAN [3] and Cancer Incidence in Five Continents Time Trends [19]. The ASIRs of Brazil, Republic of Korea, and Slovenia have been decreasing over this period (Fig. 2.1a, d, f). In contrast, the ASIRs of the USA, United Kingdom, Netherlands, and Australia have leveled off or are decreasing (Fig. 2.1b, e, g, h). As given in Table 2.2, the average annual percent change (AAPC) in cervical cancer was indicates the direction and magnitude of recent trends in the incidence and mortality in each population. Slovenia (−6.6% per year), Brazil (−6.1% per year), Republic of Korea (−4.8% per year) and the USA (−1.2% per year) showed significant decreasing trends in incidence. Although the AAPCs of Netherlands and United Kingdom were significant (both 1.7% per year), the magnitude of this increasing trend was relatively small. In contrast again, Japan showed a significant increasing trend from 2003 to 2012 (4.2% per year). Regarding mortality, Australia (−5.0%), Republic of Korea (−4.5% per year), Slovenia (−2.5% per year), United Kingdom (−2.1% per year), Netherlands

Table 2.2 The average annual percent change (AAPC) in cervical cancer incidence and mortality and cancer prevention by country

	HDI Tier[a]	AAPC in incidence (ref. [15])	AAPC in mortality (ref. [15])	Start year of HPV vaccination[b]	Type of screening[a]	Start year[a]	Target age[a]	Screening method[a]	Participation rate (%)
South America									
Brazil	High	−6.1[c] (2003–2012)	0.1 (2008–2017)	2014	Organized	1988	25–64	Cytology	NA
Northern America									
United States of America	Very high	−1.2[c] (2003–2012)	−0.6[c] (2008–2017)	2006	Organized/ opportunistic	–	21–65 30–65 30–65	Cytology HPV HPV and cytology co-testing	72.6 (2020, S[e])
Asia									
Japan	Very high	4.2[c] (2003–2012)	0.5[c] (2008–2017)	2011	Organized	1983	20+	Cytology	43.7 (2019, S[e])
Republic of Korea	Very high	−4.8[c] (2003–2012)	−4.5[c] (2008–2017)	2016	Organized	2002	20+	Cytology	57 (2020, P[d])
Nothern Europe									
United Kingdom	Very high	1.7[c] (2003–2012)	−2.1[c] (2007–2016)	2008	Organized	1988 2017	20–64 25–64	Cytology HPV	74.4 (2019, P[d])
Southern Europe									
Slovenia	Very high	−6.6[c] (2003–2012)	−2.5[c] (2008–2017)	2009	Organized	2003	20–64	Cytology	71.7 (2021, P[d])
Western Europe									
Netherlands	Very high	1.7[c] (2003–2012)	−1.8[c] (2008–2017)	2010	Organized	1970 2017	30–60 30–60	Cytology HPV	49.7 (2020, P[d])
Oceania									
Australia	Very high	0.7 (2003–2012)	−5.0[c] (2008–2017)	2007	Organized	1991 2017	20–69 25–74	Cytology HPV	55.7 (2020, P[d])

[a]IARC. CanScreen5. https://canscreen5.iarc.fr/
[b]WHO. Cervical cancer country profiles (2021). https://www.who.int/publications/m/item/cervical-cancer-country-profiles
[c]Statistically significant difference
[d]Participation rate from programme data (OECD, Health Statistics 2022, https://www.oecd.org/els/health-systems/health-data.htm)
[e]Participation rate from survey data (OECD, Health Statistics 2022, https://www.oecd.org/els/health-systems/health-data.htm)

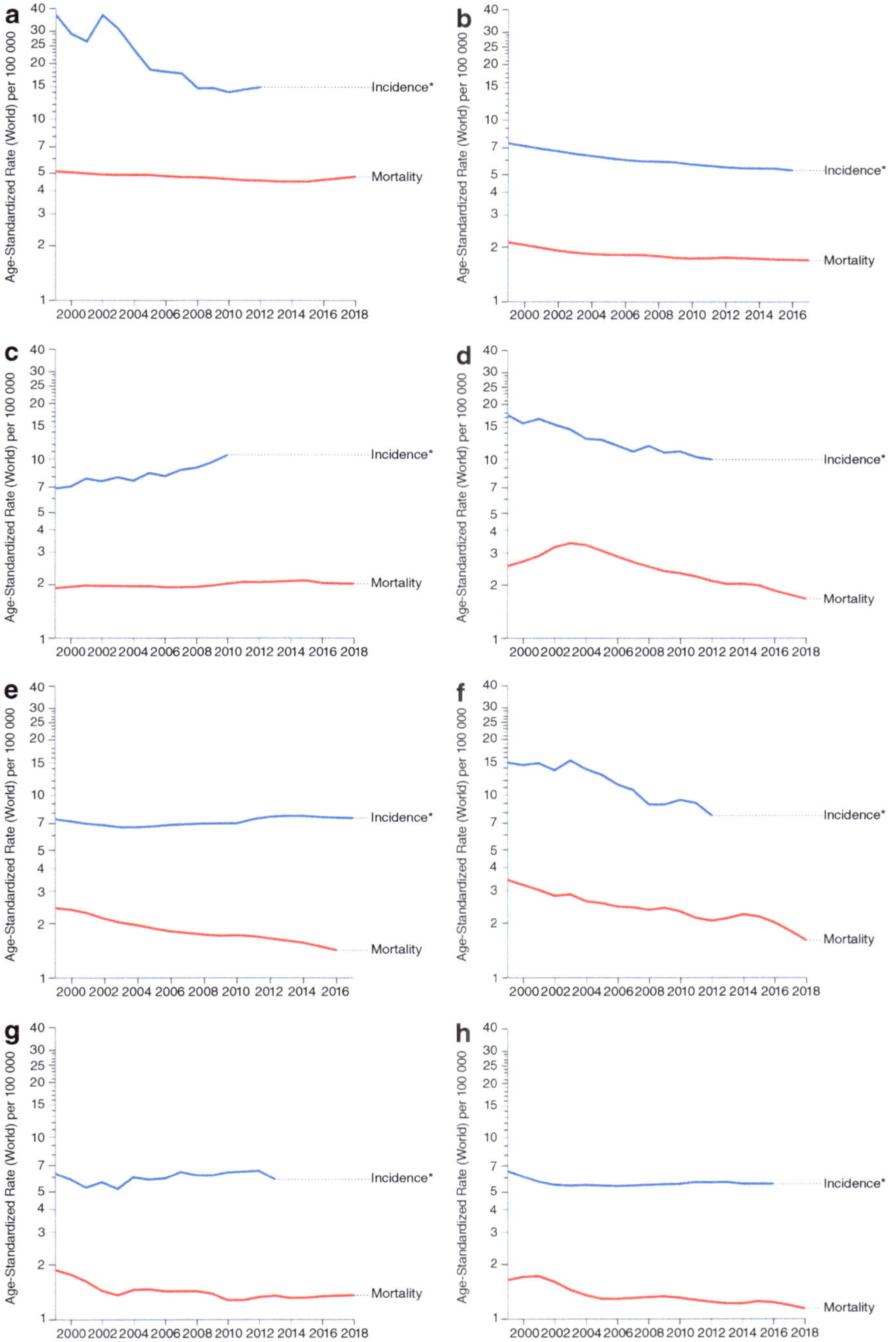

Fig. 2.1 Recent trends in age-standardized incidence (blue line) and mortality (red line) of cervical cancer by country from 1999 to 2018. All data are presented as the age-standardized rate per 100,000. (**a**) Brazil, (**b**) USA, (**c**) Japan, (**d**) Republic of Korea, (**e**) United Kingdom (England and Wales), (**f**) Slovenia, (**g**) Netherlands, (**h**) Australia

(−1.8% per year), and the USA (−0.6% per year) showed significant decreasing trends from 2008 to 2017, whereas Japan (0.5% per year) showed a significant increasing trend during this period [15].

In 2006, the quadrivalent HPV vaccine was approved by the United States Food and Drug Administration, following which all these countries implemented HPV vaccine programs to prevent HPV infection as primary prevention. Generally, the development of cervical cancer from HPV infection occurs over decades, and the lack of impact on cervical cancer incidence and mortality during these relatively short analysis periods is expected.

On the other hand, these trends in incidence and mortality might be influenced by population-based screening programs in each population. The decrease in incidence over these years, such as in the USA, might be attributable to a sustained population-based program. For example, Denmark, Finland, Sweden, and Norway instituted an organized cancer screening program in the 1960s or 1970s, which resulted in an almost 50% reduction in cervical cancer incidence [20]. Furthermore, the USA, United Kingdom, Netherlands, and Australia introduced organized screening in the 1980s and 1990s, and the trends in incidence in these countries have already decreased and then leveled off. As shown in Fig. 2.1, organized screening in the Republic of Korea and Slovenia started in the early 2000s, and a decreasing trend in incidence has been evident since. In addition to population-based screening programs, these findings might also be attributable to decreases in fertility and lower parity, and to improvements in hygiene conditions, education, and socioeconomic status. Currently, in most countries, cervical cancer incidence and mortality have been decreasing [21].

The second pattern is a continued increase in incidence, such as in Uganda and Zimbabwe [18]. Although high quality population-based cancer registries and reliable mortality data are still rare in Africa, as described above, cervical cancer incidence and mortality in sub-Saharan Africa is among the highest in the world. Furthermore, HIV was relatively prevalent in the 1990s in Uganda and Zimbabwe, and a population-based screening program has not yet been introduced in this region.

In the third pattern, the overall trend is a decrease in incidence, but an increase in younger women. One example of this pattern is China [20]. In Japan also, cervical cancer incidence has increased since the late 1990s, especially among young generation [22], although this evident increase in incidence might be associated with not only increased exposure to HPV in younger Japanese populations, but also the low coverage of screening (43.7%) or low uptake of HPV vaccination (<1%) [15]. However, it should also be considered that the Japanese Government updated the cervical cancer screening program in 2004 and changed the starting age for screening from 30 to 20 years old. Estonia also presented an increasing trend in incidence, possibly due to poor screening coverage or insufficient quality of the program [20].

2.3 Risk Factors for Cervical Cancer

2.3.1 Human Papillomavirus and Risk Factors for Cervical Cancer

Although persistent high-risk oncogenic human papillomavirus (HPV) infection can cause cervical cancer, most HPV infections are harmless and clear spontaneously. Based on a meta-analysis of one million women with normal cytology, approximately 291 million women worldwide were estimated to have HPV infection at a given point, of whom 32% were infected with HPV type 16 and 18 [23]. Genital HPV infection is one of the most common sexually transmitted diseases and most sexually active individuals of both sexes will acquire it at some point during their life [24]. Here, we discuss risk factors associated with acquiring HPV infection, impaired immune response to HPV infection and progression of cervical intraepithelial neoplasia (CIN). These factors include sexual behavior, immunodeficiency disorders such as human immunodeficiency virus (HIV) infection, a history of sexually transmitted infection, tobacco smoking, and endogenous and exogenous hormonal factors (Table 2.3).

2.3.2 Sexual Behavior and Cervical Cancer Risk

Sexual behavior such as an increasing lifetime number of sexual partners and younger age at first sexual intercourse are well-known risk factors for cervical cancer. A pooled analysis conducted by the International Agency for Research on Cancer (IARC) confirmed the relationship between cervical cancer risk and these indicators of sexual behavior, namely lifetime number of sexual partners and age at first intercourse [4]. Compared with one sexual partner, the odds ratio (OR) with 2–5 sexual partners, conditioned on age, study, and age at first intercourse, was 1.64. Similarly, the OR of $\geq$ six partners was 2.27 (95%CI, 1.98–2.61), increasing to 2.78 (95%CI, 2.22–3.47) after accounting for additional confounding by reproductive factors such as number of full-term pregnancies and age at first full-term pregnancy. A significant positive linear trend was observed (P for trend <0.001). On the other hand, cervical cancer risk increased steadily with younger age at first intercourse: compared with $\geq$25 years at first intercourse, the OR of $\leq$14 at first intercourse, adjusted for age, study, and lifetime number of sexual partners, was 3.52 (95%CI, 3.04–4.08), decreasing to 2.05 (95%CI, 1.54–2.73) after accounting for additional confounding by reproductive factors mentioned above. Regarding age at first intercourse, controlling by reproductive factors might cause over-adjustment, because first intercourse would be shortly followed by first full-term pregnancy. Despite adjusting for several confounders, these results were consistent in the positive association between cervical cancer risk and these sexual behaviors across individual studies and by study design included in the pooled analysis. In addition, a joint effect by these two indicators was indicated [4].

As expected, sexual behavior is related to the acquisition of HPV infection. Higher lifetime number of sexual partners could indicate increased exposure to HPV infection, albeit that the probability of HPV transmission per sexual act is unknown. Probably, first exposure to HPV occurs soon after first intercourse in many women [25]. Therefore, it is conceivable that younger age at first intercourse is associated with cervical cancer risk due to HPV acquisition. A second possibility is that cervical cancer risk may be associated with longer duration of HPV infection: women with an earlier sexual debut might be exposed to HPV earlier, with a resulting longer duration of HPV infection. Other possibilities are that earlier first intercourse is a marker of high-risk behavior for exposure to HPV, and that younger women are more susceptible to HPV infection. Cervical cancer might resemble other cancers caused by strong early-stage carcinogens, with incidence rates proportional to a power of time since first exposure. These possibilities therefore suggest that HPV vaccination is an important means of delaying HPV infection to prevent disease progression, without necessarily providing lifetime protection against HPV [5].

2.3.3 Immunosuppression and Cervical Cancer Risk

Immunosuppression after solid organ transplantation or HIV infection is also an important risk factor of cervical cancer (Table 2.3). HIV-infected women are reported to have higher rates of persistence of HPV infection, high-grade CIN, and cervical cancer, compared with HIV-uninfected women [6, 7, 26]. As mentioned above (2.2. Cervical Cancer Incidence and Mortality by Geographical Region), cervical cancer incidence in sub-Saharan Africa is the highest worldwide and more than 70% of HIV infections occur in sub-Saharan Africa [27]. A pooled analysis by Stelzle et al. reported that HIV prevalence among females aged ≥15 years was 29.83%, and showed a significantly elevated cervical cancer risk in women living with HIV [relative risk (RR) = 6.07, 95%CI 4.40–8.37], in which an estimated 5.8% (95%CI 4.6–7.3%) of new cancer cases in 2018 were diagnosed in women living with HIV and 4.9% were attributable to HIV infection [28]. A linkage study of HIV/acquired immunodeficiency syndrome (AIDS) and cancer registries has indicated a 2- to 22-fold increase in cervical cancer among HIV-infected compared with HIV-uninfected women [29]. It is thought that the interaction between HPV and HIV infection could be related to alterations in cell-mediated immune responses in HIV-infected women; increased susceptibility to and reactivate latent HPV infection, which is a critical component for HPV clearance [29]; and neoplastic progression [30]. Recently, the impact of antiretroviral therapy (ART) on cervical cancer incidence and mortality was investigated in South Africa: in 2004, the South Africa government rolled out a nation-wide ART program. The age-standardized incidence rate (ASIR) was 22.1 (per 100,000) in 1994 and 23.3 in 2009, and average annual percentage change (AAPC) in incidence from 1994 to 2009 was −0.9% (p-value <0.001). However, there was a slight increase in cervical cancer incidence between 2001 and 2009 (AAPC = 0.9, p-value <0.001) due to increased ART and screening.

Table 2.3 Risk factors of cervical cancer related to human papillomavirus

Risk factor	Indicators	Possible biological mechanism	Risk direction	Reference
Sexual behavior	Age at first intercourse	Early age at first intercourse might indicate longer duration of HPV infection	Increased risk	IARC_2009 [4], Plummer_2012 [5]
	Lifetime number of sexual partners	Higher lifetime number of sexual partners may increases exposure to HPV infection	Increased risk	IARC_2009 [4]
Immunosupression	Prevalence of HIV positive, HIV seropositivity, CD4 cell count, antiretroviral therapy	Immunosupression could promote the acquisition and persistence of HPV infection	Increased risk	Denny_2012 [29], Castellsague_2008 [30], Olorunfemi_2018 [31]
	After transplantation of solid organs			
History of sexually transmitted infection	Prevalence of HSV2 or C. Trachomatis, seropositivity	STD might increases susceptibiliy to HPV infection, DNA damage due to chronic inflammation, or impaired immune response to HPV	Increased risk	Smith_2002 [8], Smith_2004 [9]
Tobacco smoking	Smoking status (duration, intensity, smoking cessation)	Smoking may cause DNA damage or local immunosuppression	SCC; increasd risk, adenocarcinoma; no association	IJC_2006 [10], Jensen_2012 [34], Roura_2014 [35], IARC_2007 [36], Louie_2007 [37]
Endogenous hormonal factors	Parity Number of full-term pregnancies	Immunosuppression due to pregnancy, or increased exposure to HPV due to eversion of the squamo-columnal junction on the ectocervix during pregnancy	Increased risk	IARC_2006 [11], Roura_2016 [38], Luhn_2013 [39]
	Duration of oral contraceptive use	OC may alter hormonal receptors in cervix and then affect the natural course of HPV OC could enhance HPV E6 and E7 oncogene expression	Increased risk	IRAC_2007 [12], Roura_2016 [38], Luhn_2013 [39]

HPV human papillomavirus, *IARC* International Agency for Research on Cancer, *HIV* human immunodeficiency virus, *HSV2* herpes simplex virus-2, *C.trachomatis* Chlamidia trachomatis, *STD* sexually transmitted infection, *SCC* squamous cell carcinoma, *OC* oral contraceptives

On the other hand, the age-standardized morality rate (ASMR) decreased slightly, from 13.9 (per 100,000) in 2004 to 13.1 in 2012, as did the AAPC from 2004 to 2012, at −0.6% (p-value <0.001). Despite interventions such as ART and tobacco control in South Africa, minimal changes in temporal incidence and mortality trends were observed [31]. In a recent meta-analysis, ART was associated with a lower prevalence of high-risk HPV (adjusted OR = 0.83, 95%CI 0.70–0.99, $I^2 = 51\%$) and a significantly lowered risk of cervical cancer [crude hazard ratio (HR) = 0.40, 95%CI 0.18–0.87, $I^2 = 33\%$] among women living with HIV, compared with ART-naïve women [32]. Early ART initiation and sustained adherence are therefore likely to reduce the incidence of CIN and invasive cervical cancer. In addition, HPV vaccination also appears important, albeit that HIV may reduce the responsiveness to vaccines and also their effectiveness due to immune deficits. A systematic review and meta-analysis of the efficacy and safety of HPV vaccination in HIV-infected persons, including women, men, and children, showed a seroconversion rate almost 100% for each vaccine and significantly high antibody titers against HPV vaccine types compared with the placebo group. HPV vaccination for HIV-infected persons is safe because no differences in severe adverse events (RR = 0.60, 95%CI 0.2–1.6) or non-serious adverse events (RR = 0.60, 95%CI 0.9–1.2) were observed between vaccine and placebo group. Moreover, HPV vaccines do not affect CD4 + T cell count or HIV viral load [33]. Although these results may support HPV vaccination for HIV-infected persons, further studies are necessary to assess the effectiveness of HPV vaccines in preventing HPV infection and disease progression in people with HIV.

2.3.4 Other Sexually Transmitted Diseases and Cervical Cancer

IARC also conducted a pooled analysis to examine the effect of herpes simplex virus-2 (HSV2) infection and Chlamydia trachomatis (C. trachomatis) as HPV cofactors in the etiology of invasive cervical cancer [8, 9].

The role of HSV2 in the development of cervical cancer was questioned, because HSV2 DNA is not consistently detected in cervical cancer specimens. Several biological mechanisms have been suggested: ulcerative herpetic lesions may serve as HPV cofactors by facilitating the access of HPV to the basal cell layer; inflammatory responses by HSV2 infection may interfere with an effective immune response to HPV infection; and HSV2 infection may help the progression of cervical neoplasia. It is possible that HSV2 may act on the host's cellular DNA via a hit-and-run mechanism. In fact, a pooled analysis by IARC reported that overall HSV-2 seroprevalence was significantly higher among patients with squamous cell invasive cervical cancer (44.4%, 95%CI 41.5–47.3%) and adeno−/adenosquamous invasive cervical cancer (43.8%, 95%CI 34.2–53.5%) than among non-cancer controls subjects (25.6%, 95%CI 23.0–28.2%). When limited to HPV DNA-positive women, the association between HSV2 seropositivity and squamous cell carcinoma and adenocarcinoma was significant [OR for squamous cell carcinoma = 2.19 (95%CI, 1.41–3.40), OR for adenocarcinoma = 3.37 (95%CI, 1.47–7.74)] [8].

In a pooled analysis by IARC, overall C. trachomatis seroprevalence was similarly significantly higher among patients with squamous cell invasive cervical cancer (53.2%) and adeno−/adenosquamous invasive cervical cancer (39.4%) than among non-cancer controls subjects (30.8%) [9]. When limited to HPV DNA-positive cases and controls, C. trachomatis seropositivity was significantly associated with squamous cell cervical cancer risk (OR = 1.80, 95%CI 1.22–2.66) after adjusting for possible confounders. A dose–response relationship between C. trachomatis antibody titer and squamous cell carcinoma risk was observed (trend *p*-value <0.001). On the other hand, C. trachomatis seropositivity was not associated with adeno- or adenosquamous cell carcinoma risk (OR = 1.03, 95%CI 0.53–2.01). A possible biological mechanism is that genital C. trachomatis infection induces chronic inflammation, resulting in turn in the production of reactive oxygen species that could cause DNA damage and increase the risk of HPV-associated carcinogenesis. In vitro data also suggest that C. trachomatis infection may impair the ability to clear HPV infection or to control HPV-induced cervical neoplasia [9].

2.3.5 Tobacco Smoking and Cervical Cancer Risk

A pooled study by IARC analyzed 23 published observational studies from four continents, approximately half of which were from less-developed countries. The percentage of current smokers among non-cancer controls in the studies varied widely, from 0% to 60%. The mean number of cigarettes per day among controls who had ever smoked ranged from 3 to 19. The proportion of ever smokers and the mean number of cigarettes per day was higher in the more developed than less-developed countries (47% compared to 13%, and mean number = 14 compared to 8 per day, respectively) [10].

In several studies, tobacco smoking had been associated with increased cervical cancer and precancer risk [10, 34, 35]. In analyses restricted to women who tested positive to or with persistent HPV, there was also a significantly increased risk for cervical cancer and precancer [10, 34]. One plausible biological mechanism for these findings is the induction of a local immunosuppressive effect caused by compounds and metabolic products from smoke which could decrease the effectiveness of the immune response against HPV infection and HPV clearance. In addition, chemicals in cigarette such as nicotine, which can cause DNA damage, have been found in epithelial cells [35].

The IARC's pooled analysis included several important suggestions about tobacco smoking and cervical cancer risk [10]. Current smokers had a significantly increased risk of squamous cell carcinoma compared with never smokers [RR = 1.60, 95%CI 1.48–1.73], whereas no association was seen between smoking and cervical adenocarcinoma. Although squamous cell carcinoma and adenocarcinoma of the cervix share most risk factors, with the exception of smoking, the difference remains unexplained [36]. In current smokers, the RR of squamous cell carcinoma increased with increasing number of cigarettes per day and younger age at starting smoking [10, 35].

Past smokers were also at increased risk for squamous cell carcinoma (RR = 1.12, 95%CI 1.01–1.25), and showed no clear linear trend with time since stopping smoking (P-trend = 0.6) [10]. In contrast, the European Prospective Investigation into Cancer and Nutrition (EPIC) study showed decreasing RR with increasing time since smoking cessation compared to current smokers, albeit without statistical significance (P-trend = 0.1). For instance, women who stopped smoking 20 or more years before recruitment showed decreased risk (OR for invasive cancer = 0.3, 95%CI 0.1–1.2) and had a similar risk of disease to that of never smokers [35].

Regarding passive smoking and cervical cancer risk, the EPIC study did not show a significant association [35]. Although the pooled study by IARC showed increased risk among couples with both ever smoking men and women (OR = 2.26, 95%CI 1.40–3.64) compared to couples who were both nonsmoking, it did not show a significant association among couples with a currently smoking man and nonsmoking woman (OR = 1.34, 95%CI 0.91–1.96). Passive smoking could not be detected as an independent risk factor of cervical cancer in the absence of active smoking; nevertheless, the combined effects of active and passive smoking might suggest adverse potential for cervical carcinogenesis [37].

2.3.6 Hormonal Factors and Cervical Cancer Risk

Many studies have investigated the association between endogenous and exogenous hormonal factors and cervical carcinogenesis. Endogenous hormonal factors include various reproductive factors: the number of full-term pregnancies [11, 38, 39], age at first full-term pregnancy [11, 38], number of induced abortions [38], and cumulative years of menstrual cycles without oral contraceptives (OC) [38]. Exogenous hormonal factors include OC use [38, 39], intrauterine devices, and hormone replacement therapy (HRT) use [38].

High parity is well-known as one of the earliest risk factors identified for cervical cancer. Epidemiological studies conducted in the 1950s and 1960s indicated the association with sexual behaviors, and subsequent studies pointed to sexual transmission, specifically HPV infection. Accordingly, reproductive factors were considered as confounding factors of sexual behaviors [11]. The pooled analysis by IARC indicated a significant positive association between reproductive factors such as number of full-term pregnancies and age at first full-term pregnancy, after adjustment for study, age, lifetime number of sexual partners and age at sexual debut. The adjusted RR of invasive cervical cancer among parous women was 1.76 (95% CI 1.53–2.02) and 2.39 (2.17–2.62) for ≥7 full-term pregnancies, compared to 1–2 full-term pregnancies. In contrast, no significant trend was found between CIN3 and increasing number of births. Early age at first full-term pregnancy was also associated with invasive cervical cancer and CIN3 risk, with an adjusted RR for age at first pregnancy <17 years compared with ≥25 years of 1.77 (95%CI 1.42–2.23) for invasive cancer and 1.78 (95%CI 1.26–2.51) for CIN3. The EPIC study showed a similar positive association between number of full-term pregnancies and CIN3 risk (P for trend = 0.03). A possible biological mechanism for these associations with reproductive factors is that high concentrations of estrogen and progesterone during pregnancy or delivery-related cervical trauma are responsible for eversion of the squamo-columnal junction at the ectocervix, which in turn facilitates direct exposure to HPV infection. Another possible biological mechanism is immunosuppression due to pregnancy, which might promote the role of HPV in cervical carcinogenesis [11, 38].

Among exogenous hormonal factors, combined OC has been already classified by IARC as a cause of cervical cancer [40]. The EPIC study also showed that the multivariate HR of current OC users was 2.2 (95%CI 1.3–4.0) for invasive cervical cancer and 1.8 (95%CI 1.4–2.4) for CIN3 compared with never users [38]. In addition, a pooled reanalysis by IARC investigated the association with cervical cancer risk in relation to duration of use of combined OC and by time since last use of combined OC [12]. The proportion of ever users of OC was 32% among invasive cervical cancer cases, 57% among CIN3 cases, and 34% among non-cancer controls. The relative risk of cervical cancer increased significantly with increasing duration of OC use (P for trend <0.0001). Compared to never users, RR for ≥5 years' use was 1.90 (95%CI 1.69–2.13). Cervical cancer risk decreased with increasing years since last OC use (P for trend <0.0001), and after 10 or more years was the same as that of never users. A similar pattern was observed for invasive cervical cancer and CIN3 [12]. A possible biological mechanism of the effect of OC is that combined estrogens and progesterones may affect hormonal receptors presented in cervical tissue, especially progesterone, and change the natural course of HPV infection. Exogenous sex steroid hormones are assumed to enhance the expression of HPV E6 and E7 oncogenes, promoting the deterioration of p53 tumor suppressor genes, and thereby augment the ability of viral DNA integration and transformation of cells to induce cancer development [38]. However, the pooled analysis by IARC could not show an interaction between OC use and HPV infection, with the RR of ever users with HPV-positive testing of 1.19 (95%CI 0.92–1.52) compared with ever users with HPV-negative testing as reference [12].

2.4 Conclusion

Here, we reviewed the descriptive epidemiology of cervical cancer and evidence for risk factors related to HPV infection. For the time being, the main impact on the global cervical cancer burden may come from cancer screening programs and access to adequate treatment, while the impact of HPV vaccination on incidence and mortality must emerge in the near future. In addition, the remarkable geographical contrasts may reflect differences in risk factors and serious inequality in access to adequate medical care. In 2020, World Health Organization approved the Global Strategy for Cervical Cancer Elimination [41]. It has three main pillars to achieve this goal: vaccination, screening and treatment. Furthermore, we should consider the cofactors described in this chapter. In particular, cervical cancer control also requires lifestyle modification specified to geographical regions, such as HIV control and sexual education in Southern Africa.

Conflict of Interest The author declares no conflict of interest.

References

1. Arbyn M, Castellsague X, de Sanjose S, Bruni L, Saraiya M, Bray F, et al. Worldwide burden of cervical cancer in 2008. Ann Oncol. 2011;22(12):2675–86.
2. de Martel C, Plummer M, Vignat J, Franceschi S. Worldwide burden of cancer attributable to HPV by site, country and HPV type. Int J Cancer. 2017;141(4):664–70.
3. IARC. GLOBOCAN Lyon, France, 2022. https://gco.iarc.fr/.
4. International Collaboration of Epidemiological Studies of Cervical C. Cervical carcinoma and sexual behavior: collaborative reanalysis of individual data on 15,461 women with cervical carcinoma and 29,164 women without cervical carcinoma from 21 epidemiological studies. Cancer Epidemiol Biomark Prev. 2009;18(4):1060–9.
5. Plummer M, Peto J, Franceschi S. International collaboration of epidemiological studies of cervical C. Time since first sexual intercourse and the risk of cervical cancer. Int J Cancer. 2012;130(11):2638–44.
6. Denny L, Boa R, Williamson AL, Allan B, Hardie D, Stan R, et al. Human papillomavirus infection and cervical disease in human immunodeficiency virus-1-infected women. Obstet Gynecol. 2008;111(6):1380–7.
7. Harris TG, Burk RD, Palefsky JM, Massad LS, Bang JY, Anastos K, et al. Incidence of cervical squamous intraepithelial lesions associated with HIV serostatus, CD4 cell counts, and human papillomavirus test results. JAMA. 2005;293(12):1471–6.
8. Smith JS, Herrero R, Bosetti C, Munoz N, Bosch FX, Eluf-Neto J, et al. Herpes simplex virus-2 as a human papillomavirus cofactor in the etiology of invasive cervical cancer. J Natl Cancer Inst. 2002;94(21):1604–13.
9. Smith JS, Bosetti C, Munoz N, Herrero R, Bosch FX, Eluf-Neto J, et al. Chlamydia trachomatis and invasive cervical cancer: a pooled analysis of the IARC multicentric case-control study. Int J Cancer. 2004;111(3):431–9.
10. International Collaboration of Epidemiological Studies of Cervical C, Appleby P, Beral V, Berrington de Gonzalez A, Colin D, Franceschi S, et al. Carcinoma of the cervix and tobacco smoking: collaborative reanalysis of individual data on 13,541 women with carcinoma of the cervix and 23,017 women without carcinoma of the cervix from 23 epidemiological studies. Int J Cancer. 2006;118(6):1481–95.
11. International Collaboration of Epidemiological Studies of Cervical C. Cervical carcinoma and reproductive factors: collaborative reanalysis of individual data on 16,563 women with cervical carcinoma and 33,542 women without cervical carcinoma from 25 epidemiological studies. Int J Cancer. 2006;119(5):1108–24.
12. International Collaboration of Epidemiological Studies of Cervical C, Appleby P, Beral V, Berrington de Gonzalez A, Colin D, Franceschi S, et al. Cervical cancer and hormonal contraceptives: collaborative reanalysis of individual data for 16,573 women with cervical cancer and 35,509 women without cervical cancer from 24 epidemiological studies. Lancet. 2007;370(9599):1609–21.
13. Programme UD. Human development report 2016. Human development for everyone, 2016. https://hdr.undp.org/system/files/documents/2016humandevelopmentreportpdf1pdf.pdf.
14. Arbyn M, Raifu AO, Weiderpass E, Bray F, Anttila A. Trends of cervical cancer mortality in the member states of the European Union. Eur J Cancer. 2009;45(15):2640–8.
15. Lin S, Gao K, Gu S, You L, Qian S, Tang M, et al. Worldwide trends in cervical cancer incidence and mortality, with predictions for the next 15 years. Cancer. 2021;127(21):4030–9.
16. Bruni L, Diaz M, Castellsague X, Ferrer E, Bosch FX, de Sanjose S. Cervical human papillomavirus prevalence in 5 continents: meta-analysis of 1 million women with normal cytological findings. J Infect Dis. 2010;202(12):1789–99.
17. De Vuyst H, Alemany L, Lacey C, Chibwesha CJ, Sahasrabuddhe V, Banura C, et al. The burden of human papillomavirus infections and related diseases in sub-saharan Africa. Vaccine. 2013;31 Suppl 5(0 5):F32–46.

18. Vaccarella S, Laversanne M, Ferlay J, Bray F. Cervical cancer in Africa, Latin America and the Caribbean and Asia: regional inequalities and changing trends. Int J Cancer. 2017;141(10):1997–2001.
19. IARC. Cancer incidence in five continets time trends, 2018; https://ci5.iarc.fr/CI5plus/Default.aspx.
20. IARC. Cervical cancer screening. In: IARC handbooks of cancer prevention, vol. 18. Lyon; 2021.
21. Sung H, Ferlay J, Siegel RL, Laversanne M, Soerjomataram I, Jemal A, et al. Global cancer statistics 2020: GLOBOCAN estimates of incidence and mortality worldwide for 36 cancers in 185 countries. CA Cancer J Clin. 2021;71(3):209–49.
22. Utada M, Chernyavskiy P, Lee WJ, Franceschi S, Sauvaget C, de Gonzalez AB, et al. Increasing risk of uterine cervical cancer among young Japanese women: comparison of incidence trends in Japan, South Korea and Japanese-Americans between 1985 and 2012. Int J Cancer. 2019;144(9):2144–52.
23. de Sanjose S, Diaz M, Castellsague X, Clifford G, Bruni L, Munoz N, et al. Worldwide prevalence and genotype distribution of cervical human papillomavirus DNA in women with normal cytology: a meta-analysis. Lancet Infect Dis. 2007;7(7):453–9.
24. Crosbie EJ, Einstein MH, Franceschi S, Kitchener HC. Human papillomavirus and cervical cancer. Lancet. 2013;382(9895):889–99.
25. Schiffman M, Castle PE, Jeronimo J, Rodriguez AC, Wacholder S. Human papillomavirus and cervical cancer. Lancet. 2007;370(9590):890–907.
26. Singh DK, Anastos K, Hoover DR, Burk RD, Shi Q, Ngendahayo L, et al. Human papillomavirus infection and cervical cytology in HIV-infected and HIV-uninfected Rwandan women. J Infect Dis. 2009;199(12):1851–61.
27. HIV/AIDS JUNPo. The gap reort/UNAIDS. Geneva: HIV/AIDS JUNPo; 2014.
28. Stelzle D, Tanaka LF, Lee KK, Ibrahim Khalil A, Baussano I, Shah ASV, et al. Estimates of the global burden of cervical cancer associated with HIV. Lancet Glob Health. 2021;9(2):e161–e9.
29. Denny LA, Franceschi S, de Sanjose S, Heard I, Moscicki AB, Palefsky J. Human papillomavirus, human immunodeficiency virus and immunosuppression. Vaccine. 2012;30(Suppl 5):F168–74.
30. Castellsague X. Natural history and epidemiology of HPV infection and cervical cancer. Gynecol Oncol. 2008;110(3 Suppl 2):S4–7.
31. Olorunfemi G, Ndlovu N, Masukume G, Chikandiwa A, Pisa PT, Singh E. Temporal trends in the epidemiology of cervical cancer in South Africa (1994-2012). Int J Cancer. 2018;143(9):2238–49.
32. Kelly H, Weiss HA, Benavente Y, de Sanjose S, Mayaud P, et al. Association of antiretroviral therapy with high-risk human papillomavirus, cervical intraepithelial neoplasia, and invasive cervical cancer in women living with HIV: a systematic review and meta-analysis. Lancet HIV. 2018;5(1):e45–58.
33. Zizza A, Banchelli F, Guido M, Marotta C, Di Gennaro F, Mazzucco W, et al. Efficacy and safety of human papillomavirus vaccination in HIV-infected patients: a systematic review and meta-analysis. Sci Rep. 2021;11(1):4954.
34. Jensen KE, Schmiedel S, Frederiksen K, Norrild B, Iftner T, Kjaer SK. Risk for cervical intraepithelial neoplasia grade 3 or worse in relation to smoking among women with persistent human papillomavirus infection. Cancer Epidemiol Biomark Prev. 2012;21(11):1949–55.
35. Roura E, Castellsague X, Pawlita M, Travier N, Waterboer T, Margall N, et al. Smoking as a major risk factor for cervical cancer and pre-cancer: results from the EPIC cohort. Int J Cancer. 2014;135(2):453–66.
36. International Collaboration of Epidemiological Studies of Cervical C. Comparison of risk factors for invasive squamous cell carcinoma and adenocarcinoma of the cervix: collaborative reanalysis of individual data on 8,097 women with squamous cell carcinoma and 1,374 women with adenocarcinoma from 12 epidemiological studies. Int J Cancer. 2007;120(4):885–91.

37. Louie KS, Castellsague X, de Sanjose S, Herrero R, Meijer CJ, Shah K, et al. Smoking and passive smoking in cervical cancer risk: pooled analysis of couples from the IARC multicentric case-control studies. Cancer Epidemiol Biomark Prev. 2011;20(7):1379–90.
38. Roura E, Travier N, Waterboer T, de Sanjose S, Bosch FX, Pawlita M, et al. The influence of hormonal factors on the risk of developing cervical cancer and pre-cancer: results from the EPIC cohort. PLoS One. 2016;11(1):e0147029.
39. Luhn P, Walker J, Schiffman M, Zuna RE, Dunn ST, Gold MA, et al. The role of co-factors in the progression from human papillomavirus infection to cervical cancer. Gynecol Oncol. 2013;128(2):265–70.
40. Cogliano V, Grosse Y, Baan R, Straif K, Secretan B, El Ghissassi F, et al. Carcinogenicity of combined oestrogen-progestagen contraceptives and menopausal treatment. Lancet Oncol. 2005;6(8):552–3.
41. WHO. Global strategy to accelerate the elim-ination of cervical cancer as a public health problem. 2020; https://www.who.int/publications/i/item/9789240014107.

Topics of Histopathology and Cytology of Cervical Cancer and Screening

3

Masanori Yasuda, Tomomi Katoh, Yu Miyama, and Daisuke Shintani

Abstract

The vast majority of cervical cancers are carcinomas (99.6%)—mainly, squamous cell carcinomas (SCC) and adenocarcinomas, and very minor tumors are sarcomas (0.4%) (Acta Obstet Gynaecol Jpn 74:2345–402, 2022). SCCs are three times more common than adenocarcinomas (Acta Obstet Gynaecol Jpn 74:2345–402, 2022). Cervical cancer is the fourth most common cancer among women worldwide, after breast, colorectal, and lung cancers (Herrington et al WHO classification of tumours. Female genital tumours, Lyon, IARC Press, 2020). In Japan, cervical cancer was the 12th most common cause of death (CANCER STATISTICS IN JAPAN, 2022. https://ganjoho.jp/public/qa_links/report/statistics/2022_en.html).

According to the 2020 World Health Organization (WHO) tumor classification, cervical SCCs and adenocarcinomas have been categorized as HPV (human papillomavirus)-associated and HPV-independent cancers. Almost all cervical SCCs are HPV-associated, and a few SCCs have been reported to be HPV-independent (Casey et al Int J Gynecol Pathol 34:208–12, 2015). Although it is recommended that whether SCC is HPV-associated or HPV-independent be documented in the pathological report, there is currently no stratification in the treatment strategy between HPV-associated and HPV-independent carcinoma. A histological diagnosis of SCC—NOS without differentiating between the two categories can be an acceptable alternative. Distinguishing between

M. Yasuda (✉) · T. Katoh · Y. Miyama
Departments of Pathology, Saitama Medical University International Medical Center, Saitama, Japan
e-mail: m_yasuda@saitama-med.ac.jp

D. Shintani
Gynecologic Oncology, Saitama Medical University International Medical Center, Saitama, Japan

D. Aoki (ed.), *Recent Topics on Prevention, Diagnosis, and Clinical Management of Cervical Cancer*, Comprehensive Gynecology and Obstetrics,
https://doi.org/10.1007/978-981-99-9396-3_3

HPV-associated SCC and HPV-independent SCC is difficult based only on histologic findings; it usually requires p16 immunostaining, HPV in situ hybridization, or HPV testing. In contrast to SCCs, adenocarcinomas, whether in situ or invasive, are relatively easy to categorize as HPV-associated and HPV-independent based on histology. In this revision of the WHO classification, some minor variants such as adenoid cystic carcinoma and ground-glass carcinoma have been deleted. Adenoid cystic carcinoma is now considered a variant of HPV-associated adenocarcinoma, and ground-glass carcinoma is included in poorly differentiated adenosquamous carcinoma because of undefined diagnostic criteria. In Chap. 11, uterine neuroendocrine tumors and carcinomas in both the cervix and body are independently categorized as follows: neuroendocrine tumor, grade 1; neuroendocrine tumor, grade 2; small cell neuroendocrine carcinoma; large cell neuroendocrine carcinoma; combined small cell neuroendocrine carcinoma; and combined large cell neuroendocrine carcinoma. The low- and high-grade tumor terminologies were deleted.

The cytology of cervical cancers and their precursors has been thoroughly established based on the 2001 version of the Bethesda System, which was developed in combination with HPV testing for the triage of precursors in the 2014 version. Cytological terminologies such as squamous intraepithelial lesions (SIL) are being used as histologic terminologies along with cervical intraepithelial lesions (CIN) in the 2014 WHO tumor classification (Stoler et al WHO classification of tumours. Female genital tumours, Lyon, IARC Press, 2014).

Keywords
Cervical cancer · Precursor · HPV-associated · HPV-independent · Histopathology · Cytology

3.1 Squamous Cell Carcinoma (SCC), HPV (Human Papillomavirus)-Associated and HPV-Independent

Among SCCs, 90–95% are HPV-associated and 5–7% are HPV-independent [1–3]. Twelve types of HPV (16, 18, 31, 33, 35, 39, 45, 51, 52, 56, 58, and 59) are treated as oncogenic by WHO [4], and of these, HPV 16 and 18 are responsible for 70–80% of all SCCs [1, 5]. HPV-associated SCC shows a progression from high-grade SIL (HSIL), which is caused by high expression of the viral oncogenes E6 and E7. However, in the long term, after approximately 20–30 years of progression from HSIL to SCC, additional genetic and epigenetic alterations are thought to be required for malignant transformation [6]. In contrast, the molecular mechanism of tumorigenesis in HPV-independent SCC is poorly understood, although there are certain proven abnormalities such as mutations in *TP53*, *KRAS*, *ARID1A*, and *PTEN* [2, 7]. There is no difference in clinical treatment between these two categories.

HPV-independent SCC is generally more unfavorable in terms of prognosis because of the high stage of lymph node metastasis at diagnosis [2, 3, 8–12].

Grossly, SCCs in advanced stages are either exophytic (papillary or polypoid) and/or endophytic, showing varying degrees of admixture of both patterns, with no differences between HPV-associated SCC and HPV-independent SCC. Early or minimally invasive SCCs may be erosive or appear as slightly elevated lesions. Histologically, SCCs have traditionally been divided into non-keratinizing and keratinizing types (Fig. 3.1), according to the modified Broders' classification. Typical keratinizing SCCs are relatively minor; however, HPV-independent SCCs tend to be keratinizing. In the keratinizing type, the carcinoma cells are characterized by cancerous pearls and intercellular bridges. However, there is no apparent distinction in prognosis between the keratinizing and non-keratinizing type [13]. In the non-keratinizing type, carcinoma cells are arranged in variably sized anastomosing cords or sheets separated by a relatively narrow inflammatory or desmoplastic stroma. The nuclei are usually round with mild pleomorphism, and the cytoplasm is relatively abundant with eosinophilia, especially in the early or minimally invasive

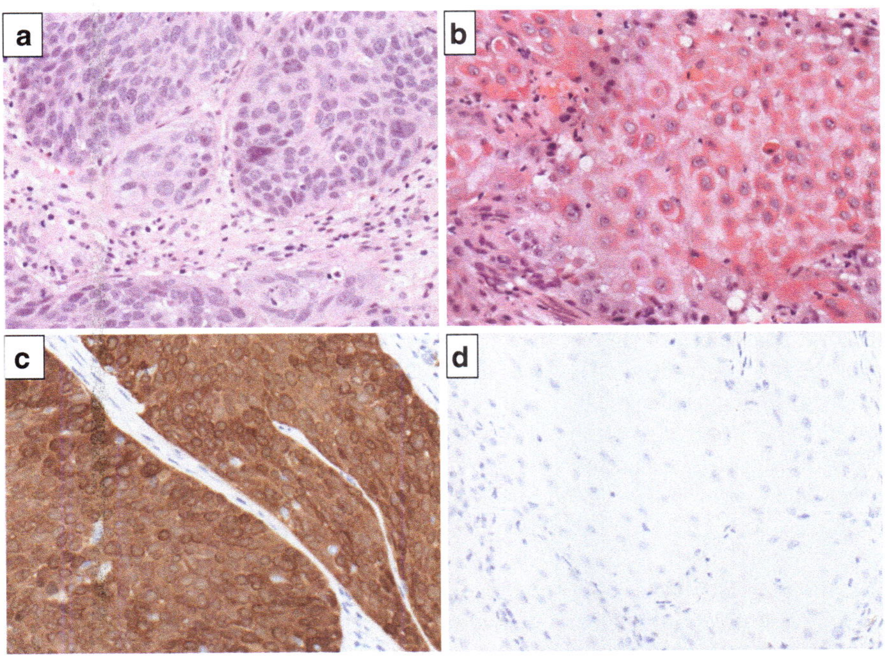

Fig. 3.1 SCC, HPV-associated and HPV-independent: (**a**) HE staining of biopsy specimen: SCC, non-keratinizing type, shows tumor cells arranged in solid and sheet-like nests. (**b**) HE staining of biopsy: SCC, keratinizing type, shows tumor cells characterized by pronounced eosinophilic cytoplasm; (**c**) Immunohistochemical staining of p16: Block-positive reaction of p16 is observed; (**d**) Immunohistochemical staining of p16: No positive reaction of p16 is observed. These findings suggest that SCC, a non-keratinizing type, is HPV-associated, and SCC, a keratinizing type, is HPV-independent

stage. In addition to the conventional type of SCC, there are several variants as follows: basaloid SCC is composed of basal-type squamous cells with scanty cytoplasm resembling HSIL, but with rare keratin pearls; warty/condylomatous type shows grossly exophytic growth and a koilocytotic appearance histologically. For the diagnosis of warty/condylomatous carcinoma to be confirmed, pure condyloma or low-grade SIL (LSIL) should be ruled out. The papillary type is characterized by multi-layered tumor cells supported by scanty fibrovascular cores, and stromal invasion may be present. Lymphoepithelioma-like SCC shows a lymphocyte-rich stroma but is not associated with EBV infection.

3.1.1 Precursor of HPV-Associated SCCs

There are two types of LSIL: exophytic and flat. The exophytic type known as condyloma acuminatum (genital wart) (Fig. 3.2) is relatively minor and is associated with low-risk HPV infection (HPV6/11). The flat type accounts for the majority (80–90%) of LSILs and are attributed to high-risk HPV infection. LSIL with high-risk HPV infection, especially HPV16/18, carries the risk of persistent infection and development of HSIL or SCC [14]. However, low-risk HPV infections rarely develop into HSIL or SCC [15]. In LSIL, the lower third of the squamous epithelium consists of basal/parabasal-like cells with occasional mitotic activity; however, abnormal mitosis is not usually observed. Koilocytosis with atypia in the upper two-thirds of the layer is characterized by nuclear enlargement, hyperchromasia, binucleation, multinucleation, and well-defined, abundant halo-like vacuoles around the centrally placed nuclei. Benign inflammatory or reactive morphologies are occasionally misinterpreted as LSIL.

In HSILs, full-thickness abnormalities such as hyperchromasia, coarse chromatin, and irregular cellular contours are observed in both CIN2 and CIN3. In CIN2, the cytoplasm accumulates in the uppermost layer and the mitotic figures extend over the lower two-thirds. However, in CIN3, there is no appreciable difference in basal-type/parabasal atypia between the uppermost and lowermost layers. Abnormal mitotic figures are also observed in CIN2 and CIN3. Notably, keratinizing HSIL differs from conventional basaloid HSIL in that its cells show more superficial differentiation with prominent keratinization but without koilocytosis. Geographical continuity with LSIL is occasionally recognized in the context of HSIL; however, whether HSIL develops from LSIL remains controversial. Simultaneous infection with different HPV types rather than the evolution of LSIL to HSIL is suggested [16].

In diagnostic practice, there are occasional problems as follows: LSIL needs to be differentiated from its mimics to avoid overdiagnoses [17, 18]; LSIL/CIN1 may be challenging to distinguish from HSIL/CIN2 even among experts [17]; the differentiation between CIN2 and CIN3 is also occasionally challenging and may result in inter-observer and intra-observer discordance. HSIL, especially CIN3, may share similar features with atrophy and/or immature squamous metaplasia.

Squamous metaplasia (Fig. 3.3) is commonly encountered at the transition between mature squamous cells and the endocervical glands. The completely

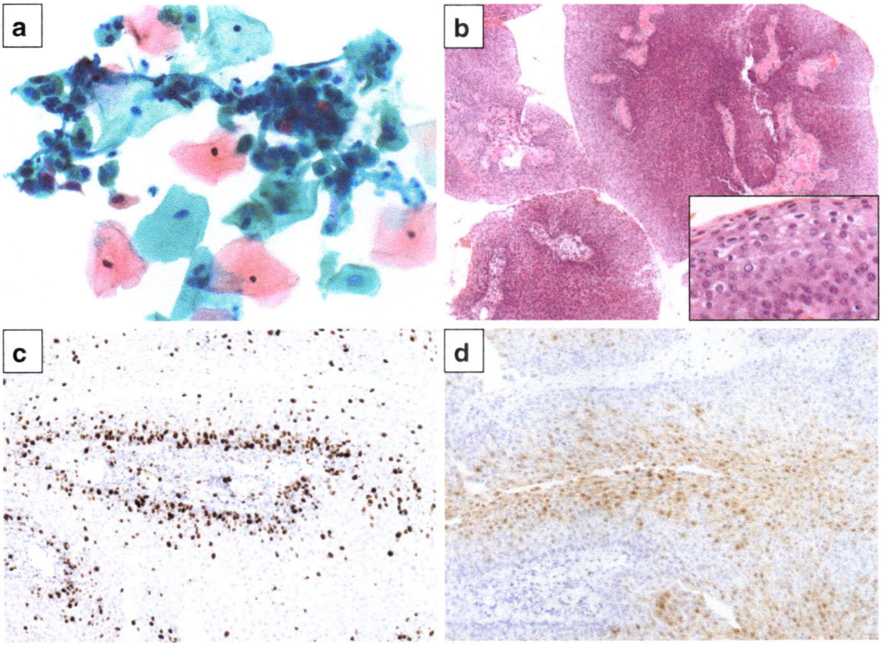

Fig. 3.2 Condyloma acuminatum: (**a**) Papanicolaou staining (LBC): Atypical cells with enlarged hyperchromatic nuclei are clustered, suggestive of HSIL/CIN2. (**b**) HE staining of biopsy specimen (inset: hyperpower view): The squamous epithelium is irregularly thickened, accompanied by a narrow stroma. In the superficial layer, atypical cells show perinuclear halos. (**c**) Immunohistochemistry of Ki-67: Positive cells are found mainly around the parabasal layer. (**d**) Immunohistochemistry of p16: Positive reaction is mild and tends to be parabasally localized

mature metaplastic squamous cells are normal and may be difficult to distinguish from the original squamous cells; however, the metaplastic area can be recognized by the presence of underlying endocervical glands. During the maturation process, the cells may be glycogenic and more eosinophilic, but show moderately high N/C ratios. Given the following features, such as nuclear enlargement lacking uniformity, high N/C ratios, irregular nuclear contours, hyperchromasia, and moderate amounts of dense eosinophilic cytoplasm, suspicion of HSIL can be raised [19]. Remnants of columnar cells containing mucin in the uppermost layer are often observed in the metaplastic process; however, remnants of mucinous columnar cells also overlie HSIL. Thus, the presence of overlying mucinous cells does not necessarily warrant the interpretation that the underlying squamous cells are metaplastic but not SIL/CIN. Some HSILs may be confused with immature squamous metaplasia with atypia and vice versa.

Atrophy of squamous cells can be caused by a deficiency or low estrogen levels, which usually occur with aging or menopause. The atrophic squamous epithelium is composed of few-layered parabasal cells that lack maturation, glycogenation, and

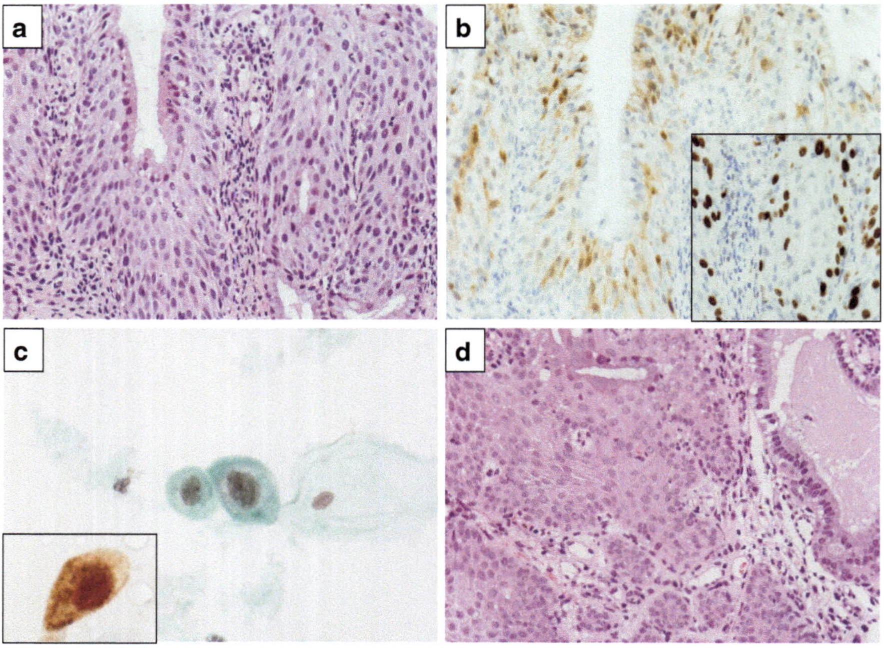

Fig. 3.3 Squamous metaplasia: (**a**) HE staining of biopsy specimen: Metaplastic squamous cells are arranged in sheet-like stratification with polarity, and columnar cells remain in the superficial layer. (**b**) Immunohistochemical staining of p16 (inset: Ki-67): Positive reaction of p16 is mild and focal/patchy. Ki-67-positive cells are irregularly distributed (inset). (**c**) Papanicolaou staining of LBC (inset: immunocytochemical dual staining of p16 and Ki-67 using CINtecPlus): A few mildly atypical cells show a moderate N/C ratio. A dual-positive reaction is detected (inset). (**d**) HE staining of biopsy specimen: Metaplastic squamous cells lack nuclear atypia and hyperchromasia and show a lobulated structure

mitosis. Pseudokoilocytosis is occasionally observed during atrophy. It should be noted that atrophic squamous cells mimic thin or atrophic HSIL.

3.1.2 Cytology of SCCs and Precursors

Non-keratinizing SCCs, including the basaloid type, show high N/C ratios, coarse chromatin, irregular nuclear shapes, and less conspicuous nucleoli. The cell borders/membranes are not clearly defined. The cytoplasm is delicate. Carcinoma cells tend to be more syncytial and hyperchromatic in liquid-based cytology (LBC) than in conventional cytology using Pap smear. HPV-associated SCC and HPV-independent SCC cannot be distinguished based on cytology.

LSIL/CIN1 is characterized by low N/C ratios, nuclei enlargement by more than three times the size of intermediate cells, hyperchromasia, coarse chromatin, and irregular nuclear contours. Many LSILs have clearly punched out perinuclear halos in the cytoplasm, which is known as koilocytosis. HSIL is divided into CIN2/moderate dysplasia, CIN3/severe dysplasia, and SCC in situ. In HSILs, especially CIN3, dysplastic cells with considerably high N/C ratios (> 80%) appear as single and/or crowded clusters. The nuclei are hyperchromatic but may be normochromic or hypochromic. The cytoplasm varies from delicate to dense or metaplastic. Typical metaplastic squamous cells have centrally placed round nuclei and dense cytoplasm with a clear cell border. According to a large population-based study, HPV-associated LSIL on cytology has a 6.1% 5-year risk of CIN3, but HPV-independent LSIL has a 2.0% risk [20]. For women with HSIL on cytology, the 5-year risk of cancer development is estimated to be 6.6–6.8% [21].

3.1.3 Surrogate Markers and Ancillary Testing

Overexpression of p16, a tumor suppressor gene protein, designated as "block-positive," is almost invariably indicative of high-risk HPV infection status in the uterine cervix and oropharyngeal cancers. Block-positive staining is defined as involving the basal keratinocytes and extending beyond the one-third layer, which is known to be a result of compensatory upregulation of p16, due to the interference of the E7 oncoprotein of high-risk HPV with RB1. As recommended by the Lower Anogenital Squamous Terminology (LAST) [22], application of p16 is useful in the following contexts: distinction of HSIL from its mimics, such as immature metaplasia, atrophy, reparative changes, or tangential sectioning; assessment of LSIL at high risk for missed HSIL on Pap; Smears for HPV testing; confirmation of the diagnosis of HSIL/CIN2 versus CIN1 in histologically equivalent cases. However, overapplication of p16 should be avoided in morphologically unequivocal cases with LSIL or HSIL. In the absence of block-positive p16 staining, HSIL is less likely. Most LSILs show mild or faint patchy or localized p16 expression. Direct HPV testing is valuable in selected cases, such as those with differential LSIL versus negative/reactive cases, because p16 immunohistochemistry is less useful in this context. Immature squamous metaplasia with some atypia can be re-evaluated as HSIL using p16. Ki-67 positive cells are diffusely distributed in two-thirds to almost the entire layer of HSILs. However, Ki-67-positive cells are usually smaller in number and irregularly distributed in immature squamous metaplasia. Atrophic squamous cells are invariably negative for p16 and show a very low Ki-67 index. Recently, dual staining biomarkers of p16 and Ki-67 have emerged as promising test [23]/objective microscopy-based triage tool [24]. The simultaneous expression of these markers in the same cell should mutually exclude each other under normal physiological conditions, and their coexpression can identify cells with an abnormal cell cycle associated with high-risk HPV infection.

3.2 Adenocarcinoma, HPV (Human Papillomavirus)-Associated and HPV-Independent

3.2.1 Adenocarcinoma In Situ (AIS), HPV-Associated

There are evidences that AIS (Figs. 3.4 and 3.5) has a precancerous potential for invasive adenocarcinoma. AIS occurs in patients 10–15 years younger than those with invasive adenocarcinoma; AIS is commonly associated with microinvasive or clinically invasive adenocarcinoma in the same specimen and occasionally AIS precedes invasive adenocarcinoma [25]. The atypical columnar cells are confined to preexisting glandular structures. Nuclei are hyperchromatic and variably enlarged with an elongated or rounded contour. These nuclei tend to be basally placed but show varying degrees of pseudostratification. Mitotic figures with basal karyorrhexis are identified in the apical portion (floating mitoses). In the so-called early or

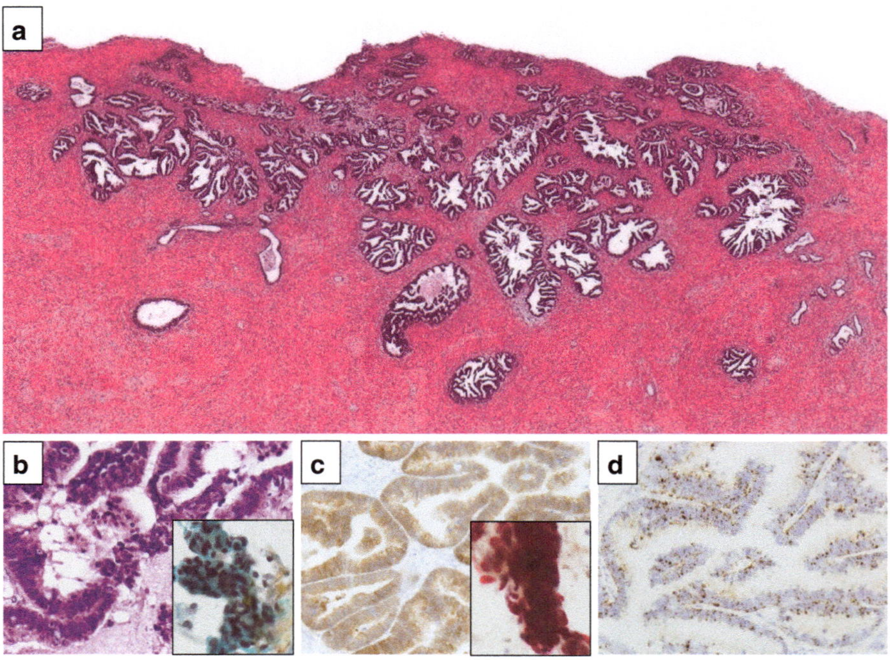

Fig. 3.4 Adenocarcinoma in situ, HPV-associated: (**a**) HE staining of hysterectomy specimen: The tumor is composed of many irregularly sized glands limited to the area of preexisting normal glands. (**b**) HE staining (hyperpower view, inset: Papanicolaou staining of LBC): The tumor cells with hyperchromatic nuclei and pseudostratification arranged in a papillary manner within the lumen. Hypercrowded tumor cell cluster looks like glandular structure). (**c**) Immunohistochemistry of p16 (inset: immunocytochemical dual staining of p16 and Ki-67 by CINtecPlus): Positive reaction of p16 is diffusely observed with moderate intensity. The tumor cells are dual-positive for these markers (inset). (**d**) High-risk HPV-DNA ISH: Many small-sized dot-like signals are observed in the nuclei

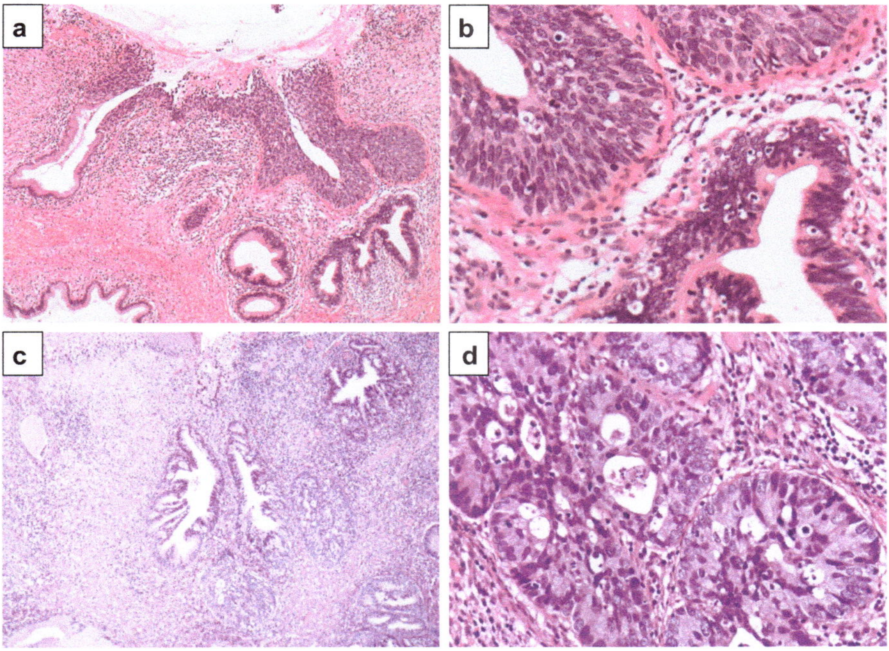

Fig. 3.5 Adenocarcinoma in situ (AIS), HPV-associated: (**a**) HE staining of conization specimen: AIS and HSIL/CIN3/severe dysplasia coexist in the neighborhood. (**b**) HE staining of conization specimens (hyperpower view): Atypical cells of HSIL extend along the cervical glands, and AIS shows an atypical glandular structure with pseudostratification. (**c**) HE staining of biopsy: AIS components of the glandular structure coexist with adjacent SMILE nests; (**d**) HE staining of biopsy specimen (hyperpower view): SMILE nests of glandular/tubular structures are composed of atypical cells with pale eosinophilic cytoplasm, indicating mucus or glycogen accumulation

superficial AIS [26], carcinoma cells with bland uniform-sized nuclei are preferentially arranged in a monolayer along the luminal surface. However, the mitotic figures and apoptotic bodies are less conspicuous. Superficial AIS occurs at a mean age that is a decade younger than typical AIS [25]. Some AISs show distinct intracytoplasmic mucin, and the goblet cell type is occasionally characteristic of intestinal differentiation, which is associated with neuroendocrine features, as demonstrated by immunostaining for chromogranin-A and synaptophysin. Typical HPV-associated AIS is characterized by mucin depletion, resembling endometrioid adenocarcinoma, and lacks confirmatory endometrioid features, such as atypical hyperplasia and squamous metaplasia. When cribriform structures and papillae are extensively observed, invasive adenocarcinoma with non-destructive invasion may be challenging as a differential diagnosis for AIS. Non-neoplastic and/or reactive columnar cells caused by inflammatory irritation, regeneration (e.g., following biopsy or conization), or metaplasia (e.g., tuboendometrioid glands) may be confused with ciliated AIS or AIS lacking overt nuclear atypia. More than half of the AIS cases are synchronous with HSIL [27]. Stratified mucin-producing intraepithelial lesions

(SMILE) are observed as a counterpart of AIS or regarded as a subtype of AIS. SMILE consists of a stratified epithelium with mucin throughout all cell layers and frequently a peripheral cuff of basaloid/reserve cells [28] and often co-exists with HSIL in 93% of cases, conventional AIS in 42%, or invasive carcinoma, including invasive stratified mucin-producing carcinoma [29] in 10% [30]. It is difficult to classify SMILE as either squamous or glandular in origin because of its mixed histological features; however, it was defined as a variant of AIS in the 2014 WHO tumor classification [31].

3.2.2 Invasive Adenocarcinoma, HPV-Associated

HPV-associated adenocarcinomas are divided into two groups: usual (Fig. 3.6) and mucinous. The usual type accounts for approximately 75% [32, 33], and cells with mucinous cytoplasm constitute approximately 50% of the tumor. Carcinoma cells show irregular confluent glands composed of mucin-depleted cells with indistinct

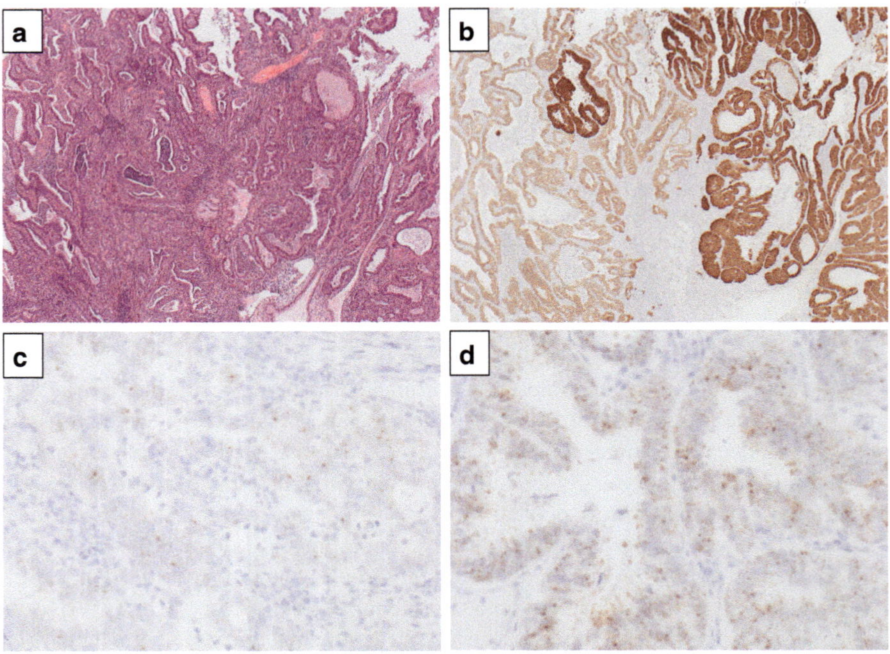

Fig. 3.6 Adenocarcinoma, HPV-associated: (**a**) HE staining of conization specimen: The tumor is composed of irregularly shaped and sized glands. (**b**) Immunohistochemistry of p16: Positive reaction is diffusely observed and clearly divided into weak and strong areas. (**c**) High-risk HPV-RNA ISH in the area of weak p16 expression shown in (**b**): Small dot-like signals are evenly dispersed. (**d**) High-risk HPV-RNA ISH in the area of strong p16 expression shown (**b**): Signals are larger in number and size compared with (**c**). The intensity of p16 may be related to HPV-DNA copy number and transcriptional activity reflected by HPV-RNA

cell borders and elongated or oval, pseudostratified, and hyperchromatic nuclei. Papillary or villoglandular pattern and micropapillary type (architecturally but not cytologically mimicking serous carcinoma) are included in the usual type. The mucinous type accounts for approximately 10% [32, 34] and is composed of cells with mucin in ≥50% of the entire tumor. The vast majority of cervical adenocarcinomas mimicking endometrioid carcinoma are considered HPV-associated adenocarcinomas with mucin depletion. True endometrioid carcinoma can be diagnosed if HPV-associated adenocarcinoma and endometrial adenocarcinoma are excluded. Based on the architectural pattern, that is, the proportion of tubular or papillary structures and solid components, as well as the nuclear grade, the tumor can be graded as grades 1, 2, or 3. This grading system is considered to be in good agreement with clinical outcomes [35]. In the 2020 WHO classification, grade 1 usual type endocervical adenocarcinoma has solid component <10% and mild to moderate nuclear atypia; grade 2 has 11–50% solid component and nuclear atypia intermediate between grade 1 and 3; grade 3 has solid component >50% and marked nuclear atypia [36]. The International Society of Gynecological Pathologists [37] and the International Collaboration on Cancer Reporting (ICCR) [37] recommend the application of this grading system for HPV-associated adenocarcinoma. However, when the areas with high-grade nuclear atypia are more than 50%, the grade increases from 1 to 2 and from 2 to 3. A confluent microglandular pattern is regarded as a solid component, and the presence of micropapillary pattern, signet ring cells, and invasive SMILE are regarded as G3. Gastric-type and clear cell types are classified as high-grade [38].

The histological pattern-based classification (Silva system), which focuses on the invasive pattern and is closely associated with nodal metastasis, recurrence, and survival, has been proposed for HPV-associated adenocarcinoma, and is as follows [39, 40]: pattern A, non-destructive invasion (well-demarcated glands with rounded contour; no lymphovascular invasion; complex intraglandular growth acceptable, i.e., cribriform growth, papillae; lack of solid growth, i.e. architecturally well to moderately differentiated); pattern B, early/focally destructive invasion (individual or small groups of tumor cells, separated from the rounded glands, focally desmoplastic or inflamed stroma; foci may be single, multiple, or linear at base of tumor; lymphovascular invasion +/−; lack of solid growth, i.e., architecturally well to moderately differentiated); pattern C, diffusely invasion (diffusely infiltrative glands with associated extensive desmoplastic response; glands often angulated or with canalicular pattern, with interspersed open glands; confluent growth filling a 4x field (5 mm), glands, papillae (stroma only within papillae) or mucin lakes; solid, poorly differentiated component (architecturally high-grade); nuclear grade is disregarded; lymphovascular invasion +). This system is valuable in terms of reproducibility, particularly in distinguishing between indolent tumors with pattern A and potentially aggressive tumors with patterns B and C [39, 40]. The hallmarks of HPV-associated adenocarcinoma architecture include apical mitoses and karyorrhexis, which are conspicuous and identifiable under low-power magnification [32].

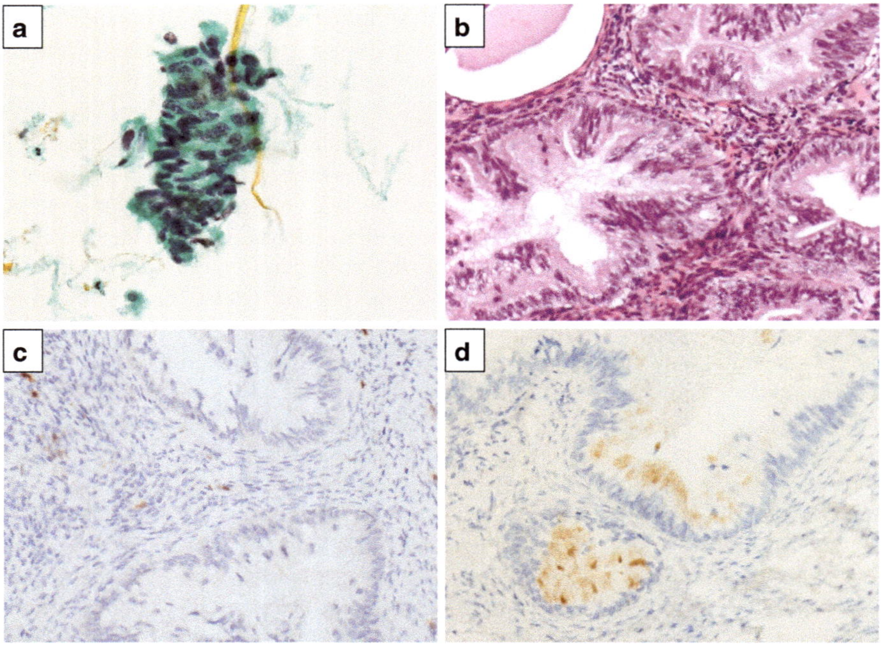

Fig. 3.7 Adenocarcinoma in situ, HPV-independent/gastric-type: (**a**) Papanicolaou staining (LBC): A tumor cell cluster shows round to short spindle-shaped nuclei with mild stratification and irregular arrangement. (**b**) HE staining of hysterectomy specimen: The tumor cells are replacing proper glands and arranged in a papillary manner protruding into the luminal space. (**c**) Immunohistochemistry of p16: The tumor cells show negative reaction. (**d**) Immunohistochemistry of HIK1083: The tumor cells focally show positive reaction

3.2.3 Adenocarcinoma, In Situ (AIS), HPV-Independent

Gastric-type differentiation is a characteristic of HPV-independent AIS (Fig. 3.7). The preexisting endocervical glands replaced by tumor cells are architecturally complex with cribriform or papillary patterns. The tumor cells are cuboidal to columnar with distinct cell borders, round nuclei with mild to moderate atypia, and eosinophilic to pale and/or foamy vacuolated cytoplasm. Mitosis and apoptotic bodies are less prominent. Intestinal features or goblet cells are often observed to varying degrees. Lobular endocervical glandular hyperplasia (LEGH) with atypia is a related lesion, belonging to the spectrum of gastric-type adenocarcinomas.

3.2.4 Invasive Adenocarcinoma, HPV-Independent

Adenocarcinomas with gastric (pyloric) differentiation are HPV-independent and characteristically impart a barrel shape to the cervix [41] (Fig. 3.8). Tumor cells can be well-differentiated or poorly differentiated. Minimal deviation adenocarcinoma

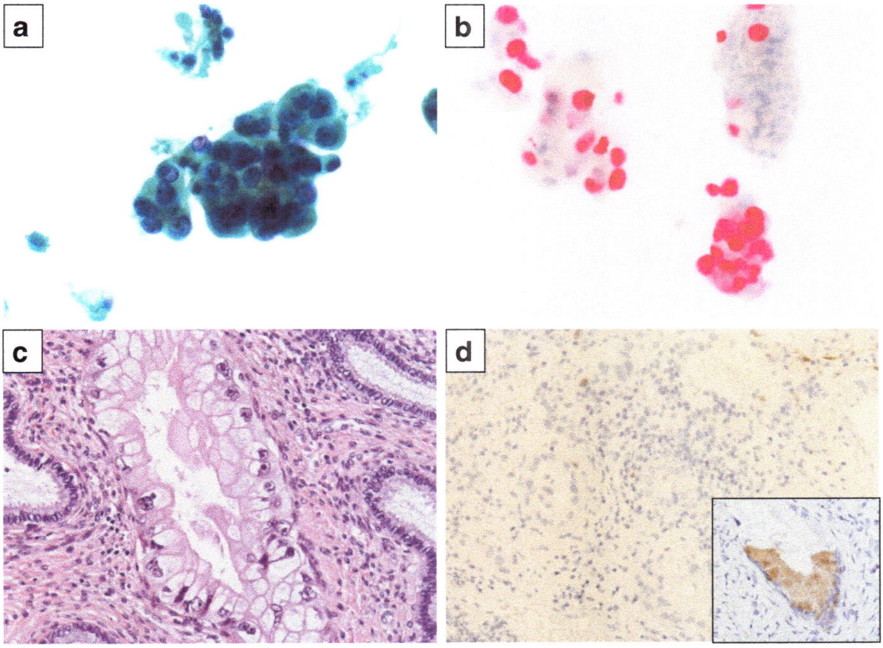

Fig. 3.8 Adenocarcinoma, HPV-independent/gastric-type: (**a**) Papanicolaou staining (LBC): The tumor cells having irregularly enlarged nuclei with hyperchromasia are arranged in stratified cluster. (**b**) Immunocytochemical dual staining of p16 and Ki-67 (CINtecPlus): The tumor cells are positive for Ki-67, which stain red with fast red, but negative for p16. These findings demonstrate that the tumor is independent of HPV infection. (**c**) HE staining of hysterectomy specimen: Glandular tumor cells are characteristic of abundant clear cytoplasm and nuclei with prominent nucleoli. (**d**) Immunohistochemistry of p16 (inset: HIK1083): No positive expression of p16 is observed. The tumor cells are focally positive for HIK1083. *HE* hematoxylin and eosin, *HPV* human papillomavirus, *SCC* squamous cell carcinoma, *LBC* liquid-based cytology, *ISH* in situ hybridization, *N/C* nucleus-to-cytoplasmic

or adenoma malignum has been traditionally considered as an extremely well-differentiated counterpart of gastric-type adenocarcinoma. Carcinoma cells typically have distinct cell borders and abundant clear or pale eosinophilic cytoplasm [42, 43], with neutral mucins that stain pinkish-red with alcian blue/PAS staining [44]. The mucins of normal endocervical glandular cells are acidic and stain dark purple. The well-differentiated glands of the minimal deviation type have smooth contours and a haphazard distribution. The glands are composed of tall columnar cells with abundant pale and foamy cytoplasm and distinct cell borders that lack desmoplasia. In the poorly differentiated type, the glands are irregularly shaped, irregularly sized, and angular. The nuclei are atypical, pleomorphic, and vesicular, with prominent nucleoli. The cytoplasm is abundant, eosinophilic, and vacuolated.

HPV-independent adenocarcinomas other than gastric-type include endometrioid carcinoma, clear cell carcinoma, and mesonephric carcinoma. However, serous carcinoma has been excluded because of a recent consensus that most or all serous carcinomas detected in the uterine cervix represent direct invasion of endometrial serous carcinomas or metastasis of adnexal serous carcinoma [45].

3.2.5 Cytology

HPV-associated AIS shows strips and clusters of crowded or overlapping atypical columnar cells that are arranged in a palisading manner. The nuclear protrusion is known as feathering. Nuclei with increased N/C ratios are enlarged and elongated and have typically coarse or granular nuclei. The honeycomb pattern of the normal endocervical glandular arrangement is lost. When atypia overlaps with benign mimics, the glandular abnormalities are categorized as atypical glandular cells/AGC, NOS or favored neoplastic. AIS and HSIL can be encountered in the same preparation [27]. Compared to AIS, invasive adenocarcinoma cells tend to appear in more syncytial-aggregated clusters. The nuclei are enlarged and pleomorphic, with considerably coarse chromatin and macronucleoli. In LBC, granular and apoptotic debris clinging to the edges of cell clusters are observed [6]. Gastric-type HPV-independent AIS can be diagnosed by the presence of yellowish gastric-type mucin. However, in LBC, mucin produced by neoplastic cells is usually difficult to distinguish from normal endocervical mucin. The two-toned yellow gastric-type and pink normal endocervical type mucins on conventional Pap smear are regarded as a diagnostic clue to identify gastric-type adenocarcinoma [46]. Other diagnostic hallmarks include monolayered sheets of atypical glandular cells with foamy vacuolar cytoplasm, distinct cell borders, intracytoplasmic neutrophils, and vesicular nuclei with prominent nucleoli. Gastric-type adenocarcinoma may mimic reactive endocervical cells, and identification of glandular cells with uniform nuclear enlargement in conjunction with any of the other cytologic features may help avoid false-negative Pap results [47].

3.2.6 Surrogate Marker and Ancillary Testing

In terms of reproducibility, p16 is the most convenient and useful surrogate marker for the diagnostic confirmation of adenocarcinoma and SCCs. Recently, immunocytochemical double staining of p16 and Ki-67 can be helpfully applied for detection of adenocarcinoma as well as SIL/CIN [48]. p16 is strongly expressed in almost all HPV-associated adenocarcinomas both in situ and invasive. Unlike the patchy staining observed in hyperplastic, reactive, or metaplastic cells, the strong positive expression in both the nucleus and cytoplasm (i.e., block-positive) confirms HPV infection. However, some adenocarcinomas with high-grade atypia, such as endometrial serous carcinoma, clear cell carcinoma, and high-grade endometrioid, also show block-positive p16 expression. Direct HPV testing and high-risk HPV-RNA or DNA in situ hybridization are helpful to confirm the diagnosis of these problematic cases. Rare p16-negative cases may be due to methylation-induced inactivation [49]. Immunohistochemically, cervical adenocarcinomas show p53 normal/

wild-type staining and are positive for CK7, PAX8, and CDX2 (particularly intestinal type) [50], but negative for ER, PgR, vimentin, CK20, and STAB2 [45, 51]. AIS is typically PAX8+/PAX2−, unlike normal endocervical glands which are PAX8+/PAX2 + [52].

HPV-independent adenocarcinoma of the gastric type and lobular endocervical hyperplasia are specifically and focally positive for HIK1083 (gastric pyloric gland marker) and MUC6 (not specific) [53]. PAX8, CAIX, and CEA are usually positive, but ER and PgR are negative. p16 is either negative or patchy-positive, but its overexpression can be seen [54–56]. Some gastric-type adenocarcinomas are related to Peutz-Jeghers syndrome and frequently show *STK11* mutations [57] and *TP53* alterations [58]. Expressions of HNF-1β and napsin A are sensitive for clear cell adenocarcinoma, but not specific [45, 54]. Mesonephric adenocarcinoma is positive for GATA3, CD10, and TTF-1 but negative for ER, AMACR, and napsin A [54, 59–66].

In terms of differentiation between cervical adenocarcinoma and endometrial adenocarcinoma, representative diagnostic immunohistochemical markers include p16, ER, vimentin, and CEA. p16 is strongly expressed in HPV-associated cervical adenocarcinomas and high-grade endometrial carcinomas, such as serous carcinoma, with no distinct differences in their staining patterns. However, in differentiated endometrioid adenocarcinomas, a patchy or mosaic pattern of p16 expression is observed. ER is clearly expressed in differentiated endometrial endometrioid carcinoma; however, cervical adenocarcinomas, whether HPV-associated or -independent, are negative or mildly positive for ER. Vimentin is expressed in endometrial endometrioid carcinomas to some extent; however, it is usually absent in cervical adenocarcinomas. CEA expression is more apparent in cervical adenocarcinoma than in endometrial adenocarcinoma.

3.3 Reporting of Cervical Cancer

The fourth edition of updated dataset for the reporting of carcinoma of the cervix by ICCR [37, 67] was undertaken to incorporate the major changes based on International Federation of Gynecology and Obstetrics (FIGO) in 2018 [68] and WHO 2020 tumor classification. The maximum depth of invasion is taken from the base of epithelium, but there are some situations where it is impossible to measure the depth. The pathologist and clinician should equate the tumor thickness with invasion for staging and management purposes. Uncommonly, SCC and adenocarcinoma and other histologic types take predominantly polypoid/exophytic growth pattern. ICCR recommends some examples of staging criteria for polypoid/exophytic tumor ≤20 mm in largest dimension:

- With a total thickness of 15 mm, the portion of destructive stromal invasion into the cervical wall (nonexophytic component) measures 4 mm in depth—Stage IB1.

- With a total thickness of 4 mm, the portion of the tumor with true destructive stromal invasion into the cervical wall (nonexophytic component) measures 1 mm in depth—Stage IA2.
- With a total thickness of 2.5 mm, the portion of the tumor with true destructive stromal invasion into the cervical wall (nonexophytic component) measures 1 mm in depth—Stage IA1.

References

1. de Sanjose S, WGV Q, Alemany L, et al. Retrospective International Survey and HPV Time Trends Study Group: human papillomavirus genotype attribution in invasive cervical cancer: a retrospective cross-sectional worldwide study. Lancet Oncol. 2010;11:1048–56.
2. Nicolás I, Marimon L, Barnadas E, et al. HPV-negative tumors of the uterine cervix. Mod Pathol. 2019;32:1189–96.
3. Rodríguez-Carunchio L, Soveral I, Steenbergen RDM, et al. HPV-negative carcinoma of the uterine cervix: a distinct type of cervical cancer with poor prognosis. BJOG. 2015;122:119–27.
4. McBride AA. Oncogenic human papillomaviruses. Philos Trans R Soc Lond B Biol Sci. 2017;372:20160273.
5. Clifford GM, Smith JS, Plummer M, et al. Human papillomavirus types in invasive cervical cancer worldwide: a meta-analysis. Br J Cancer. 2003;88:63–73.
6. Herrington CS, Kim K-R, Kong CS, et al. Tumours of the uterine cervix. In: Lokuhetty D, White VA, Cree IA, editors. WHO classification of tumours. Female genital tumours. 5th ed. Lyon: IARC Press; 2020. p. 335–89.
7. Cancer Genome Atlas Research Network, Albert Einstein College of Medicine, Analytical Biological Services, et al. Integrated genomic and molecular characterization of cervical cancer. Nature. 2017;543:378–84.
8. Feng D, Hui X, Li X, et al. An association analysis between mitochondrial DNA content, G10398A polymorphism, HPV infection, and the prognosis of cervical cancer in the Chinese Han population. Tumour Biol. 2016;37:5599–607.
9. Pilch H, Günzel S, Schäffer U, et al. The presence of HPV DNA in cervical cancer: correlation with clinico-pathologic parameters and prognostic significance: 10 years experience at the Department of Obstetrics and Gynecology of the Mainz University. Int J Gynecol Cancer. 2001;11:39–48.
10. Riou G, Favre M, Jeannel D, et al. Association between poor prognosis in early-stage invasive cervical carcinomas and non-detection of HPV DNA. Lancet. 1990;335:1171–4.
11. Cole L, Stoler MH. Issues and inconsistencies in the revised gynecologic staging systems. Semin Diagn Pathol. 2012;29:167–73.
12. Araújo Catão Zampronha R, Freitas-Junior R, Murta EFC, et al. Human papillomavirus types 16 and 18 and the prognosis of patients with stage I cervical cancer. Clinics. 2013;68:809–14.
13. Pirog EC, Wright TC, Ronnett BR, et al. Carcinoma and other tumors of the cervix. In: Kurman RJ, Ellenson LH, Ronnett BM, editors. Blaustein's pathology of the female genital tract. 7th ed. Switzerland: Springer; 2019. p. 315–74.
14. Rodríguez-Trujillo A, Martí C, Angeles MA, et al. Value of HPV 16/18 genotyping and p16/Ki-67 dual staining to predict progression to HSIL/CIN2+ in negative cytologies from a colposcopy referral population. Am J Clin Pathol. 2018;150:432–40.
15. Guimerà N, Lloveras B, Lindeman J, et al. The occasional role of low-risk human papillomaviruses 6, 11, 42, 44, and 70 in anogenital carcinoma defined by laser capture microdissection/PCR methodology: results from a global study. Am J Surg Pathol. 2013;37:1299–310.

16. van der Marel J, Berkhof J, Ordi J, et al. Attributing oncogenic human papillomavirus genotypes to high-grade cervical neoplasia: which type causes the lesion? Am J Surg Pathol. 2015;39:496–504.
17. Stoler MH, Schiffman M. Atypical squamous cells of undetermined significance-low-grade squamous intraepithelial lesion triage study (ALTS) group: interobserver reproducibility of cervical cytologic and histologic interpretations: realistic estimates from the ASCUS-LSIL triage study. JAMA. 2001;285:1500–5.
18. Mills AM, Coppock JD, Willis BC, et al. HPV E6/E7 mRNA in situ hybridization in the diagnosis of cervical low-grade squamous intraepithelial lesions (LSIL). Am J Surg Pathol. 2018;42:192–200.
19. van der Marel J, Baars R, Alonso I, et al. Oncogenic human papillomavirus-infected immature metaplastic cells and cervical neoplasia. Am J Surg Pathol. 2014;38:470–9.
20. Katki HA, Schiffman M, Castle PE, et al. Five-year risks of CIN 2+ and CIN 3+ among women with HPV-positive and HPV-negative LSIL pap results. J Low Genit Tract Dis. 2013;17:S43–9.
21. Katki HA, Schiffman M, Castle PE, et al. Five-year risks of CIN 3+ and cervical cancer among women with HPV-positive and HPV-negative high-grade pap results. J Low Genit Tract Dis. 2013;17:S50–5.
22. Darragh TM, Colgan TJ, Cox JT, et al. Members of LAST project work groups: the lower anogenital squamous terminology standardization project for HPV-associated lesions: background and consensus recommendations from the College of American Pathologists and the American Society for Colposcopy and Cervical Pathology. Arch Pathol Lab Med. 2012;136:1266–97.
23. Luttmer R, Dijkstra MG, Snijders PJF, et al. p16/Ki-67 dual-stained cytology for detecting cervical (pre)cancer in a HPV-positive gynecologic outpatient population. Mod Pathol. 2016;29:870–8.
24. McMenamin M, McKenna M, Andrew MD. Clinical utility of CINtec PLUS triage in equivocal cervical cytology and human papillomavirus primary screening. Am J Clin Pathol. 2018;150:512–21.
25. Costa S, Venturoli S, Negri G, et al. Factors preceding the outcome of conservatively treated adenocarcinoma in situ of the uterine cervix: an analysis of 166 cases. Gynecol Oncol. 2012;124:490–5.
26. Witkiewicz A, Lee KR, Brodsky G, et al. Superficial (early) endocervical adenocarcinoma in situ: a study of 12 cases and comparison to conventional AIS. Am J Surg Pathol. 2005;29:1609–14.
27. Jaworski RC, Pacey NE, Greenberg ML, et al. The histologic diagnosis of adenocarcinoma in situ and related lesions of the cervix uteri. Adenocarcinoma in situ. Cancer. 1988;61:1171–81.
28. Park JJ, Sun D, Quade BJ, et al. Stratified mucin-producing intraepithelial lesions of the cervix: adenosquamous or columnar cell neoplasia? Am J Surg Pathol. 2000;24:1414–9.
29. Onishi J, Sato Y, Sawaguchi A, et al. Stratified mucin-producing intraepithelial lesion with invasive carcinoma; 12 cases with immunohistochemical and ultrastructural findings. Hum Pathol. 2016;55:174–81.
30. Boyle DP, McCluggage WG. Stratified mucin-producing intraepithelial lesion (SMILE): report of a case series with associated pathological findings. Histopathology. 2015;66:658–63.
31. Stoler M, Bergeron C, Colgan TJ, et al. Tumours of the uterine cervix. In: Kurman RJ, Carcangiu ML, Herrington CS, Young RH, editors. WHO classification of tumours. Female genital tumours. 4th ed. Lyon: IARC Press; 2014. p. 169–206.
32. Stolnicu S, Barsan I, Hoang L, et al. International endocervical adenocarcinoma criteria and classification (IECC): a new pathogenetic classification for invasive adenocarcinomas of the endocervix. Am J Surg Pathol. 2018;42:214–26.
33. Young RH, Clement PB. Endocervical adenocarcinoma and its variants: their morphology and differential diagnosis. Histopathology. 2002;41:185–207.
34. Hodgson A, Olkhov-Mitsel E, Howitt BE, et al. International endocervical adenocarcinoma criteria and classification (IECC): correlation with adverse clinicopathological features and patient outcome. J Clin Pathol. 2019;72:347–53.

35. Baalbergen A, Ewing-Graham PC, Hop WCJ, et al. Prognostic factors in adenocarcinoma of the uterine cervix. Gynecol Oncol. 2004;92:262–7.
36. Association of Directors of Anatomic and Surgical Pathology. Recommendations for the reporting of surgical specimens containing uterine cervical neoplasms. Mod Pathol. 2000;13:1029–33.
37. International collaboration on cancer reporting. Carcinomas of the cervix. https://www.iccr-cancer.org/datasets/published-datasets/female-reproductive/carcinomas-of-the-cervix/.
38. Talia KL, Oliva E, Rabban JT, et al. Grading of endocervical adenocarcinomas: review of the literature and recommendations from the international society of gynecological pathologists. Int J Gynecol Pathol. 2021;40(Suppl 1):S66–74.
39. Parra-Herran C, Taljaard M, Djordjevic B, et al. Pattern-based classification of invasive endocervical adenocarcinoma, depth of invasion measurement and distinction from adenocarcinoma in situ: interobserver variation among gynecologic pathologists. Mod Pathol. 2016;29:879–92.
40. Rutgers JKL, Roma AA, Park KJ, et al. Pattern classification of endocervical adenocarcinoma: reproducibility and review of criteria. Mod Pathol. 2016;29:1083–94.
41. Kwon SY, Choe MS, Lee HW, et al. Minimal deviation adenocarcinoma of the cervix and tumorlets of sex-cord stromal tumor with annular tubules of the ovary in Peutz-Jeghers syndrome. J Gynecol Oncol. 2013;24:92–5.
42. Kojima A, Mikami Y, Sudo T, et al. Gastric morphology and immunophenotype predict poor outcome in mucinous adenocarcinoma of the uterine cervix. Am J Surg Pathol. 2007;31:664–72.
43. Kawakami F, Mikami Y, Kojima A, et al. Diagnostic reproducibility in gastric-type mucinous adenocarcinoma of the uterine cervix: validation of novel diagnostic criteria. Histopathology. 2010;56:551–3.
44. Kondo T, Hashi A, Murata S-I, et al. Gastric mucin is expressed in a subset of endocervical tunnel clusters: type A tunnel clusters of gastric phenotype. Histopathology. 2007;50:843–50.
45. Stolnicu S, Barsan I, Hoang L, et al. Diagnostic algorithmic proposal based on comprehensive immunohistochemical evaluation of 297 invasive endocervical adenocarcinomas. Am J Surg Pathol. 2018;42:989–1000.
46. Omori M, Kondo T, Nakazawa K, et al. Interpretation of endocervical cells with gastric-type mucin on pap smear; a proposal for a cytologic category "atypical endocervical cells with gastric-type mucin". Am J Clin Pathol. 2018;150:259–66.
47. Schwock J, Starova B, Khan ZF, et al. Cytomorphologic features of gastric-type endocervical adenocarcinoma in liquid-based preparations. Acta Cytol. 2021;65:56–66.
48. Ryu A, Honma K, Shingetsu A, et al. Utility of p16/Ki67 double immunocytochemistry for detection of cervical adenocarcinoma. Cancer Cytopathol. 2022;130:983–92.
49. Nuovo GJ, Plaia TW, Belinsky SA, et al. In situ detection of the hypermethylation-induced inactivation of the p16 gene as an early event in oncogenesis. Proc Natl Acad Sci U S A. 1999;96:12754–9.
50. McCluggage WG, Shah R, Connolly LE, et al. Intestinal-type cervical adenocarcinoma in situ and adenocarcinoma exhibit a partial enteric immunophenotype with consistent expression of CDX2. Int J Gynecol Pathol. 2008;27:92–100.
51. Hodgson A, Park KJ, Djordjevic B, et al. International endocervical adenocarcinoma criteria and classification: validation and interobserver reproducibility. Am J Surg Pathol. 2019;43:75–83.
52. Shukla A, Thomas D, Roh MH. PAX8 and PAX2 expression in endocervical adenocarcinoma in-situ and high-grade squamous dysplasia. Mod Pathol. 2012;25:296A.
53. Hodgson A, Parra-Herran C, Mirkovic J. Immunohistochemical expression of HIK1083 and MUC6 in endometrial carcinomas. Histopathology. 2019;75:552–8.
54. Ordi J, Romagosa C, Tavassoli FA, et al. CD10 expression in epithelial tissues and tumors of the gynecologic tract: a useful marker in the diagnosis of mesonephric, trophoblastic, and clear cell tumors. Am J Surg Pathol. 2003;27:178–86.
55. Carleton C, Hoang L, Shatrughan S, et al. A detailed immunohistochemical analysis of a large series of cervical and vaginal gastric-type adenocarcinomas. Am J Surg Pathol. 2016;40:636–44.

56. Wada T, Ohishi Y, Kaku T, et al. Endocervical adenocarcinoma with morphologic features of both usual and gastric types: clinicopathologic and immunohistochemical analyses and high-risk HPV detection by in situ hybridization. Am J Surg Pathol. 2017;41:696–705.
57. Kuragaki C, Enomoto T, Ueno Y, et al. Mutations in the STK11 gene characterize minimal deviation adenocarcinoma of the uterine cervix. Lab Invest. 2003;83:35–45.
58. Garg S, Nagaria TS, Clarke B, et al. Molecular characterization of gastric-type endocervical adenocarcinoma using next-generation sequencing. Mod Pathol. 2019;32:1823–33.
59. Goyal A, Yang B. Differential patterns of PAX8, p16, and ER immunostains in mesonephric lesions and adenocarcinomas of the cervix. Int J Gynecol Pathol. 2014;33:613–9.
60. Howitt BE, Emori MM, Drapkin R, et al. GATA3 is a sensitive and specific marker of benign and malignant mesonephric lesions in the lower female genital tract. Am J Surg Pathol. 2015;39:1411–9.
61. Pors J, Cheng A, Leo JM, et al. A Comparison of GATA3, TTF1, CD10, and calretinin in identifying mesonephric and mesonephric-like carcinomas of the gynecologic tract. Am J Surg Pathol. 2018;42:1596–606.
62. Pors J, Segura S, Cheng A, et al. Napsin-A and AMACR are superior to HNF-1β in distinguishing between mesonephric carcinomas and clear cell carcinomas of the gynecologic tract. Appl Immunohistochem Mol Morphol. 2020;28:593–601.
63. Silver SA, Devouassoux-Shisheboran M, Mezzetti TP, et al. Mesonephric adenocarcinomas of the uterine cervix: a study of 11 cases with immunohistochemical findings. Am J Surg Pathol. 2001;25:379–87.
64. Bagué S, Rodríguez IM, Prat J. Malignant mesonephric tumors of the female genital tract: a clinicopathologic study of 9 cases. Am J Surg Pathol. 2004;28:601–7.
65. Kenny SL, McBride HA, Jamison J, et al. Mesonephric adenocarcinomas of the uterine cervix and corpus: HPV-negative neoplasms that are commonly PAX8, CA125, and HMGA2 positive and that may be immunoreactive with TTF1 and hepatocyte nuclear factor 1-β. Am J Surg Pathol. 2012;36:799–807.
66. Roma AA, Goyal A, Yang B. Differential expression patterns of GATA3 in uterine mesonephric and nonmesonephric lesions. Int J Gynecol Pathol. 2015;34:480–6.
67. Park KJ, Selinger CI, Alvarado-Cabrero I, et al. Dataset for the reporting of carcinoma of the cervix: recommendations from the International Collaboration on Cancer Reporting (ICCR). Int J Gynecol Pathol. 2022;41(Suppl 1):S64–89.
68. Bhatla N, Berek JS, Cuello FM, et al. Revised FIGO staging for carcinoma of the cervix uteri. Int J Gynaecol Obstet. 2019;145:129–35.

Part II

Strategies of Cancer Screening and Prevention of Cervical Cancer

Assessment and Management of Cervical Cancer Screening Programs in Japan

4

Tohru Morisada and Daisuke Aoki

Abstract

In recent years, the implementation of HPV test as a new modality of cervical cancer screening has been discussed in Japan. Cancer screening, however, does not mean simply a screening test for examinees, but a series of programs conducted for a large population of subjects, including post-test medical treatment, follow-up management, and monitoring of the outcome of the screening. Although the choice of effective screening modality is important, its role is only a small part of the screening program. Meanwhile, evaluating the operation of the screening program and repeatedly improving it is a major part of the program and leads to minimizing the harms to the examinees while ensuring the effectiveness of cancer screening. The importance of quality control of screening (management), which evaluates and improves the operation of cancer screening, needs to be clearly distinguished from that of efficacy evaluation (assessment), which uses mortality reduction effects to select test modality. Here, we present information on the current status of population-based screening in Japan and outline the concept of quality control of cancer screening, including its relationship to assessment of the efficacy of cancer screening.

Keywords

Cervical cancer screening · Population-based screening · Assessment · Management · Effectiveness of screening · Quality control · Benefit · Harm

T. Morisada
Department of Obstetrics and Gynecology, Faculty of Medicine, Kyorin University, Tokyo, Japan

D. Aoki (✉)
Akasaka Sanno Medical Center, International University of Health and Welfare Graduate School, Tokyo, Japan
e-mail: aoki@z7.keio.jp

D. Aoki (ed.), *Recent Topics on Prevention, Diagnosis, and Clinical Management of Cervical Cancer*, Comprehensive Gynecology and Obstetrics,
https://doi.org/10.1007/978-981-99-9396-3_4

In medical strategies for uterine cervical cancer, cancer screening plays an important role as a form of secondary prevention through early detection and treatment of patients with cancer. In Japan, attention of health providers has been focused on the development and introduction of new screening methods to improve the effectiveness of cancer screening. However, to improve the effectiveness of screening, the environment in which the selected screening method is implemented its important in terms of keeping the quality of screening programs; therefore, it is essential to evaluate and improve the environment. The establishment of a system to manage this environment is referred to as the "Establishment of a management system for a screening program." Moreover, international standards require this system to be in place prior to the implementation of a new screening method [1]. This paper describes the screening management system, which is the foundation of screening, and the importance of quality control and assurance in cancer screening.

4.1 Purpose of Cancer Screening

The purpose of cancer screening is to reduce the mortality rate of the target cancer; hence, it is of great benefit to the individuals who are screened. Objective numerical indicators are often used to assess whether the screening objectives have been met. The most reliable indicator is a comparison of the reduction in mortality rates between the group of individuals screened for the target cancer and the group of individuals who were not screened. Generally, the purpose of cervical cancer screening is to reduce the incidence and mortality of cervical cancer. Cervical intraepithelial neoplasia (CIN) is a precursor lesion; however, these lesions could develop into invasive cancers. CIN can be detected through cervical cancer screening and therapeutic interventions can prevent the development of invasive cancer. In some cases, such as stomach and lung cancers, which are the targets of screening programs in Japan, precancerous lesions may not be detected, and the efficacy of screening is assessed not only by a reduction in incidence but also by a reduction in mortality rates. In Japan, there have been inappropriate opinions regarding the effectiveness of cervical cancer screening that focuses on fertility preservation or pregnancy rates. Because cervical cancer screening includes individuals across a broad age range; moreover, there is no evidence supporting the efficacy of assessing screening using preservation of fertility in all eligible subjects as an indicator. In addition, it is inappropriate to use the pregnancy rate of the population as an indicator of the effectiveness of screening because it is significantly influenced by other inevitable confounding factors.

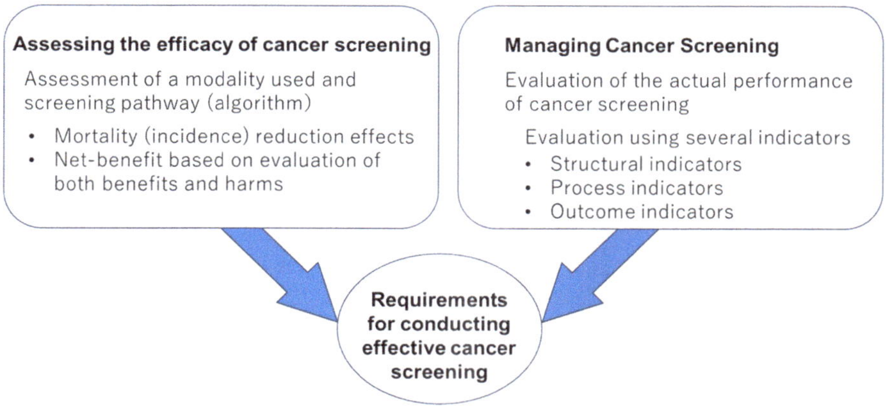

Fig. 4.1 Relationship between efficacy assessment and management in cancer screening. To improve the effectiveness of cancer screening, it is necessary to conduct both efficacy assessment and management based on quality indicators. The efficacy assessment is conducted prior to the implementation of the screening program, while the management is required while screening is ongoing. *Incidence reduction can be used to assess the efficacy of cervical cancer screening as a surrogate outcome

4.2 Relationship Between Assessment and Management

To reduce the mortality rates of target cancers through cancer screening (incidence reduction is also used for cervical cancer screening), screening assessment and management systems are necessary (as shown in Fig. 4.1), and require an understanding of the relationship between the two [2].

4.2.1 Assessment: Assessing the Efficacy of Cancer Screening

The most effective screening method, the cut-off value for a positive screening result (indicating the need for further detailed examination), and the flow of detailed examinations should be determined. If there are several effective screening methods, the one that best fits the prevailing medical infrastructure in the country should be selected after considering whether it is possible to establish a sufficiently effective delivery system (capacity) and a quality control system. To outline the flow of medical procedures, including the detailed examination method, determining when a screen-negative individuals should return for the next screening, a flowchart known as an "algorithm" is used. In the algorithm for cervical cancer screening using cervical cytology, all cases other than those with a negative cytology result (negative for intraepithelial lesion or malignancy [NILM]) are designated as requiring detailed examinations. All examinees are assigned to either " detailed examination and subsequent management" by a physician or "next screening." Screening is evaluated not only based on whether the screening test provides accurate screening results but also based on the entire algorithm. Even if the screening method is the same, the presence or absence and size of the screening effect may differ if the algorithm is different. The presence or absence of the effect of screening is evaluated using objective numerical values, such as whether mortality or incidence is reduced; this is called an efficacy assessment. This assessment is conducted before a decision is made to implement a new cancer screening modality. Specifically, a randomized controlled trial or cohort study is conducted in which the individuals to be screened are divided into two groups: one group is screened using the new screening modality and the other group is not screened, or one group is screened using the conventional screening modality whose efficacy and effectiveness have already been established, and the efficacy of each group in reducing incidence or mortality is compared. High-quality studies should be conducted in each country, and the results of national and international studies should be comprehensively reviewed, assessed, and judged, including the validity of individual studies. The process and results can then be compiled and published as guidelines. Guidelines based on the efficacy assessment of various types of cancer screening have been published in Japan. The guidelines include not only the benefits in terms of reducing mortality and incidence but also the evaluation of harm.

The targets of cancer screening are healthy individuals, unlike those who attend medical institutions for disease treatment. Therefore, minimizing the harm caused by cancer screening is necessary. Harm that may occur during cervical cancer screening includes the detection of precancerous lesions and cancers that could have gone undetected and would not be life-threatening if they had not undergone screening (overdiagnosis). For example, in Japan the 2015 fiscal year report showed that regarding cervical cancer screening, up to 9996 per 10,000 persons were cancer-free and 9985 per 10,000 persons did not have CIN3 or worse (less than 4 per 10,000 persons were diagnosed with cancer during the screening and 15 per 10,000 persons had CIN3 or worse) [3], indicating that no significant immediate benefit in terms of reduction in cancer incidence or death is expected for the majority of the population screened. However, if the harm occurs at a frequency that is not exceptional, it is not negligible for the entire population. Finally, the screening methods were assessed by weighing the benefits of reduced mortality and incidence against harm. Even if the benefit of reduced mortality and incidence can be demonstrated, screening should not be implemented if the harm is evaluated to be relatively large.

4.2.2 Management: Required for Quality Control in Screening

This was done to evaluate whether screening tests and subsequent medical procedures were actually performed in compliance with the algorithm and whether they were successful. Screening can be ineffective when conducted in the real world, although it is effective at the research setting. This is because the operational status of screening differs between research and practice. In the study, the participants were individuals who voluntarily agreed to adhere to the algorithm. Moreover, the physicians and medical institutions that conducted screening tests and provided subsequent medical care were obligated to comply with the research protocol. Overall, the management of the study was well guaranteed. However, the management situation would be poor if concerted efforts are not made at the actual screening sites. The scope of cancer screening for which quality control should be performed includes not only screening tests but also all the following processes.

- Selection of participants prior to screening.
- Invitation of screening for each person.
- Recall those who have not undergone screening and encourage them to return for screening.
- Detailed examinations and follow-up management should be conducted according to an algorithm for those who tested positive.
- Recall screen-positive individuals who did not undergo a detailed examination.
- Track and monitor the results of detailed examinations and follow-ups.
- The next screening should be based on the results of the above procedures.
- A survey should be conducted to determine whether cancer ultimately developed in the entire target population and whether there were cancer deaths.
- Screening performance should be evaluated based on these data.

Despite the substantial amount of work involved in these processes, they are feasible and essential for collecting, managing, and evaluating data, which is the essence of quality control. In other words, screening cannot be performed simply by adopting screening modalities that have proven to be effective in research (assessment only); moreover, the environment for operating screening (screening program) must be improved. For the latter, there are screening programs in Japan that evaluate the state of management as part of the quality control of screening.

4.3 Types of Cancer Screening and Quality Control: A Comparison of Population-Based Screening and Opportunistic Screening

Although quality control is the basis of screening, its implementation differs significantly depending on the type of screening. The types of screening provided in Japan can be largely divided into population-based and opportunistic screening (Table 4.1). In Japan, screening conducted by local governments is an example of population-based screening. Cancer screening provided in workplace should be conducted in a setting of population-based screenings, but largely not. Opportunistic screening is not categorized within the definition of population-based screening and is conducted based on individuals' free will, without specifying the target population for screening [4–6].

Table 4.1 Types of cancer screenings and their management status in Japan

Population-based screening			Opportunistic screening
	Provided by municipalities	Provided offered by employers in workplace	Provided based on personal requests or recommendation from the medical professionals
Target population for screening	Stipulated	Partly to fully stipulated or not	Not stipulated
Specified test morality	Specified	Not specified	Not specified
Screening algorithm	Determined	None	None
Basis of cancer screening management	Guidelines for cancer prevention focused health education and cancer screening [4] issued by Ministry of Health, labour and Welfare[a]	Manual on cancer screening in the workplace issued by Ministry of Health, labour and Welfare[b]	None
Systematic management of cancer screening and reports on its performance status	Yes	No	No

Tabulated based on references [4–6]
[a]Stipulated to be legally complied
[b] Not stipulated legally

4.3.1 Population-Based Screening

Cancer screening is based on a public policy aimed at reducing the mortality rate of a specific group of people. A person in charge of implementation (e.g., the municipality) decides who is to be screened and the method of the screening and implements the screening. Screening modalities that are effective in reducing mortality rates, as determined by the efficacy assessment, are used. The municipality, which is in charge of implementation, invites all eligible persons for screening, and monitors whether they have undergone screening and detailed examinations, as well as their results. An algorithm is then established to determine the need for a detailed examination, what is performed as a detailed examination, and under what conditions those who had a detailed examination are sent back for the next screening.

In population-based screening, the target age group, screening intervals, and screening modalities are defined in the "Guidelines for Implementation of Cancer-Focused Health Education and Cancer Screening" (hereafter referred to as the National Guidelines) [4]. When a municipality entrusts screening to a screening organization or medical institution, it enters into a contract with the organization or medical institution by including the details of the contract in its specifications. The status of quality control is also evaluated, and the evaluation for each municipality is made public according to structural and process indicators. Structural indicators are provided in the national guidelines and evaluated based on whether each item should be complied with in each municipality. Process indicators are calculated and evaluated based on the number of examinees, persons requiring detailed examinations, persons undergoing detailed examinations, and cancers detected. Finally, outcome indicators, such as the mortality and incidence rates of invasive cancer are calculated [2], as these data are required for matching in cancer registries.

4.3.2 Opportunistic Screening

The screening is often performed at a medical institution. These usually included health checkups. Even for opportunistic screening, it is desirable to use a screening modality that has been proven to reduce the mortality rate of the target cancer; however, there are no restrictions on the adoption of screening modalities. In opportunistic screening, the individual examinee decides whether to undergo screening after receiving the appropriate information from the screening provider. There is no obligation or authority to collect information on screening performance, such as whether a detailed examination has been performed or the examinee has been informed of the results; moreover, there is no obligation to undergo inspection or make improvements. Furthermore, in many cases, the algorithms for detailed examinations and examination modalities are not clearly indicated. In European countries, where the cervical cancer mortality rate has been reduced at the national level, opportunistic screening may have already been discontinued, and only organized screening is provided as a national program.

4.4 Quality Control of Cervical Cancer Screening in Population-Based Screening

The only population-based screening program implemented in Japan is conducted by local governments. Over 1700 municipalities in Japan provide population-based screening. This health promotion program is based on the Health Promotion Act, which requires quality control. Quality control is conducted in accordance with the actual status of cancer screening, management, and outcomes based on national guidelines.

Screening methods (test modality, target age groups, and screening intervals) that are recognized as effective and specified in the guidelines provided by the Ministry of Health, Labor, and Welfare (MHLW) are currently being implemented, However, it is unclear whether screening methods that are not specified in the guidelines are being provided. The screening methods that should be implemented are based on scientific evidence and updated by the Commission on Cancer Screening, and authorized by the MHLW. Currently (as of July 2023), only biennial cervical cytology screening is permitted for population-based screening of cervical cancer in individuals aged ≥20 years. The MHLW conducts a survey on the actual performance status of cancer screening in municipalities [7] and published these results annually.

Data on structural and process indicators of the screening program are collected and published. The contents of the structural indicators are checklists for prefectures, municipalities, and screening institutes [8]. These checklists are used to analyze and evaluate the status of screening operations. The National Cancer Center surveys the results of checklists [9] and publishes the performance status (whether the items on the checklist have been met) of each prefecture and municipality. The process indicator data were obtained from the Report on Regional Public Health Services and Health Promotion Services [3]. Each local government compiles the number of target populations, number of examinees, number of examinees by examination result, number of examinees requiring detailed examination, number of examinees by result, and number of serious accidents that occurred in the process of screening and detailed examination from the list of examinees prepared for each fiscal year, and reports this information to the prefectural government. Prefectures combine reports from local governments and report them to the national government, which officially announces the number of reports published by municipalities and prefectures [10]. The following are the structural and process indicators for quality control of population-based screening.

4.4.1 Structural Indicators

The government recommends the following items as "minimum screening systems to be provided": (1) securing the necessary systems (screening facilities, physicians, technicians, etc.) and (2) establishing the operational procedures of screening institutions. Specific details are described in the checklists of screening institutes, municipalities, and prefectures. The checklists are used to establish an operational system, and the compliance rate of the items on the checklists are used to evaluate the quality control status. The checklist for screening institutions describes what they should do. For example, the checklist includes an explanation for examinees, which states that examinees who are judged to require detailed examination must undergo detailed examination. It also includes details of the detailed examinations and explains the benefits and harms of screening. These details should be presented to examinees in writing.

Cytological specimens are taken by a physician, who follows specific procedures for cell sample collection, and specimen preparation. Additionally, there are set requirements for the qualifications of cytotechnologists and cytopathologists performing the cytological evaluations and the standards for the cytological evaluation facility. In cervical cancer screening, there are many cases in which the facilities that perform cytological sample collection and the facility that conducts cytological evaluation differ. In such cases, the medical facility, which is the sample collection facility, is required to monitor and report the status of the cytological evaluation facility.

4.4.2 Process Indicators

Cancer screening uptake rate, referral rate (positive rate of screening test), rate of screen-positive examinees who undergo detailed examination (referral rate), positive predictive value, and cancer detection rate national standard values were set, and the achievement rate was evaluated for quality control. In this case, a positive screening test indicates cases where cytological evaluations other than NILM, and a detailed examination are performed. In the case of ASC-US (atypical squamous cells of undetermined significance), the work-up was not limited to a biopsy. The detailed examination rate is the percentage of examinees who undergo a detailed examination. If a detailed examination is performed outside the guidelines, the examinee is classified as not having undergone this examination. The positive predictive value refers to the percentage of those who actually had cancer among those who were required to undergo referral, and the cancer detection rate is the percentage of those who were detected as having cancer among all those who underwent screening [2]. In addition, in recent years, the number of cancer cases has been on the increase in Japan. Data on CIN3 and invasive cancer compiled in Japan are published from fiscal years 2014.

4.5 Quality Control of Opportunistic Screening (Management)

Quality control, which is the basis for opportunistic screening, has not been systematically implemented. In opportunistic screening, methods of screening (testing modalities, age, interval, etc.) that have not been evaluated for their effectiveness in reducing mortality are often provided, and informed consent after disclosing this information must be obtained from the examinee.

4.6 Cancer Screening Offered in the Workplace

In Japan, cancer screening in the workplace is primarily provided to workers by health insurers and employers, and the scale cannot be ignored. Cancer screening in the workplace is provided to specific groups, such as employees. Therefore, it is necessary to consider the benefits and harms to the target group (employees). Furthermore, the design of the screening system should be similar to that of population-based screening systems. However, cancer screening provided in workplaces in Japan has no legal basis. In many cases, it is provided as a welfare program and does not involve quality control. Even if opportunities for cancer screening are provided, screening providers often do not capture the results of screening and detailed examinations. In addition, instructions regarding detailed examinations are left to the discretion of the screening or medical institutions, and some cases are comparable to those of optimistic screening. MHLW released the "Manual for Cancer Screening in the Workplace" [6] in March 2018, which requires the same quality control in the workplace as in population-based screening. However, this is not legally mandated; hence, it is considered optional.

4.7 Cervical Cancer Screening Using HPV Testing as a Cancer Screening Modality

Between 2000 and 2015, the efficacy of cancer screening using HPV testing (a test to detect high-risk HPV from collected cervical cells), which is more sensitive than cervical cytology, was demonstrated [10]. In July 2020, the National Cancer Center published the "Cervical Cancer Screening Guidelines Based on Efficacy Assessment 2019" [11], which lists the HPV test alone (recommended Grade A) and the HPV test plus cytology (recommended Grade C) as screening modalities, along with the current cytology alone (recommended Grade A). This guideline assessed the benefits of HPV screening by integrating six randomized controlled trials conducted mainly in Europe. The main focus was on assessing the reduction in mortality as a beneficial outcome and the potential harm associated with false positives. The guidelines also state that the establishment of a precision control system, including long-term follow-up for HPV-positive examinees, is a prerequisite for the establishment of a unified algorithm, and that the burden of additional referrals for HPV-positive examinees and compliance with the timing of the next examination is inevitable in screening with HPV testing [12]. Currently, an algorithm that minimizes the burden on municipalities and minimizes the harm of the increasing number of false positives is being considered, given that HPV testing has inferior specificity compared to cytological examination.

In Japan, approximately four million people are screened for cervical cancer using the population-based screening program annually, and the screening system is monitored [3]. In addition, follow-up management is required for those who need to be screened. The operational status of screening is repeatedly checked using process indicators; furthermore, the evaluation of screening quality using checklists is repeated annually. Therefore, a quality control system has been established for population-based screening. Many gynecologists are involved in this screening program and play significant roles. Although some issues need to be resolved in population-based screening, Health providers including gynecologists should have a deeper understanding of the screening system and proactive involvement in quality control. In addition, when involved in opportunistic screening, understanding the problems of quality control will not only enable examinees to provide appropriate information, but may also serve as basic platform for reform toward the ideal system for cervical cancer screening in Japan.

References

1. Andermann A, Blancquaert I, Beauchamp S, Déry V. Revisiting Wilson and Jungner in the genomic age: a review of screening criteria over the past 40 years. Bull World Health Organ. 2008;86:317–9.
2. Committee on the Evaluation of Cancer Screening Programs. Report on the future evaluation of cancer screening programs in Japan. Ministry of Health, Labour and Welfare; 2008; https://www.mhlw.go.jp/shingi/2008/03/s0301-4.html.
3. Report on regional public health services and health promotion services. https://www.e-stat.go.jp/stat-search/files?page=1&toukei=00450025&tstat=000001030884&cycle=8&cycle_facet=tclass1&metadata=1&data=1.
4. Guidelines for cancer prevention focused health education and cancer screening. https://www.mhlw.go.jp/file/06-Seisakujouhou-10900000-Kenkoukyoku/0000111662.pdf.
5. Advisory Panel Committee for Improving Cancer Screening, Cancer Screening Improvement Guidance Project, Ministry of Health, Labour and Welfare. Cancer screening handbook for family physicians: aiming to improve the screening uptake rate. 2010; Chrome-extension://efaidnbmnnnibpcajpcglclefindmkaj/https://www.mhlw.go.jp/file/06-Seisakujouhou-10900000-Kenkoukyoku/0000059965_1.pdf.
6. Manual on cancer screening in the workplace. https://www.mhlw.go.jp/file/05-Shingikai-10901000-Kenkoukyoku-Soumuka/0000204422.pdf.
7. FY 2017 survey on cancer screening in municipalities: results. https://www.mhlw.go.jp/file/05-Shingikai-10901000-Kenkoukyoku-Soumuka/0000208400.pdf.
8. "Checklists for project evaluation" and "Minimum necessary quality control items to be written in specifications". https://ganjoho.jp/med_pro/pre_scr/screening/check_list.html.
9. Saito H, Machii R, Kasuya K, Zoga K, Matsuda K. Cancer screening in Japan. In: National cancer screening data book—the health promotion act. National Cancer Center, National Cancer Center; 2017.
10. Ronco G, Dillner J, Elfström KM, et al. Efficacy of HPV-based screening for prevention of invasive cervical cancer: follow-up of four European. Lancet. 2014;383:524–32.
11. Guidelines based on the efficacy assessment of cervical cancer screening. 2019. http://ncc.go.jp/shikyukeiguide2019.pdf.
12. Health and Labor Sciences Research Grant for Comprehensive Research Project for the Promotion of Cancer Control, "Investigation of Problems and Specific Operation Methods of Introducing HPV Testing for Cervical Cancer Screening in Japan," Research Report, Daisuke Aoki, 2021. https://mhlw-grants.niph.go.jp/project/156458.

Evidence and Implementation of HPV Vaccination

5

Etsuko Miyagi

Abstract

Due to the combination of effective cervical screening and prophylactic vaccination by the HPV (human papillomavirus) vaccines, cervical cancer has become a preventable cancer. In May 2018, the WHO announced a global call for action to eliminate cervical cancer. The evolution and implementation of cervical cancer screening and HPV vaccines and the global strategy instigated by the WHO are moving humankind toward the elimination of cervical cancer, although there are still many challenges to overcome. This chapter summarizes the status of HPV vaccination in the world, including the effectiveness and safety of HPV vaccines available at present. Real-world data from three countries with successful national HPV vaccine programs show that elimination of cervical cancer is no longer impossible through regional efforts and international cooperation.

Keywords
HPV vaccine · Implementation · Herd immunity · Effectiveness · Safety

5.1 Prophylactic Vaccination Against Human Papillomavirus (HPV Vaccines)

5.1.1 Types of HPV Vaccines and Vaccination Schedules

Three types of HPV vaccines are currently available globally (Table 5.1). These inactivated vaccines produced by recombinant DNA technology use multiple major

E. Miyagi (✉)
Department of Obstetrics and Gynecology, Yokohama City University School of Medicine, Yokohama, Japan
e-mail: emiyagi@yokohama-cu.ac.jp

D. Aoki (ed.), *Recent Topics on Prevention, Diagnosis, and Clinical Management of Cervical Cancer*, Comprehensive Gynecology and Obstetrics,
https://doi.org/10.1007/978-981-99-9396-3_5

papillomavirus capsid protein L1 virus-like particles (VLPs) to induce high titers of HPV-neutralizing antibodies. Since 2006, bivalent (2-valent), quadrivalent (4-valent), and nonavalent (9-valent) vaccines have been widely distributed, and, as of 2020, more than 100 of the 194 WHO Member States have introduced HPV vaccination [1, 2].

The FDA approved the 4-valent HPV vaccine (Gardasil®4) in 2006 for females aged 9–26 years for the prevention of diseases caused by HPV types 6, 11, 16, and 18 (the L1 VLP of HPV 6 and 11 can prevent benign lesions such as condyloma acuminatum). The 2-valent HPV vaccine (Cervarix™) was approved by the European Medicines Agency in 2007 and by the FDA in 2009, and it is highly effective and protective against the most common HPV 16 and 18 oncogenic genotypes. The 9-valent HPV vaccine (Gardasil®9, Silgard®9) was approved in 2014 by the FDA; this vaccine uses the same expression system and production method as Gardasil®4 but covers five other hrHPV types, protecting against HPV 6, 11, 16, 18, 31, 33, 45, 53, and 58. At present, the 4-valent HPV vaccine is not available for use in the USA but remains included in the national HPV vaccine programs in many countries.

The standard inoculation schedule for these HPV vaccines is three doses; however, two-dose HPV vaccination schedules with 6- or 12-month intervals for young people below 15 years have already been adopted in many countries, based on evidence regarding the high immunogenicity of HPV vaccines among young boys and girls [1]. Moreover, recently, the WHO Strategic Advisory Group of Experts on

Table 5.1 Characteristics of three HPV vaccines

	Bivalent HPV vaccine (Cervarix™)	Quadrivalent HPV vaccine (Gardasil®4)	Nonavalent HPV vaccine (Gardasil®9, Silgard®9)
Manufacturer	GlaxoSmithKline	Merck, sharp & dome	Merck, sharp & dome
Adjuvant	AS04: 500 μg aluminum hydroxide, 50 μg 3-deacylated monophosphoryl lipid A (MPL)	225 μg amorphous aluminum hydroxyl-phosphate sulfate	500 μg amorphous aluminum hydroxyl-phosphate sulfate
Recombinant technology	Baculovirus in Trichoplusia in insect cells	Saccharomyces cerevisae	Saccharomyces cerevisiae
L1-VLP antigens	HPV16 (20 μg)HPV18 (20 μg)	HPV6 (20 μg) HPV11 (40 μg) HPV16 (40 μg) HPV18 (20 μg)	HPV6 (30 μg)HPV11 (40 μg)HPV16 (60 μg) HPV18 (40 μg) HPV31/33 /45 /52 /58 (20 μg each)
Single inoculation dose	0.5 mL	0.5 mL	0.5 mL
Standard vaccination schedule (3 doses)	Day 1, month 1 and month 6	Day 1, month 2 and month 6	Day 1, month 2 and month 6

VLP virus-like particle

Immunization concluded that single-dose schedules provide comparable efficacy to two- or three-dose regimens. The WHO updated its recommendations regarding HPV vaccination schedules in December 2022 as follows [3]:

- One- or two-dose schedule for girls aged 9–14 years.
- One- or two-dose schedule for girls and women aged 15–20 years.
- Two doses with a 6-month interval for women older than 21 years.

This recommendation also highlighted the vaccination of immunocompromised individuals as a priority, stating that these individuals should receive two doses at minimum, and three doses where possible.

5.1.2 Implementation of HPV Vaccines

The introduction rates of HPV vaccination in the national immunization program differ significantly between high-income (HICs) and low- and middle-income countries (LMICs). It is reported that the rates are only about 30% in Africa and 40% in Asia, on the other hand, they are about 80% in America and Europe. As for the HPV vaccination for the target populations, Australia, New Zealand had the highest (about 80%), and Latin America also achieved 60% coverages. However, the vaccination rates in Europe and North America were about 35% in 2019. In addition, Northern Africa, Oceania, excluding Australia and New Zealand, and Asia had very low coverage rates [2, 4]. Estimated coverage of HPV vaccination reported through the WHO/UNICEF Joint Reporting Form on Immunization (JRF) [4] is shown in Fig. 5.1.

To prevent other HPV-related cancers (including anal, vulvar, vaginal, penal, and oropharyngeal cancers) as well as cervical cancer, gender-neutral HPV vaccine programs have been adopted in high- and upper-middle-income countries. Around 60%

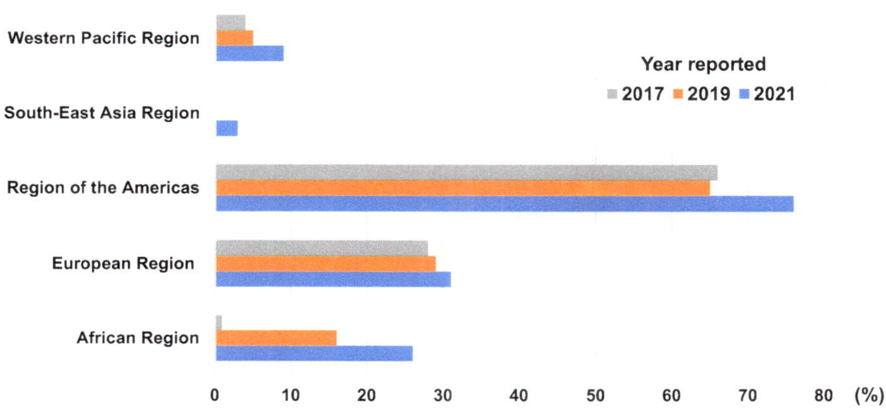

Fig. 5.1 Estimated regional HPV Vaccination coverage by age 15 (first dose, females)

of such programs deliver HPV vaccines through schools, either as the main strategy or in combination with facility-based delivery. In 2019, gender-neutral HPV vaccine program was introduced in 44% of HICs and only 5% of LMICs [2].

5.2 Efficacy and Effectiveness of HPV Vaccines

5.2.1 Evidence from Clinical Trials

The estimation for the 2-valent and 4-valent HPV vaccines was that they would prevent 60%–70% of cervical cancer cases, based on the contribution of HPV 16/18. According to the Cochrane Review, which compared the effects of the monovalent HPV 16 vaccine and 2-valent/4-valent HPV vaccines [1] with those of placebos, the vaccines reduced the numbers of HPV 16/18-associated cervical intraepithelial neoplasia (CIN) 2+, CIN3+, and AIS cases in adolescent girls and women aged 15–26. The review showed high-certainty evidence that vaccines lowered CIN2+ case numbers from 164 to 2/10,000 (relative risk, RR, 0.01 [0 to 0.05]) and CIN3+ numbers from 70 to 0/10,000 (RR 0.01 [0.00 to 0.10]). Moderate-certainty evidence that vaccines reduced the risk of AIS from 9 to 0/10,000 [RR 0.10 (0.01 to 0.82)] was also demonstrated. For women vaccinated between 24 and 45 years of age, there was moderate-certainty evidence that the risks of any CIN2+, including HPV 16/18-associated CIN2+, were similar in vaccinated and unvaccinated women (RR 0.74 [0.52 to 1.05] and RR 1.04 [0.83 to 1.30], respectively).

Regarding the efficacy and immunogenicity of the 9-valent vaccine in women aged 16–26 years, compared with the 4-valent vaccine, non-inferior immune responses to HPV 6, 11, 16, and 18, were demonstrated. Furthermore, this vaccine demonstrated 96.7% efficacy against CIN2+, vulvar intraepithelial neoplasia (VIN) 2+, and vulvar and vaginal lesions caused by HPV 31, 33, 45, 52, and 58 (95% CI, 80.9–99.8) [5]. The final clinical trial data of the 9-valent HPV vaccine revealed 97.4% protection against high-grade cervical, vulvar, and vaginal lesions in women aged 16–26 [6].

These clinical trial results clarified that adolescent ages—when most girls are not sexually active—should be the target of national HPV vaccine programs.

5.2.2 Real-World Data

Since 2006, countries such as Australia, the United Kingdom, the USA, and Northern European countries have achieved high HPV vaccination rates through national vaccine programs that have been running for over 10 years; real-world data showing significant reductions in the incidence of CIN2+ cases have been reported from these countries [7]. Moreover, in Australia, where 4-valent HPV vaccination

(9-valent vaccine at present) has been thoroughly promoted, a 2014 study reported significantly reduced infection rates for vaccine-related HPV types among unvaccinated women in urban areas, indicating a herd immunity effect [8].

In Scotland, a school-based 2-valent HPV vaccine program has also been successful, with almost 90% of women born in 1995–96 having received the HPV vaccine. In comparison with unvaccinated women born in 1988, CIN3+ prevalence was reduced by 89% in the vaccinated women (95% confidence interval [CI], 81%–94%). The evidence of herd protection against CIN2+ in unvaccinated women was also confirmed in this cohort [9].

In the 2020s, three countries published epidemiological evidence of the effects of the HPV vaccine on invasive cervical cancer incidence. In Sweden, the 4-valent HPV vaccine has been a routine vaccination since 2006, with a free catch-up vaccination period by age 18 (now ended). A two-dose vaccination schedule was implemented in 2015 as a school-based program, and vaccination for 10–12-year-olds has since become established. In a follow-up survey of around 1.67 million women aged 10–30 years, invasive cervical cancer occurred in 19 of the approximately 530,000 women who received at least one dose of the vaccine, compared with 538 of approximately 1.15 million unvaccinated individuals. After adjusting for age at follow-up and other factors, the incidence ratio was 0.37 (95% CI, 0.21–0.57). Furthermore, the HPV vaccine was highly protective among women who were vaccinated before 17 years of age, as recommended, with an incidence ratio of 0.12 (95% CI, 0.00–0.34) [10].

In England, where 2-valent HPV vaccination was introduced in 2008 and achieved a high vaccination rate, drastic reductions in high-grade cervical precancerous lesions and cervical cancer in vaccinated women have also been reported, based on the population-based cancer registry (2006–2019). The estimated relative reductions in cervical cancer rates by age at vaccine offer were 34% (95% CI, 25–41) for 16–18 years, 62% (95% CI, 52–71) for 14–16 years, and 87% (95% CI, 72–94) for 12–13 years (school year 8), compared with the reference unvaccinated cohort [11].

The study in Denmark included women aged 17–30 years between 2006 and 2019, with cervical cancer incidence rate ratios (IRRs) according to vaccination status estimated from nationwide registries. The data were adjusted for age, education, and ethnicity, and the cohort comprised 867,689 women. The IRRs of cervical cancer for women vaccinated at 16 years of age or younger or at 17–19 years of age were 0.14 (95% CI, 0.04–0.53) and 0.32 (95% CI, 0.08–1.28), respectively, compared with unvaccinated women. By contrast, in women aged 20–30 years at the time of vaccination, the incidence rate was higher than among unvaccinated women (IRR, 1.19; 95% CI, 0.80–1.79) [12]. This report indicates the importance of HPV vaccination at a young age as well as the limitations of catch-up vaccination. The effectiveness of catch-up HPV vaccination may vary by country, region, and targeted age.

The summary of three real-world epidemiological reports is given in Table 5.2.

Table 5.2 Cohort-specific incidence rate ratios of cervical cancer

Ages at vaccination	Adjusted IRRs (95% CI)
Sweeden	
10–16 years	0.12 (0.00–0.34)
10–30 years	0.37 (0.21–0.57)
17–39 years	0.47 (0.27–0.75)
England	
12–13 years	0.13 (0.03–0.28)
14–16 years	0.38 (0.29–0.48)
16–18 years	0.66 (0.59–0.75)
Denmark	
12–16 years	0.14 (0.04–0.53)
16–19 years	0.32 (0.08–1.28)
20–30 years	1.19 (0.80–1.79)

Real-world effectiveness of HPV vaccination against cervical cancer. *IRRs* incidence rate ratios, *95% CI* 95% confidence interval

5.3 Safety of HPV Vaccines

An updated review focusing on special populations and adverse events of special interest following the widespread use of the 9-valent HPV vaccine evaluated 109 studies, including 15 population-based studies covering over 2.5 million vaccinated individuals across six countries [13]. The review concluded that all vaccines demonstrated an acceptable safety profile. Although injection-site reactions (redness, swelling, and pain) were more common for the 9-valent HPV vaccine than for the 4-valent HPV vaccine, there was no consistent evidence of increased risk of any adverse events of special interest. In particular, neither demyelinating syndromes nor neurological conditions (such as complex regional pain and postural orthostatic tachycardia syndromes) showed a direct causal relationship with the HPV vaccines issued in Japan, Denmark, or other countries. There was also no increased risk of spontaneous abortion, stillbirth, or infant mortality following unintended HPV vaccination during pregnancy; however, it should be noted that insufficient evidence was available from randomized control studies to prove definitive vaccination influences for women who became pregnant during the vaccination period [1].

5.4 The WHO's Cervical Cancer Elimination Strategy

As a result of the combination of effective cervical screening and prophylactic vaccination, cervical cancer has become a preventable cancer. In May 2018, the director-general of the WHO announced a global call for action to eliminate cervical cancer, with all stakeholders urged to unite behind this common goal. The World Health Assembly then adopted the global strategy for cervical cancer elimination in 2020 [14]. According to this strategy, all countries must reach and maintain a threshold of 4 per 100,000 women: achieving this goal rests on three key pillars, the 90-70-90 targets as shown in Fig. 5.2.

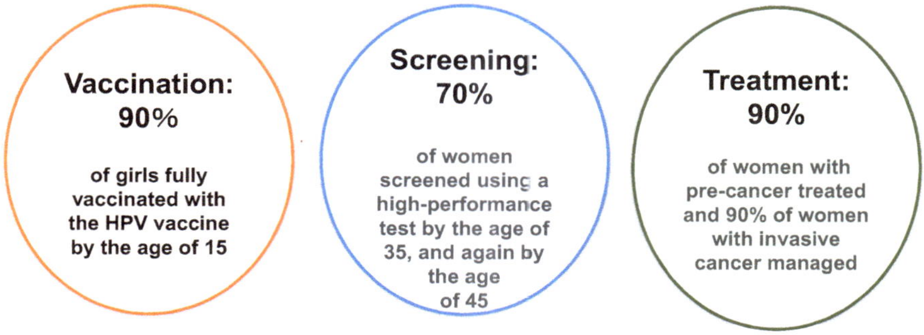

Fig. 5.2 Cervical cancer elimination strategy by the WHO

The WHO says that each country must meet the 90-70-90 targets by 2030 to be on the path to eliminating cervical cancer within the next century. With the realization of a global health strategy for the elimination of cervical cancer as a public health problem, the WHO also stated that the market must be reshaped to reduce cost as a barrier to prevention and treatment in the world's poorest countries. In addition, an alliance consisting of the International Agency for Research on Cancer and the United Nations Development Programme, as well as other bodies, including the Union for International Cancer Control, Gavi, and the Vaccine Alliance, are contributing to the global distribution of HPV vaccines and introduction of new technologies. The development of new, affordable, high-sensitivity HPV testing kits to detect precancerous lesions and invasive cervical cancers is vital to enable LMICs to conduct this strategy.

References

1. Arbyn M, et al. Prophylactic vaccination against human papillomaviruses to prevent cervical cancer and its precursors. Cochrane Database Syst Rev. 2018;5:CD009069.
2. Bruni L, et al. HPV vaccination introduction worldwide and WHO and UNICEF estimates of national HPV immunization coverage 2010–2019. Prev Med. 2021;144:106399.
3. Departmental News. WHO updates recommendations on HPV vaccination schedule. 2022; https://www.who.int/news/item/20-12-2022-WHO-updates-recommendations-on-HPV-vaccination-schedule. Accessed 21 Feb 2023.
4. WHO Human Papillomavirus (HPV) vaccination coverage. https://immunizationdata.who.int/pages/coverage/hpv.html?GROUP=WHO_REGIONS&ANTIGEN=15HPV1_F&YEAR=&CODE=. Accessed 10 Mar 2023.
5. Joura EA, et al. A 9-valent HPV vaccine against infection and intraepithelial neoplasia in women. N Engl J Med. 2015;372:711–23.
6. Huh WK, et al. Final efficacy, immunogenicity, and safety analyses of a nine-valent human papillomavirus vaccine in women aged 16-26 years: a randomised, double-blind trial. Lancet. 2017;390:2143–59.
7. Garland SM, et al. Impact and effectiveness of the quadrivalent human papillomavirus vaccine: a systematic review of 10 years of real-world experience. Clin Infect Dis. 2016;63:519.

8. Tabrizi SN, et al. Assessment of herd immunity and cross-protection after a human papillomavirus vaccination programme in Australia: a repeat cross-sectional study. Lancet Infect Dis. 2014;14:958.
9. Palmer T, et al. Prevalence of cervical disease at age 20 after immunization with bivalent HPV vaccine at age 12-13 in Scotland: retrospective population study. BMJ. 2019;365:1161.
10. Lei J, et al. HPV vaccination and the risk of invasive cervical cancer. N Engl J Med. 2020;383:1340.
11. Falcaro M, et al. The effects of the national HPV vaccination programme in England, UK, on cervical cancer and grade 3 cervical intraepithelial neoplasia incidence: a register-based observational study. Lancet. 2021;398:2084.
12. Kjaer SK, et al. Real-world effectiveness of human papillomavirus vaccination against cervical cancer. J Natl Cancer Inst. 2021;113:1329.
13. Phillips A, et al. Safety of human papillomavirus vaccines: an updated review. Drug Saf. 2018;41:329.
14. Global strategy to accelerate the elimination of cervical cancer as a public health problem. World Health Organization 2020. Global strategy to accelerate the elimination of cervical cancer as a public health problem. Accessed 21 Feb 2023.

Part III

Diagnosis and Clinical Management of Cervical Intraepithelial Neoplasia (CIN)

6 Diagnosis of Cervical Intraepithelial Neoplasia with Special Reference to Roles of Cervical Cytology and Colposcopy

Takuma Fujii

Abstract

With the integration of cytology into the cervical cancer screening, the mortality rate of cervical cancer has dramatically decreased. Cytology has since been incorporated into the cervical cancer screening. The revised Bethesda System for cervical cancer screening now includes sections that address the quality of cytological specimens and that highlight the limitations of cytology. The most significant topic, especially in the revised 2001 edition, is the introduction of the concept of human papillomavirus (HPV) infection into cytology. However, cytology is significantly less sensitive than the molecular biological method, PCR. Initial screening using a highly sensitive method followed by a high-specificity cytology triage is therefore an appropriate screening algorithm.

Aging and pregnancy pose two specific issues with regard to cytology in Japan. As the Japanese population is aging rapidly, the interpretation of cytology must take into account aging-dependent factors that modulate readouts. With regard to pregnancy, it is often the case that cytology tests are first performed in women once they become pregnant; younger women are rarely offered such tests.

Colposcopy is performed as a workup test for patients who have received abnormal results following cervical cancer screening or for those individuals in whom abnormal cervical morphologies are detected following visual inspection. Colposcopy is predominantly used for detecting high-grade squamous intraepithelial lesions rather than overt invasive carcinoma. Inter-observer bias is also common. It has also been reported that different levels of cytology knowledge

T. Fujii (✉)
Department of Gynecology, Fujita Health University, School of Medicine, Toyoake, Aichi, Japan

Fujita Health University Okazaki Medical Center, Okazaki, Aichi, Japan
e-mail: fujiit44@fujita-hu.ac.jp

D. Aoki (ed.), *Recent Topics on Prevention, Diagnosis, and Clinical Management of Cervical Cancer*, Comprehensive Gynecology and Obstetrics,
https://doi.org/10.1007/978-981-99-9396-3_6

and experience between colposcopists can lead to diverse interpretations of colposcopy results. This had led to the creation of a system that standardizes the grading of lesion severity so that results are concordant between examiners. Most CIN3 lesions are flat. In contrast, nodular, papillary, or have outgrowing contours and are indicators of the precursors to invasive cancer. Ulcers are associated with invasive carcinoma. The highest grade lesion, an opaque white color, often described as a deep white or oyster gray, may be where the acetic acid-induced white coloration is most persistent. The distance between vessels in CIN3 lesions is heterogeneous compared to CIN1. The timing of the colposcopy during pregnancy is important for accurate diagnosis. Ideally, colposcopy and histology results should be obtained in the first 20 weeks of gestation to yield robust and concordant data.

Keywords
Cytology · Colposcopy · Cervical intraepithelial neoplasia · Screening · Swede score · Pregnancy · Elderly women

6.1 Cytology

6.1.1 Significance of Cytology

With the introduction of cytology into the screening system, the mortality rate of cervical cancer has decreased by more than 70% [1]. It is estimated that 60% of all invasive cervical cancers detected are in women who have never been examined in the past or who underwent their last examination more than 5 years prior to diagnosis. Sponsored by the National Cancer Institute, cytology was first implemented as a cervical cancer screening in Kentucky, Jefferson County, USA [2]. After 4 consecutive years of screening, the incidence of invasive cervical cancer was reportedly reduced to zero. Although this finding underscored the utility of cytology screening, quality control in cytology in the USA became an issue over the following decade. Subsequently, the so-called Pap scandal, which was characterized by repeated missed detection of cervical cancer by cytology, developed into a social problem. To resolve this issue, the Bethesda System of Cytology was published in 1988, and it was revised in 2001. The revised Bethesda System now includes sections that address the quality of cytology specimens and that highlight the limitations of cytology. The most significant topic, especially in the revised 2001 edition, is the introduction of the concept of human papillomavirus (HPV) infection into cytology. That is, a low-grade squamous intraepithelial lesion (LSIL) indicates HPV infection and a high-grade squamous intraepithelial lesion (HSIL) indicates neoplastic changes; atypical squamous cells of undermined significance (ASC-US) can now be further triaged with the advent of HPV testing.

The revised Bethesda System was deployed in Japan in 2008. In terms of screening performance based on an endpoint of cervical intraepithelial neoplasia (CIN2) or worse, the sensitivity and specificity of detection within a large cohort study were 70.9% and 97.3%, respectively [3].

There is an interesting relationship between HPV infection and abnormal cellular morphology in the general population of Costa Rica [4]. In their study, Kovacic and colleagues compared the results of PCR and cytology: even if PCR indicates HPV infection is present, cytology only picks up morphological abnormalities in 38% of cases for HPV 16 and 31% for HPV 18. Therefore, although the Bethesda System is a useful method for inferring HPV infection and associated abnormalities, its sensitivity is significantly lower than that of the molecular biological method, PCR.

Currently, HPV testing is gaining attention as a screening method. The use of highly sensitive method and follow-up triage by cytology with high specificity is a logical process to introduce into the screening workflow. In Japan, the current method of triage for individuals with cytology; ASC-US is, however, HPV testing. This is because the accuracy of HPV test was uncertain at the end of the 90's, and in today's clinical practice it is not reasonable to use the least sensitive screening method first and the most sensitive method for triage [5]. It is an ideal strategy that the HPV test is the first followed with cytology as a triage.

6.1.2 Risk-Based Management

The new American Society of Colposcopy and Cervical Pathology (ASCCP) risk-based consensus management guidelines describe six clinical actions that providers can use when managing patients with abnormal screening results. These are treatment, optional treatment or colposcopy/biopsy, colposcopy/biopsy, 1-year surveillance, 3-year surveillance, and return to 5-year regular screening [6]. The risk benchmarks have been updated to reflect the management guidelines for CIN3+ observed in a cohort from Kaiser Permanente Northern California, a large integrated health care organization with a population of over 1.5 million women screened over 10 years. Exploration of numerous potential risk factors revealed that a patient's CIN3+ risk can be estimated based on current HPV and cytology test results and previous test results, colposcopy impressions, biopsy results and treatments [6, 7]. The CIN3+ immediate risk is 4.4% if the patient's current status is ASC-US, HPV-positive, with an unknown history of prior HPV infection. The recommended management is colposcopy. However, the CIN3+ immediate risk is 2.0% in patients whose status is ASC-US, HPV-positive, but with a history of testing HPV-negative. The recommended management for these groups is a 1-year follow-up. Notably, a 1-year follow-up is also recommended for patients with LSIL status but who are HPV-positive with a history of testing HPV-negative. This was a different algorithm compared with the previous guideline.

6.1.3 Significance of P16 Immunocytochemistry in ASC-US and LSIL Triage

In Japan, the current management guidelines recommend HPV testing as the follow-up procedure in patients with a cytology, ASC-US, whereas colposcopy is recommended for those patient with LSIL [8]. In real world clinical practice, are ASC-US and LSIL patients really distinguishable? In fact, ASC-US/LSIL triage studies have shown no difference between these two categories [9]. Handling patients who have been categorized based on ASC-US/LSIL criteria is sometimes difficult in clinical practice in Japan. Patients may be recommended for a follow-up cytology several months later, or may sometimes be referred for a colposcopy without any significant reason. Performing colposcopy on all of these patients is not only disadvantageous to the patient, but also has a negative impact on medical economics and medical resources. In contrast, to follow-up with cytology alone without workup may miss CIN2+ lesions. To address these issues, a dual immunostaining kit containing anti-p16 and ki-67 antibodies (CINtec PLUS kit; Roche Corporation) has been developed as a triage test for ASC-US/LSIL. In the case of ASC-US, the Japanese guidelines recommend triage with HPV testing and follow-up with colposcopy in HPV-positive patients. In practice, however, it is difficult to distinguish between ASC-US and LSIL (as mentioned above), and the CINtec PLUS kit is a breakthrough in this regard. Specimens collected for liquid-based cytology (LBC) are advantageous, since the residual specimen can be used for the HPV test, and both tests can be performed with a single specimen collection, which minimizes patient discomfort. A clinical trial for ASC-US/LSIL triage (JGOG-1073) using this kit has therefore been conducted in Japan [10].

The sensitivity and specificity with which CIN2+ can be diagnosed by ASC-US/LSIL triage using this reagent were 87% and 76%, respectively. In contrast, the HPV test yielded a sensitivity and specificity of 94% and 33%, respectively. Analysis of these results using the McNemar method showed that this reagent was superior to the HPV test as a triage method, and the results were comparable to those obtained in the United States and Europe. I therefore believe that the triage test using the CINtec PLUS kit will attract increasing attention as LBCs become more widespread in Japan in the future. Recently, HPV testing has been introduced in cervical cancer screening, and further triage based on dual immunocytochemical staining with p16 and Ki67 has been considered. Wentzensen and colleagues [11] have proposed that colposcopy should be performed in patients who are HPV16- or HPV18-positive, or in patients with a high risk of being HPV-positive and in whom the dual staining result is positive.

6.1.4 Characteristics of Cytology in the Elderly Women

The Bethesda System of cervical cytology requires collection of both squamous and columnar cells, including metaplastic cells derived from the squamo-columnar junction (SCJ), which is the natal site of cervical cancer. While these cells are easily collected in women of reproductive age, their collection from post-menopausal women is challenging due to the anatomical migration of the physiologic SCJ. Failure to collect the endocervical cells from elderly women compromises the validity of any cytological examination. The difference among countries is significant, as 30% of the elderly women in Japan are 65 years of age or older, while in Latin America only a few percent of women are over 65 [12]. If the proportion of elderly women continues to increase in society, this may render the cytology screening system non-viable.

Most women with cytology, HSIL will have been diagnosed with histological HSIL following a colposcopically-directed punch biopsy. In the case of cytology, HSIL, the corresponding diagnosis by biopsy is different for those under 65 years of age versus those older than 65 [13]. Elderly patients are more likely to be diagnosed with benign or invasive cancer than those under 65 years of age, so differences due to age should be taken into account in the determination of cytology, HSIL. Depending on the situation, it may be necessary to administer estrogen (to remove the confounding variable of age-related atrophic changes) and repeat the cytology [14].

6.1.5 Screening and Management of Abnormal Cytology in Pregnancy

In Japan, cytology is actively performed even in early pregnancy due to the low screening rate among young women. For this reason, pregnancy is the first time that some women have a screening test. Taking cervical samples from pregnant women is associated with some specific challenges. For example, the abundant mucus excreted from the cervix interferes with the collection of cells. Also, physicians tend to deploy the collection brush much more gently for fear of inducing bleeding after cell collection. This means that extremely low numbers of cells are collected, which may contribute to under diagnosis of disease in this population. Once cells are collected, there are other challenges related to the screening step. Specifically, decidual cells under the microscope can mimic the cell morphology of LSIL, tissue repair, HSIL or cancer. Since cellular changes unique to pregnancy can cause overdiagnosis, determination of pre (malignancy) in pregnant women should be carried out with caution.

In the case of ASC-US at the time of pregnancy, no workup should be performed until after delivery [7, 15]. In contrast, there have been case reports of invasive carcinoma being found even in ASC-US at the time of pregnancy, so checking for abnormalities in the cervix at least by visual inspection (or, if possible, by colposcopy) could be essential [16].

6.2 Colposcopy

6.2.1 The Role of Colposcopy

By the late 1970s, colposcopy had become widely used in the USA for workup of abnormal cytology results. Before then, high-grade SIL of cytology results (including those suspected of being cancerous) were managed by conization or hysterectomy. As a direct consequence of colposcopy, therefore, the number of conization and hysterectomy procedures was dramatically decreased [17]. Colposcopy is performed as a workup test for patients who have received abnormal results during cervical cancer screening or in whom abnormal cervical morphologies were discovered upon visual inspection. Mainly, the colposcopy is used for detecting high-grade SILs rather than overt invasive carcinoma because obvious tumors are visible to the naked eyes. Although the purpose of the colposcopy is to obtain biopsies at sites of the colposcopic abnormality to guide the final histological diagnosis, colposcopic findings are not always accurate. Therefore, multiple colposcopic directed biopsies are recommended for more accurate diagnosis. Unlike cytology, colposcopy can identify lesions of abnormality. Furthermore, if there is abnormal cytology but the ectocervix and vagina are normal, the endocervix may be abnormal. Colposcopy is safe and can be used to detect cervical abnormalities during pregnancy. The decision to perform a colposcopic directed biopsy is based on age or colposcopic findings. Colposcopy is extremely important in the evaluation of pretreatment lesions, as it can determine the appropriate extent of resection to avoid over-resection, especially in younger patients and in patients requiring fertility preservation. Although final diagnosis by cone resection is the gold standard, it is difficult to calculate the accuracy of the colposcopy in practice. For example, if the worst lesion only occupies a tiny area, it may not be detected in a cone resection specimen. Inter-observer bias is also common. Whereas CIN1 is uniformly recognized as HPV infection and CIN3 as a neoplastic lesion, the histologic diagnosis of CIN2 is highly variable. Furthermore, the problem is exacerbated by the fact that biopsies of seemingly normal lesions are sometimes diagnosed as immature metaplasia, which resembles CIN 2 or 3 (CIN2/3), and diagnoses often vary between pathologists. Colposcopy is used to make a diagnosis by targeting biopsies where a worst lesion is likely to be present. However, confirmation of the final histology by performing a cone resection revealed that the worst lesion is missed by colposcopy in 41% of patients [18]. In other words, there is a strong possibility of underdiagnosis if clinicians rely on the results of colposcopy directed biopsy alone. In contrast, small CIN3 lesions may be collected during colposcopy directed biopsy, but not detected in the following cone resection; thus, histology derived from the cone resection is not always the gold standard. Additionally, the amount of cytology expertise and knowledge varies between colposcopists, which can lead to different interpretations of colposcopy results.

6.2.2 Characteristics of Colposcopic Findings

6.2.2.1 Normal Findings

At reproductive age, stratified squamous epithelia containing glycogen cover the stromal surface [19]. In colposcopy, this epithelial layer appears pink or slightly reddish. Before puberty and after menopause, the epithelia are thin and lacks cytoplasmic glycogen due to estrogen deficiency. The blood supply to the stroma is also reduced, and the tissue appears light red in colposcopy. The columnar epithelia contain mucin and appears transparent and bright red because of its single layer. The metaplastic epithelia are thinner than normal squamous epithelia and contains no glycogen, so it is relatively transparent and appears bright red. The atypical cells in the intraepithelial neoplastic lesions contain little or no glycogen. The density of proliferating cells is increased and the cellular nucleus: cytoplasm ratio is higher. The proliferated cells appear grayish-white or white. The repair cells are thinner than normal epithelia and contains no glycogen. Accompanied by keratinization, the colposcopic appearance is grayish-white. The keratinized lesions are opaque and gray.

6.2.3 Abnormal Findings

One of the characteristics of SIL is a sharp border (Fig. 6.1). Mosaic and punctation patterns are usually found on the outer side of the transformation zone (TZ) when normal. The grade of mosaic and punctation were classified into fine and coarse. Fine indicates for metaplasia or LSIL, whereas coarse for HSIL. The thicker, shorter, and longer duration of color of change after application of acetic acid is generally indicative of a higher grade lesion. The lesions are dull to yellow-red color before application of acetic acid, and become white after application. Cuffed gland openings are present. A sharp white margin inside a less opaque area in the TZ region after application of acetic acid is called an inner border, whereas a prominent opaque white area is called a ridge sign (Fig. 6.2); both observations are consistent with HSIL. Erosion is a condition in which the epithelium is peeled off (Fig. 6.3), while

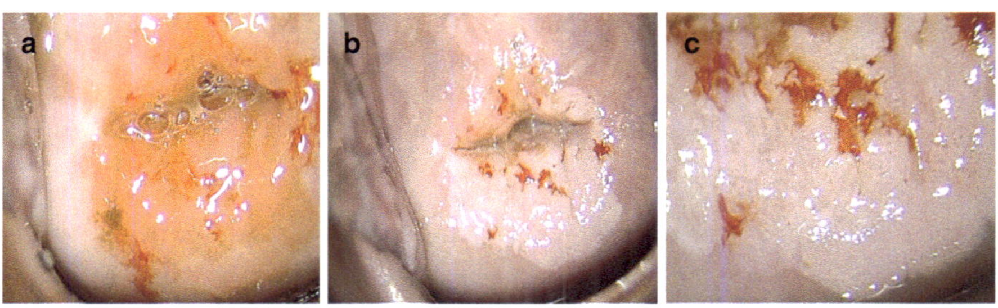

Fig. 6.1 A 30's-year-old patient with CIN3, sharp border. Left, before application of acetic acid. Middle, after application of acetic acid. Right, after application of acetic acid, posterior position

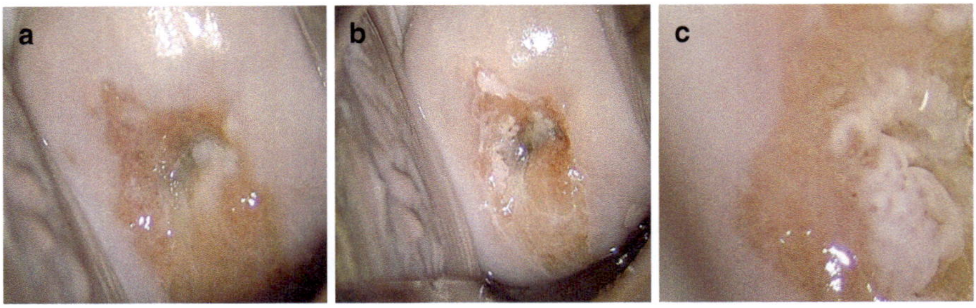

Fig. 6.2 A 30's-year-old patient with CIN3, ridge sign in the area of the columnar cells. Left, before the application of acetic acid. Middle, after the application of acetic acid. Right, after the application of acetic acid, 7 o'clock position

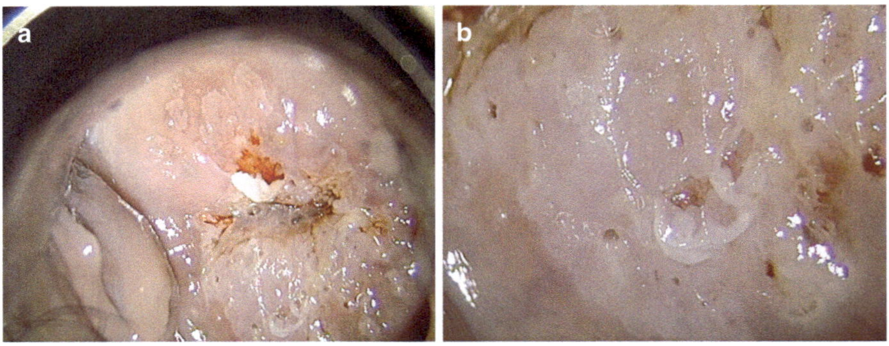

Fig. 6.3 A 30's-year-old patient with CIN3, peeling of the white epithelia after application of acetic acid

ulceration extends into the laceration to the stroma. Erosion can be caused by a trauma, which can be either scarring or dysplasia (Fig. 6.1). There are no typical colposcopic findings for microinvasive carcinoma. However, if the HSIL lesion is large, microinvasion may be present [19]. Conversely, a small HSIL lesions are unlikely to be invasive. In the case of microinvasive carcinoma, colposcopic examination is appropriate for cases related to the ectocervix, but not for those related to the endocervix. Hypervascularity may indicate invasion. A finding of adenocarcinoma in situ (AIS) is challenging in colposcopy; it may be associated with HSIL, but not necessarily adjacent to the SCJ. The characteristics of AIS is expressed as large glandular orifices, papillary areas and budding epithelia.

6.2.4 Associations Between Epithelial Thickness, Age, and HPVs

In the case of CIN2/3, the epithelia are thinner in patients over 35 years of age than they are in younger patients [20, 21]. Epithelial thickness is generally thicker in high-grade intraepithelial lesions, although thinner epithelia are sometimes observed

[20]. The difference in thickness is due to the nature of the abnormal epithelia, not the colposcopic technique. It is easy to detect HPV16 infection by colposcopy because viral infection engenders broad lesions [22–24]. It is anticipated that in the future, colposcopy will be less important for this type of diagnosis, because vaccination is dramatically reducing the number of HPV-induced cervical carcinomas. Therefore, colposcopy training will have to change as the vaccine becomes more prevalent.

6.2.5 Taking More Biopsies to Increase Sensitivity

To find more CIN, more biopsies are needed. A trained oncologist will fulfill the sensitivity requirement on the first biopsy. In contrast, nurses and general gynecologists may take more biopsies to achieve an acceptable level of sensitivity [25].

Endocervical curettage (ECC) can increase sensitivity by 13% for diagnosis of CIN2+ in patients over 40 years of age. In contrast, the detection rate of CIN2+ is only 2% for those under 40 years of age [26]. There is some debate as to when ECC should be performed, but at the very least, ECC is recommended in cases where colposcopic findings are inconclusive. The American Society of Cervical Colposcopy and Pathology (ASCCP) guidelines also state that ECC is recommended for atypical glandular cells (AGC) in non-pregnant women over 35 years of age, and in women under 35 years of age and at risk for endometrial cancer [7].

6.2.6 Benefits of a Colposcopy Grading System

Although the diagnosis is made by colposcopic directed biopsy, clinical colposcopy findings can help prevent diagnostic errors that arise when incomplete or inaccurate specimens are obtained from lesions. The diagnostic agreement among pathologists for both cytology and histology was moderate at $k = 0.46$ [27]. For example, one pathologist may make a diagnosis of CIN2 while other diagnoses the same patient with CIN1 or CIN3. Hence, the agreement between colposcopists is far from perfect. Therefore, a grading system has been created to evaluate the severity of the lesion in a way that maximizes the likelihood of agreement between examiners. This system takes into account the color and transparency of the epithelium before and after application of acetic acid as well as the shape and border of abnormal lesions, and also the diameter, pattern, branch characteristics and distance between vessels, size, location, and surface contour of the lesion. The colposcopy grade system is a useful method of systematically analyzing the observed findings. The severity of the lesion is estimated by scoring parameters related to the epithelia and vasculature. Familiarity with this grading system among colposcopists can greatly reduce the possibility of missed observations and can help standardize the observations and interpretations made by colposcopists. It is also useful as an educational method, as colposcopy skills can be improved by retrospectively examining colposcopy findings after a histologic diagnosis has been obtained. If there is a discrepancy between the colposcopic findings and the histopathology or cytology, the colposcopists should review these data.

6.2.7 Characteristic Colposcopic Findings According to CIN Classification

6.2.7.1 CIN1

In general, it is difficult to distinguish immature metaplasia from HPV infection [28]. Whereas CIN2/3 lesions are adjacent to the SCJ, CIN1 lesions are found in various locations. The margin is irregular and asymmetric. The contours of CIN1 (including those associated with HPV infection) are varied. For example, they can be micropapillary, papillary, papule, with a flat or raised contour. Occasionally they can appear gyrate. Some are tumors are indistinguishable from benign or malignant lesions on visual inspection and require biopsy. The color classification is subjective. The white color change after application of acetic acid recovers fastest in CIN1 and slowest in CIN3 [29]. Although the white color of CIN1 is the most transparent, some CIN1 lesions have a dark white epithelium [20]. Blood vessels are thin, narrow, and uniform.

6.2.7.2 CIN2

The diagnosis of CIN2 is sometimes challenging [30, 31]. Histology and colposcopic findings are difficult to reconcile because of inter-observer variation. A small CIN2 lesion may be present within a larger CIN1 lesion. CIN2 lesions are located adjacent to the SCJ. Contour appears as macular. The margins are smooth and circular. A broad and irregular outer side is characteristic of CIN1, but since there is an inner border adjacent to the inner SCJ, it is possible to find CIN2 lesions within a CIN1 lesion. The color of a CIN1 lesion is not as purely white as CIN3. Transparency is also intermediate between CIN1 and CIN3. The vascularity of a CIN2 lesion is intermediate between CIN1 and CIN3. The lesion may be adjacent to the SCJ at the external cervix or in the cervical canal; CIN2 lesions are rarely found as satellite lesions. If the cytology is interpreted as ASC-US or LSIL, the colposcopic observations are generally interpreted as CIN1. However, if the cytology indicates HSIL, colposcopy may classify the lesion as CIN3. Thus, there is a bias in the judgment depending on the cytology results, which highlights the difficulty in differentiating CIN2 from CIN1 and CIN3.

6.2.7.3 CIN3

CIN3 lesions tend to be larger than CIN1 and CIN2 lesions, with a greater concentration of abnormal characteristic findings. Unlike CIN1, CIN3 is solitary. If CIN3 is located in a large area, potential microinvasive carcinoma (MIC) may be missed. Therefore, when performing vaporization, multiple biopsies should be performed to rule out the possibility of MIC in advance. When cytology is determined to be ASC-US, LSIL, colposcopic directed biopsy often indicates CIN3. However, the final diagnosis of invasive carcinoma is rare. Invasion is generally associated with larger CIN3 lesions, and rarely with small CIN3 lesions. CIN3 lesions are adjacent to the inside of the SCJ or in the cervical canal. The margins are smooth, circular, or straight. Epithelial peeling and inner borders are also features of CIN3 lesions. Most lesions of CIN3 are flat. Nodular, papillary, or outgrowing contours are indicators of invasive cancer. Ulcers are associated with invasive carcinoma. As an opaque white, it is described as a deep white or oyster gray. The worst lesions may be located in those where the white change is most persistent after application of acetic acid. The distance between vessels is heterogeneous compared to CIN1. CIN3 lesions often present without vascular abnormalities. Indeed, atypical vessels suggest cancer rather than CIN3, while it has been reported that 2–6% of patients with atypical vessels are cancer-free [32, 33].

6.2.8 Characteristic Colposcopy Observations in Pregnant Women

In pregnant women, the cervix is dark purple due to increased blood flow (Chadwick's sign) [34].

Use of an ultrasound probe cover is recommended to block the expanded vaginal wall in order to gain the visual field for the entire cervix. It is difficult to remove the highly viscous mucus; therefore, it is useful to put aside mucus using the cotton swab or tweezers. If a TZ is not clear in the first trimester, it is again recommended to examine with colposcopy in the mid-trimester [34]. As the pregnancy progresses, the TZ in the cervical canal migrates outward physiologically.

During pregnancy, the component of Swede score including vessel patterns, lesion size and margins plus surface is a useful index for estimation of CIN [35]. The timing of the colposcopy during pregnancy is important for accurate diagnosis. For the best correlation between colposcopy and histology results, it is preferable that both procedures are carried out in the first 20 weeks of gestation [36]. Biopsies during pregnancy tend to be postponed if invasiveness is not suspected [37]. However, some physicians are prepared to accept additional risk and perform the biopsy in the second trimester instead of the first trimester [38, 39]. Recent guidelines recommend that cone resection for CIN should be postponed until delivery [7, 40, 41]. If invasive cancer cannot be ruled out, or a patient is diagnosed with AIS, diagnostic cone resection is recommended during pregnancy. In the postpartum period, cervical inflammation subsides at 8 weeks postpartum; examination after this time is therefore preferable [39, 42]. The U.S. guidelines require examination by 6 weeks postpartum because of the insurance reimbursement system [7]. Patients with CIN 2/3 whose lesions are in the visible zone during pregnancy and whose cytologic diagnosis is consistent with colposcopy findings and histologic diagnosis by biopsy should undergo colposcopy and cytology every 6–8 weeks; additional biopsies should be performed only if invasion is suspected. It is important to reevaluate at 8 weeks postpartum and to minimize the rate of patient follow-up dropouts [43] alternatively, deferring colposcopy to the post-partum period is acceptable [7].

References

1. Frable WJ. Error reduction and risk management in cytopathology. Semin Diagn Pathol. 2007;24:77–88.
2. Christopherson WM, Parker JE, Drye JC. Control of cervical cancer. Preliminary report on community program. JAMA. 1962;182:179–82.
3. Kurokawa T, Onuma T, Shinagawa A, et al. The ideal strategy for cervical cancer screening in Japan: result from the Fukui cervical cancer screening study. Cytopathology. 2018;29:361–7.
4. Kovacic MB, Castle PE, Herrero R, et al. Relationships of human papillomavirus type, qualitative viral load, and age with cytologic abnormality. Cancer Res. 2006;66:10112–9.
5. Tota JE, Bentley J, Blake J, et al. Introduction of molecular HPV testing as the primary technology in cervical cancer screening: acting on evidence to change the current paradigm. Prev Med. 2017;98:5–14.
6. Egemen D, Cheung LC, Chen X, et al. Risk estimates supporting the 2019 ASCCP risk-based management consensus guidelines. J Low Genit Tract Dis. 2020;24:132–43.
7. Perkins RB, Guido RS, Castle PE, et al. 2019 ASCCP risk-based management consensus guidelines for abnormal cervical cancer screening tests and cancer precursors. J Low Genit Tract Dis. 2020;24:102–31.
8. Kawaguchi R, Matsumoto K, Ishikawa T, et al. Guideline for gynecological practice in Japan: Japan Society of Obstetrics and Gynecology and Japan Association of Obstetricians and Gynecologists 2020 edition. J Obstet Gynaecol Res. 2021;47:5–25.
9. Dona MG, Vocaturo A, Giuliani M, et al. p16/Ki-67 dual staining in cervico-vaginal cytology: correlation with histology, human papillomavirus detection and genotyping in women undergoing colposcopy. Gynecol Oncol. 2012;126:198–202.
10. Fujii T, Saito M, Hasegawa T, et al. Performance of p16/Ki-67 immunocytochemistry for identifying CIN2+ in atypical squamous cells of undetermined significance and low-grade squamous intraepithelial lesion specimens: a Japanese gynecologic oncology group study. Int J Clin Oncol. 2015;20:134–42.
11. Wentzensen N, Clarke MA, Bremer R, et al. Clinical evaluation of human papillomavirus screening with p16/Ki-67 dual stain triage in a large organized cervical cancer screening program. JAMA Intern Med. 2019;179:881–8.
12. Department of Economic and Social Affairs Population Dynamics. World population prospects key findings & advance tables 2017 revision. New York, NY: United Nations; 2017.
13. Miki M, Imaeda Y, Takahashi H, et al. Lower accuracy of cytological screening for high-grade squamous intraepithelial neoplasia in women over 50 years of age in Japan. Int J Clin Oncol. 2021;27:427–33.
14. Bateson DJ, Weisberg E. An open-label randomized trial to determine the most effective regimen of vaginal estrogen to reduce the prevalence of atrophic changes reported in postmenopausal cervical smears. Menopause. 2009;16:765–9.
15. Korenaga TK, Tewari KS. Gynecologic cancer in pregnancy. Gynecol Oncol. 2020;157:799–809.
16. Ribeiro F, Correia L, Paula T, et al. Cervical cancer in pregnancy: 3 cases, 3 different approaches. J Low Genit Tract Dis. 2013;17:66–70.
17. Cox JT. The road to cervical cancer prevention: historical perspective. In: Mayeaux J, Cox JT, et al., editors. Modern colposcopy: textbook & atlas. 3rd ed. Lippincott Williams & Wilkins (LWW); 2012. p. 1–13.
18. Buxton EJ, Luesley DM, Shafi MI, et al. Colposcopically directed punch biopsy: a potentially misleading investigation. Br J Obstet Gynaecol. 1991;98:1273–6.
19. Girardi F, Reich O, Tamussino K, et al. Histology and histopathology. In: Girardi F, Reich O, Tamussino K, et al., editors. Burghardt's colposcopy and cervical pathology: textbook and atlas. Thieme; 2015. p. 24–61.
20. Yang B, Pretorius RG, Belinson JL, et al. False negative colposcopy is associated with thinner cervical intraepithelial neoplasia 2 and 3. Gynecol Oncol. 2008;110:32–6.

21. Zahm DM, Nindl I, Greinke C, et al. Colposcopic appearance of cervical intraepithelial neoplasia is age dependent. Am J Obstet Gynecol. 1998;179:1298–304.
22. Jeronimo J, Massad LS, Schiffman M. Visual appearance of the uterine cervix: correlation with human papillomavirus detection and type. Am J Obstet Gynecol. 2007;197:47.e41–8.
23. Sherman ME, Wang SS, Tarone R, et al. Histopathologic extent of cervical intraepithelial neoplasia 3 lesions in the atypical squamous cells of undetermined significance low-grade squamous intraepithelial lesion triage study: implications for subject safety and lead-time bias. Cancer Epidemiol Biomark Prev. 2003;12:372–9.
24. Stellato G, Paavonen J. A colposcopic scoring system for grading cervical lesions. Eur J Gynaecol Oncol. 1995;16:296–300.
25. Gage JC, Hanson VW, Abbey K, et al. Number of cervical biopsies and sensitivity of colposcopy. Obstet Gynecol. 2006;108:264–72.
26. Solomon D, Stoler M, Jeronimo J, et al. Diagnostic utility of endocervical curettage in women undergoing colposcopy for equivocal or low-grade cytologic abnormalities. Obstet Gynecol. 2007;110:288–95.
27. Stoler MH, Schiffman M. Interobserver reproducibility of cervical cytologic and histologic interpretations: realistic estimates from the ASCUS-LSIL triage study. JAMA. 2001;285:1500–5.
28. Ferris DG, Mayeaux J, Cox JT. Colposcopy of cervical intraepithelial neoplasia. In: Mayeaux J, Cox JT, et al., editors. Modern colposcopy: textbook & atlas. 3rd ed. Lippincott Williams & Wilkins (LWW); 2012. p. 235–305.
29. Sakuma T, Hasegawa T, Tsutsui F, et al. Quantitative analysis of the whiteness of the atypical cervical transformation zone. J Reprod Med. 1985;30:773–6.
30. Schiffman M, Castle PE, Jeronimo J, et al. Human papillomavirus and cervical cancer. Lancet. 2007;370:890–907.
31. Dalla Palma P, Giorgi Rossi P, Collina G, et al. The reproducibility of CIN diagnoses among different pathologists: data from histology reviews from a multicenter randomized study. Am J Clin Pathol. 2009;132:125–32.
32. Sillman F, Boyce J, Fruchter R. The significance of atypical vessels and neovascularization in cervical neoplasia. Am J Obstet Gynecol. 1981;139:154–9.
33. Sugimori H, Matsuyama T, Kashimura M, et al. Colposcopic findings in microinvasive carcinoma of the uterine cervix. Obstet Gynecol Surv. 1979;34:804–7.
34. Ferris DG, Cox JT, Mayeaux J, et al. Colposcopy and pregnancy. In: Mayeaux J, Cox JT, et al., editors. Modern colposcopy: textbook & atlas. 3rd ed. Lippincott Williams & Wilkins (LWW); 2012. p. 343–75.
35. Kärrberg C, Ryd W, Strander B, et al. Histological diagnosis and evaluation of the swede score colposcopic system in a large cohort of pregnant women with atypical cervical cytology or cervical malignancy signs. Acta Obstet Gynecol Scand. 2012;91:952–8.
36. Ciavattini A, Serri M, Di Giuseppe J, et al. Reliability of colposcopy during pregnancy. Eur J Obstet Gynecol Reprod Biol. 2018;229:76–81.
37. Fader AN, Alward EK, Niederhauser A, et al. Cervical dysplasia in pregnancy: a multi-institutional evaluation. Am J Obstet Gynecol. 2010;203:113.e111–6.
38. Stonehocker J. Cervical cancer screening in pregnancy. Obstet Gynecol Clin N Am. 2013;40:269–82.
39. Hunter MI, Monk BJ, Tewari KS. Cervical neoplasia in pregnancy. Part 1: screening and management of preinvasive disease. Am J Obstet Gynecol. 2008;199:3–9.
40. Jeronimo J, Castle PE, Temin S, et al. Secondary prevention of cervical cancer: ASCO resource-stratified clinical practice guideline. J Glob Oncol. 2017;3:635–57.
41. Amant F, Halaska MJ, Fumagalli M, et al. Gynecologic cancers in pregnancy: guidelines of a second international consensus meeting. Int J Gynecol Cancer. 2014;24:394–403.
42. Levitt C, Shaw E, Wong S, et al. Systematic review of the literature on postpartum care: selected contraception methods, postpartum Papanicolaou test, and rubella immunization. Birth. 2004;31:203–12.
43. Van Calsteren K, Vergote I, Amant F. Cervical neoplasia during pregnancy: diagnosis, management and prognosis. Best Pract Res Clin Obstet Gynaecol. 2005;19:611–30.

Clinical Management of CIN Including Recent Therapeutic Strategies

7

Kei Kawana

Abstract

CIN is clearly caused by HPV infection, but the pathogenesis is thought to differ between CIN1 and CIN2/3. A recent morphological definition classifies CIN1 (LSIL) as a lesion indicating HPV infection and CIN2/3 (HSIL) as a neoplastic lesion. No treatment is needed for CIN1 because it has no symptoms and mostly regresses spontaneously. However, CIN2/3 is a precancerous lesion of cervical cancer and is therefore considered to be a candidate for treatment intervention to reduce the risk of cervical cancer. The only treatment available for CIN2/3 at present is surgical treatment. However, it is not clear why a therapeutic drug remains undeveloped for CIN2/3. In this review, we discuss the current progress in drug discovery for CIN2/3.

Keywords

Cervical intraepithelial neoplasia · Cervical cancer · Human papillomavirus (HPV) · High-risk HPV · HPV-targeting therapeutics · Immunotherapy · Mucosal immunity · *Lactobacillus*-based vaccine

K. Kawana (✉)
Department of Obstetrics and Gynecology, Nihon University School of Medicine, Tokyo, Japan
e-mail: kawana.kei@nihon-u.ac.jp

D. Aoki (ed.), *Recent Topics on Prevention, Diagnosis, and Clinical Management of Cervical Cancer*, Comprehensive Gynecology and Obstetrics,
https://doi.org/10.1007/978-981-99-9396-3_7

7.1 Current Treatments for CIN2/3 and Their Subjects

The incidence of CIN2/3 is increasing in low-income developing countries in which HPV prophylactic vaccines remain unavailable. In Japan, approximately 15,000 people are diagnosed with CIN2/3 annually, and the peak age of cervical cancer, including precancerous lesions, is 30–40 years old [1]. Because proactive recommendation of HPV vaccination had been suspended for more than 8 years, the incidence of both cervical cancer and CIN2/3 continues to increase in Japan [2].

HPV vaccination coverage in the worldwide population eligible for vaccination is estimated to be approximately 40%, and the catch-up vaccination coverage is approximately 10% [3]. This suggests that the HPV vaccine is too expensive for low-income countries to adopt, and there are many countries globally in which it is difficult to implement national HPV immunization programs as a policy. Simulations by the World Health Organization indicate that cervical cancer will eventually be eliminated by HPV vaccination and cervical cancer screening by 2060 [4]. However, its simulations set the global vaccination rate of HPV vaccination at 90%. At the current vaccination coverage rates noted above, the elimination of cervical cancer will take at least 50 years. Until then, for women infected with high-risk HPVs, cervical cancer remains a threat.

Although numerous studies regarding the management of CIN have been undertaken to explore new biomarkers to predict the risk of progression, there have been no novel findings directly related to clinical applications in the past decade, and there have been no new developments in the management of CIN. As a result, the only way to detect CIN lesions is by cancer screening, such as HPV testing, followed by continued periodic follow-up. When CIN progresses to CIN2/3 during follow-up, therapeutic intervention is used to reduce the risk of cervical cancer. Although HPV genotyping allows for risk assessment of CIN progression, it does not go so far as to personalize the management of CIN by HPV genotypes.

Currently, the only treatment for CIN2/3 is surgical resection or vaporization, and there is no non-invasive therapy. A total hysterectomy eliminates fertility, and cervical conization or loop electrosurgical excision procedure (LEEP) lead to poor obstetric outcomes in subsequent pregnancies. In pregnancies following conization to treat CIN2/3, the risk of preterm delivery is approximately three times higher, and the cesarean delivery rate and low birth weight rate are also approximately three times higher [5]. Because the peak age at which CIN2/3 occurs coincides with the age at which an individual becomes pregnant and gives birth, poor obstetric outcomes resulting from surgical treatment for CIN2/3 are a problem for the entire field of obstetrics and gynecology. However, laser vaporization, the least invasive treatment, does not worsen the obstetric outcome [5], although the recurrence rate after treatment is 20%–25% per year [6], and there is a limit to the radical cure. While LEEP does not increase the rate of preterm birth, the surgery must be performed under anesthesia, and postoperative bleeding often occurs. Curative and non-invasive treatment modalities are ideal treatment for women with CIN2/3, and therapeutic agents for CIN2/3 are an unmet clinical need.

7.2 Development Status of Therapeutic Agents for CIN2/3

The efficacy of immune checkpoint inhibitors against cervical cancer, which is caused by HPV, is promising. In the KEYNOTE 158 study of pembrolizumab [7] and the GOG 3016/ENGOT En-Cx9 study of cemiplimab [8], PD-1-blocking antibodies were demonstrated to improve the prognosis of recurrent cervical cancer when administered in combination or as single agents, and have already been used in clinical practice. However, CIN is well-known to spontaneously regress via the host immunity against HPV antigens [9]. In cohort studies of patients with CINs, approximately 70% of CIN1, 50%–60% of CIN2, and 20% of CIN3 regress spontaneously [10, 11]. HPV viral proteins E2 and E6/E7 are expressed ubiquitously in the lesions of CIN1 and CIN2/3 or cervical cancer, respectively, and are also thought of as tumor antigens. They are virus-derived allogenic antigens and are likely to be targets for the host's immune response. Patients in whom the immune response to HPV viral proteins has been elicited are likely to have a spontaneous regression. This leads to the idea that immunization with these viral antigens could be a promising therapeutic strategy for CINs, mimicking spontaneous regression.

In the last two decades, a number of immunotherapies targeting the HPV viral proteins have been developed for therapeutics against CIN2/3 (Table 7.1) [12–21], and the target lesions for most clinical trials are CIN2/3. All the agents currently in development aim to elicit host immune responses against E6 and/or E7 of HPV types 16 and/or 18. E6/E7 proteins/peptides are transported as vaccine antigens by fusion proteins, expression plasmid, or microbes. In some trials, imiquimod or fungus body are used as adjuvant agents [12, 17]. It is clear that treatment to induce immunity against E6/E7 (immunotherapy) is a well-understood concept that is a strategy for the development of novel therapeutics for CIN2/3.

For therapeutic agents, the routes of administration can be grouped into muscular or subcutaneous injections and oral administration. Most are injected intramuscularly or subcutaneously, and orally administered agents are being developed in Japan and Korea. GLBL101c and BLS-ILB-E710c are the same agent, although the code numbers vary from country to country. Two clinical trials conducted in Japan were followed up by other trials in Korea. Another oral agent, IGMKK16E7, is newly developed by Japanese researchers and is a second-generation drug that was optimized from GLBL101c.

The development of VGX-3100, Pepcan (E6 peptides) + Candin, VB10.16/atezolizumab, and IGMKK16E7 is currently ongoing. All these agents have advanced to the development stage of phase II–III clinical trials. Among them, the most advanced therapeutic vaccine currently in development is VGX-3100 (Inovio Inc.), which is a plasmid DNA vaccine that is injected intramuscularly [15]. In a phase IIb study of 167 patients with HPV16-positive CIN2/3, the rate of histopathological regression and viral clearance was 40% in the VGX-3100 group and 12% in the placebo group in a modified intention-to-treat analysis. Although there was a significant difference in efficacy, inoculation site adverse events occurred in 98% of patients [16]. In addition, the results of a phase III study of 201 patients with CIN2/3 as a modified intention-to-treat population were also reported. The primary

Table 7.1 Summary of clinical trials for therapeutics targeting CIN2/3

Code	Phase	Agent	No. ClinicalTrials. gov	Country	Main facility	Disease	Trial period	No. of enrolled patients	Endpoint	Bind	Placebo	Randomization	No. of dose	Route	Publicaion no.
MILACLE study	Phase 1/2	IGMKK16E7	UMIN000034253	Japan	Nihon University	CIN2/3	2019.6-2022.7	164	24w	Double-blind	Placebo-controlled	Randomized	Weeks 1, 2, 4, 8	p.o.	(-)
E6 peptides/ Candin®2	Phase 2	Pepcan(E6 peptides)+ Candin®	NCT02481414	USA	University of Arkansas	CIN2/3	2015.11-2025	125	48w	Double-blind	Placebo-controlled	Randomized	Weeks 0, 3, 6, 9	S.C.	(-)
VB10.16	Phase2a	VB10.16/ Atezolizumab	NCT04405349	EU	Nykode	Cervical cancer	2020.7-2024.3	50	52w	No	No	No	Every 6wks for VB10.16/every 3 wks for Atezolizumab	i.m. for VB10.16/i.v. for Atezolizumab	(-)
VGX-3100-3	Phase3 (REVEAL 2)	VGX-3100	NCT03721978	USA	Inovio Pharmaceuticals	CIN2/3	2019.4-2022.9	203	36w	Double-blind	Placebo-controlled	Randomized	Weeks 0, 4, 12	i.m.	(-)
VGX-3100-2	Phase3 (REVEAL 1)	VGX-3100	NCT03185013	USA	Inovio Pharmaceuticals	CIN2/3	2017.6-2021.4	201	36w	Double-bilnd	Placebo-controlled	Randomized	Weeks 0, 4, 12	i.m.	(-)
BLS-ILB-E710c-2	Phase2b	BLS_ILS_E710c	NCT03274206	Korea	BioLeaders Corporation	CIN2/3	2017.8-2020.8	126	16w	Double-blind	Placebo-controlled	Randomized	Weeks 1, 2, 4, 8	p.o.	(-)
GX-188E-2	Phase2	GX-188E+ imiquimode	NCT03206138	Korea	Genexine, Inc.	CIN3	2017.5-2018.10	50	36w	No	No	Randomized	NA	i.m.+local	(-)
GX-I7	Phase1	GX-I7	NCT03144934	Korea	Genexine, Inc.	HPV infection	2017.2-2018.3	32	4w	Double-blind	Placebo-controlled	Randomized	Weeks 0, 4	Local	(-)
GX-188E-1	Phase2	GX-188E	NCT02139267	Korea	Genexine, Inc.	CIN3	2014.7-2016.3	72	20w	No	No	Randomized	Weeks 0, 4, 12	i.m.	[21]
BLS-ILB-E710c-1	Phase 1/2a	BLS_ILS_E710c	NCT02195089	Korea	BioLeaders Corporation	CIN3	2014.3-2016.4	18	16w	No	No	No	Weeks 1, 2, 4, 8	p.o.	[20]
GLBL101c-2	Phase 2b	GLBL101c	UMIN000012229	Japan	University of Tokyo	CIN2	2014.3-2017.9	40	16w	Double-blind	Placebo-controlled	Randomized	Weeks 1, 2, 4, 8	p.o.	[19]
E6 peptides+ Candin®	Phase 1	Pepcan(E6 peptides) +Candin®	NCT01653249	USA	University of Arkansas	CIN2/3	2012.8-2015.7	34	21w	No	No	No	Weeks 0, 3, 6, 9	s.c.	[17, 18]
VGX-3100-1	Phase2	VGX-3100	NCT01304524	USA	Inovio Pharmaceuticals	CIN2/3	2011.4-2015.4	167	36w	Double-blind	Placebo-controlled	Randomized	Weeks 0, 4, 12	i.m.	[16]
pNGVL4a-CRT/ E7(detox)	Phase1	pNGVL4a-CRT/ E7(detox)	NCT00988559	USA	Johns Hopkins	CIN2/3	2009.11 ~ 2013.9	27	15w	No	No	No	weeks 0, 4,8	i.m.	[15]
Tipapkinogen sovacivec (TS) vaccine	Phase2b	Tipapkinogen sovacivec (TS) vaccine (RO5217790)	NCT01022346	USA	University of Missouri	CIN2/3	2009.8 ~ 2013.9	192	24w	Double-blind	Placebo-controlled	Randomized	Days 1, 8, 15	s.c.	[14]
GLBL101c-1	Phase 1/2a	GLBL101c	UMIN000001686	Japan	University of Tokyo	CIN3	2009.2– 2013.11	17	9w	No	No	No	Weeks 1, 2, 4, 8	p.o.	[13]
TA-HPV	Phase1	pNGVL4a-sig/ E7(detox)/ HSP70 DNA vaccine+ imiquimod	NCT00788164	USA	Johns Hopkins	CIN3	2008.11 ~ 2023.7	75	41w	No	No	No	Days 1, 29, 57	i.m.	[12]

endpoint was a histologically confirmed LSIL/normal that was negative for HPV16 and/or HPV18 DNA at week 36. The percentage of patients with LSIL/normal and viral clearance was 22.5% with VGX-3100 and 11.1% with placebo, which were not significantly different. Comparison of the primary endpoint results of the phase IIb and III studies showed that the efficacy of VGX-3100 was lower in the phase III trial, although the results in the placebo group were similar. These results suggested promising therapeutic candidates for CIN2/3 have been not yet developed at present.

Most CIN2/3 drug therapies developed to date are administered via intramuscular or subcutaneous routes. Sufficient E7-specific cellular immunity is induced in the peripheral blood, but the rate of regression to normal was not high. Because the placebo group also regresses approximately 20%–30% of CIN2/3, the true efficacy of the investigational drug cannot be determined without comparison to the placebo group. Of the clinical trials listed in Table 7.1, nine were placebo-controlled, and three of these trials have been published. As discussed above, among clinical trials conducted to date, the phase IIb trial of VGX-3100 showed the largest difference between the VGX-3100 and placebo groups (40% vs. 12%) [16]. The response rate of the VGX-3100 group will be a milestone for the development of therapeutics for CIN2/3.

7.3 Host and Mucosal Immunity in the Cervix

Because CIN2/3 is an intraepithelial lesion arising in the cervical mucosa (squamous epithelium), induction of mucosal immunity against tumor antigens is considered to be favorable for immunological regression. The mechanism is as follows: in mucosal immunity of the cervical epithelium, Peyer's patches on the intestinal mucosa (GALT, gut-associated lymphoid tissues) or mesenteric lymph nodes are known to be inductive tissue (Fig. 7.1). Antigen-specific memory T cells are educated in GALT and mesenteric lymph nodes, and lymphocytes that have acquired the recognition of viral antigens possess unique characteristics as "mucosal lymphocytes." Mucosal lymphocytes have surface receptors called integrin β7 and CCR9 as homing receptors. Mucosal lymphocytes home to all of the mucosa via peripheral circulation by binding their homing receptors to natural ligands on the endothelial cells of the submucosal vessels.

In our study, we found that approximately 20%–40% of the lymphocytes that presented in the cervical epithelium of patients with CIN were gut-derived integrin β7+/CCR9+ T cells. Furthermore, we found that patients with CIN were likely to exhibit spontaneous regression when the gut-derived T cells residing in the CIN lesions were detected by flow cytometry at high rates [22]. In this way, gut-derived memory T cells, especially TH1 cells, are thought to play a role as tumor-infiltrating lymphocytes that accumulate into the CIN2/3 lesions.

Therefore, we considered inducing E7-specific TH1 mucosal T cells at GALT by oral administration of HPV16 E7 in patients with CIN2/3 caused by HPV16. The mechanism is that when T cells induced in the intestinal mucosa and homing to the cervical epithelium recognize E7, which is highly expressed in the CIN2/3 lesions, and E7-specific TH1 cells produce IFN-γ, causing a TH1 response including NK cell activity, this leads to an anti-tumor effect (Fig. 7.2).

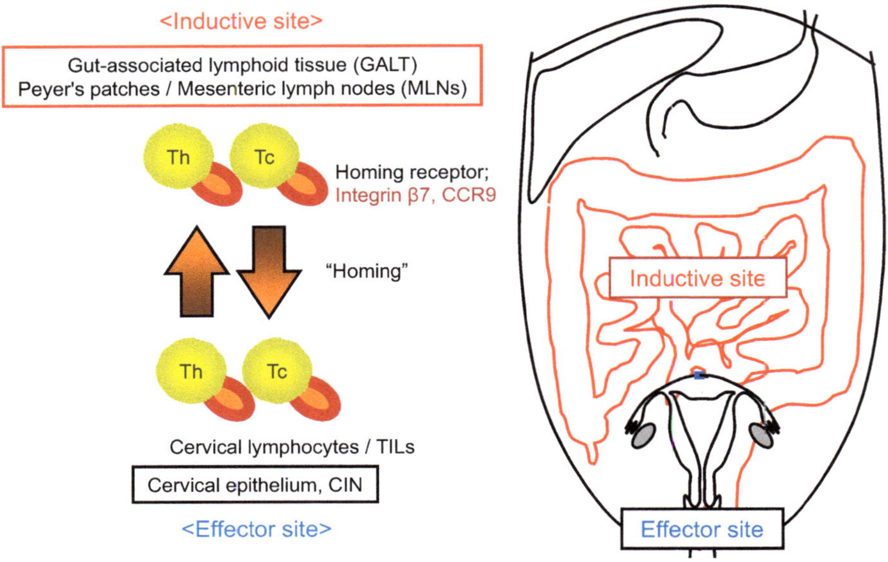

Fig. 7.1 Mechanisms of mucosal immune system at the cervix. The mechanism of mucosal immune responses at the cervix is as follows: In mucosal immunity of the cervical epithelium, Peyer's patches on the intestinal mucosa (GALT, gut-associated lymphoid tissues) or mesenteric lymph nodes are known to be inductive tissue

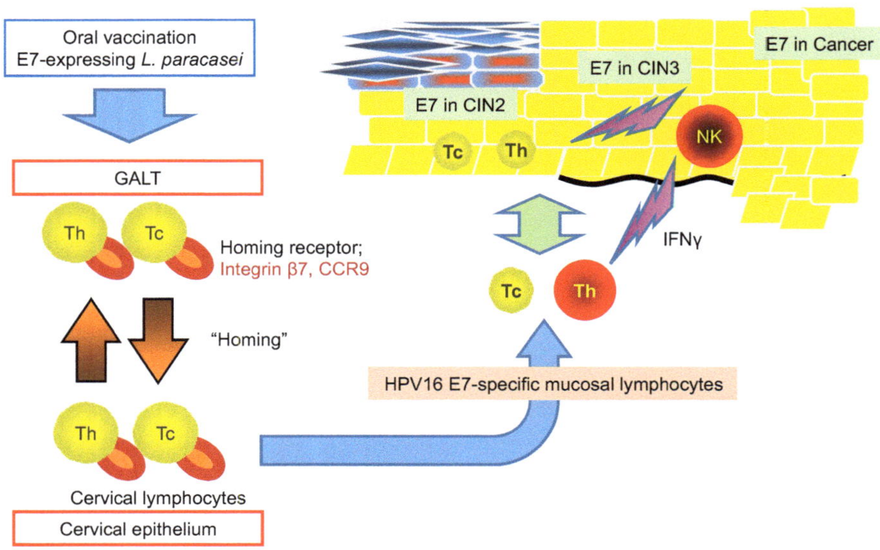

Fig. 7.2 Mechanisms of oral immunization for treatment of CIN2/3. The mechanism of IGMKK16E7 is that when T cells induced in the intestinal mucosa and homing to the cervical epithelium recognize E7, which is highly expressed in the CIN2/3 lesions, and E7-specific TH1 cells produce IFN-γ, causing a TH1 response including NK cell activity, this leads to an antitumor effect

7.4 Development of Therapeutic Agents Via Anti-HPV Mucosal Immunity

We developed IGMKK16E7 (HPV16 full-length E7-expressing *Lacticaseibacillus paracasei: L. paracasei*) as a therapeutic agent for CIN2/3. First, in a pre-clinical study using mice, we confirmed that oral administration of an E7-expressing *L. paracasei* preferentially induced E7-specific cellular immunity via the mucosal immune system in the gut compared with intramuscular or subcutaneous injection [23]. Based on these results, we conducted a proof of concept study at our hospital (Table 7.1) [13]. Subjects were CIN3 patients with HPV16 single-positive, and E7-expressing *L. paracasei*, GLBL101c, the first-generation drug based on this concept, was administered orally once a day for 5 days/week at weeks 1, 2, 4, and 8. No adverse events of grade 2–3 occurred in any of the 17 patients recruited in the study. In total, 62% of patients treated with 1.0–1.5 g/day GLBL101c had a partial regression at 2 months after the first dose, and 38% of them had a CR at 12 months after the first dose. Because the incidence of spontaneous regression from CIN3 was approximately 10% during the 4-month follow-up period, the regression rate by treatment may be higher than that of no treatment. E7-specific IFN-γ-producing T cells in patients with pathological regression were elicited in cervical lesions at a higher rate than in those of patients with non-regression, suggesting that the pathological regression occurred through the infiltration of high levels of E7-specific IFN-γ-producing T cells into the cervical epithelium [13]. We next conducted a randomized, double-blind, placebo-controlled study of GLBL101c in patients with HPV16 single-positive CIN2 (Table 7.1). This study showed that the pathological regression to normal was 10% and 0% in the GLBL101c and placebo groups, respectively, with no significant difference, and that there was no difference in adverse events between the two groups, confirming the safety of the E7-expressing *L. paracasei* [19].

The first-generation E7-expressing *L. paracasei*, GLBL101c, used in these two exploratory clinical studies was considered to have limited pharmacological efficacy. Then, we developed a new agent (IGMKK16E7), which showed four-times higher pharmacological effects on the induction of E7-specific IFN-γ-producing mucosal T cells [24]. We obtained an international patent and conducted a phase I/II investigator-initiated clinical trial of IGMKK16E7 in June 2019. This was a parallel-group randomized controlled multicenter trial with four groups: placebo, low dose, intermediate dose, and high dose (1:1:1:1 allocation) in patients with HPV16-positive CIN2/3 (Table 7.1). The target enrollment was 164 cases (124 for CIN3 and 40 for CIN2), and the primary endpoint was pathological regression (CR = normal, PR = CIN1, SD=CIN2–3, PD = invasive cancer) at 16 and 24 weeks after the first dose [25]. The patient registration closed in July 2022. The final analysis of the results has finished and IGMKK16E7 showed expected efficacy and safety. We plan to start a phase III trial in the summer of 2023.

7.5 Future Prospects

HPV-associated neoplasm is a tumor that expresses the allogenic antigens E6 and E7, and thereby is susceptible to host immune responses. However, some women infected with HPV cannot acquire HPV-specific cellular immunity, depending on the immune repertoire that each individual harbors. The strategy of HPV-specific active immunotherapy using immunization by other routes may overcome the personal limitation of immune response to antigens. Furthermore, we might use a combination of immune checkpoint inhibitors to further increase the efficacy of active immunotherapy, following future research of biomarkers that inhibit local immune responses in the cervix. Otherwise, the development of companion diagnostics using biomarkers to show the profile of non-responders for the immunotherapy may be expected. Non-invasive treatment for CIN2/3 would be of greatest benefit for women, especially for those of child-bearing age.

Acknowledgments We thank H. Nikki March, PhD, from Edanz (https://jp.edanz.com/ac) for editing a draft of this manuscript.

References

1. Sakakibara A, Nakayama T, Uchida H, Odagiri Y, Ito Y, Katayama T, Ueda Y, Higuchi T, Terakawa K, Matsui K, Miyazaki K, Konishi I. Trends and future projections of cervical cancer-related outcomes in Japan: what happens if the HPV vaccine program is not implemented? Int J Cancer. 2022;152:1863. https://doi.org/10.1002/ijc.34391; Online ahead of print.
2. Yagi A, Ueda Y, Nakagawa S, Ikeda S, Tanaka Y, Sekine M, Miyagi E, Enomoto T, Kimura T. Potential for cervical cancer incidence and death resulting from Japan's current policy of prolonged suspension of its governmental recommendation of the HPV vaccine. Sci Rep. 2020;10(1):15945. https://doi.org/10.1038/s41598-020-73106-z.
3. Bruni L. Global estimates of human papillomavirus vaccination coverage by region and income level: a pooled analysis. Lancet Glob Health. 2016;4(7):e453–63.
4. A global strategy for elimination of cervical cancer—PAHO/WHO. Pan American Health Organization. https://www.paho.org/en/towardshealthier-generations-free-diseases/global-strategy-elimination-cervical-cancer. Accessed 3 May 2022.
5. Kyrgiou M, Athanasiou A, Kalliala IEJ, et al. Obstetric outcomes after conservative treatment for cervical intraepithelial lesions and early invasive disease. Cochrane Database Syst Rev. 2017;11(11):CD012847. https://doi.org/10.1002/14651858.CD012847.
6. Inaba K, Nagasaka K, Kawana K, Arimoto T, Matsumoto Y, Tsuruga T, Mori-Uchino M, Miura S, Sone K, Oda K, Nakagawa S, Yano T, Kozuma S, Fujii T. High-risk human papillomavirus correlates with recurrence after laser ablation for treatment of patients with cervical intraepithelial neoplasia 3: a long-term follow-up retrospective study. J Obstet Gynaecol Res. 2014;40(2):554–60. https://doi.org/10.1111/jog.12196.
7. Chung HC, Ros W, Delord JP, Perets R, Italiano A, Shapira-Frommer R, Manzuk L, Piha-Paul SA, Xu L, Zeigenfuss S, Pruitt SK, Leary A. Efficacy and safety of Pembrolizumab in previously treated advanced cervical cancer: results from the phase II KEYNOTE-158 study. J Clin Oncol. 2019;37(17):1470–8. https://doi.org/10.1200/JCO.18.01265.
8. Tewari KS, Monk BJ, Vergote I, Miller A, de Melo AC, Kim HS, Kim YM, Lisyanskaya A, Samouëlian V, Lorusso D, Damian F, Chang CL, Gotovkin EA, Takahashi S, Ramone D, Pikiel J, Maćkowiak-Matejczyk B, Guerra Alía EM, Colombo N, Makarova Y, Rischin D, Lheureux S, Hasegawa K, Fujiwara K, Li J, Jamil S, Jankovic V, Chen CI, Seebach F, Weinreich DM,

Yancopoulos GD, Lowy I, Mathias M, Fury MG, Oaknin A, Investigators for GOG protocol 3016 and ENGOT protocol En-Cx9. Survival with cemiplimab in recurrent cervical cancer. N Engl J Med. 2022;386(6):544–55. https://doi.org/10.1056/NEJMoa2112187.

9. Loopik DL, Bentley HA, Eijgenraam MN, IntHout J, Bekkers RLM, Bentley JR. The natural history of cervical intraepithelial neoplasia grades 1, 2, and 3: a systematic review and meta-analysis. J Low Genit Tract Dis. 2021;25(3):221–31. https://doi.org/10.1097/LGT.0000000000000604.
10. Matsumoto K, Oki A, Furuta R, Maeda H, Yasugi T, Takatsuka N, Mitsuhashi A, Fujii T, Hirai Y, Iwasaka T, Yaegashi N, Watanabe Y, Nagai Y, Kitagawa T, Yoshikawa H; Japan HPV And Cervical Cancer Study Group, Predicting the progression of cervical precursor lesions by human papillomavirus genotyping: a prospective cohort study., Int J Cancer 2011;128(12):2898–2910. doi: https://doi.org/10.1002/ijc.25630.
11. Einstein MH, Kadish AS, Burk RD, Kim MY, Wadler S, Streicher H, Goldberg GL, Runowicz CD. Heat shock fusion protein-based immunotherapy for treatment of cervical intraepithelial neoplasia III. Gynecol Oncol. 2007;106:453–60.
12. Maldonado L, Teague JE, Morrow MP, Jotova I, Wu TC, Wang C, Desmarais C, Boyer JD, Tycko B, Robins HS, Clark RA, Trimble CL. Intramuscular therapeutic vaccination targeting HPV16 induces T cell responses that localize in mucosal lesions. Sci Transl Med. 2014;6(221):221ra13. https://doi.org/10.1126/scitranslmed.3007323.
13. Kawana K, Adachi K, Kojima S, Taguchi A, Tomio K, Yamashita A, Nishida H, Nagasaka K, Arimoto T, Yokoyama T, Wada-Hiraike O, Oda K, Sewaki T, Osuga Y, Fujii T. Oral vaccination against HPV E7 for treatment of cervical intraepithelial neoplasia grade 3 (CIN3) elicits E7-specific mucosal immunity in the cervix of CIN3 patients. Vaccine. 2014;32:6233–9. https://doi.org/10.1016/j.vaccine.2014.09.020.
14. Harper DM, Nieminen P, Donders G, EinsteinMH GF, Huh WK, Stoler MH, Glavini K, Attley G, Limacher JM, Bastien B, Calleja E. The efficacy and safety of Tipapkinogen Sovacivec therapeutic HPV vaccine in cervical intraepithelial neoplasia grades 2 and 3: randomized controlled phase II trial with 2.5 years of follow-up. Gynecol Oncol. 2019;153(3):521–9. https://doi.org/10.1016/j.ygyno.2019.03.250.
15. Alvarez RD, Huh WK, Bae S, Lamb LS Jr, Conner MG, Boyer J, Wang C, Hung CF, Sauter E, Paradis M, Adams EA, Hester S, Jackson BE, Wu TC, Trimble CL. A pilot study of pNGVL4a-CRT/E7(detox) for the treatment of patients with HPV16+ cervical intraepithelial neoplasia 2/3 (CIN2/3). Gynecol Oncol. 2016;140(2):245–52. https://doi.org/10.1016/j.ygyno.2015.11.026.
16. Trimble CL, Morrow MP, Kraynyak KA, Shen X, Dallas M, Yan J, Edwards L, Parker RL, Denny L, Giffear M, Brown AS, Marcozzi-Pierce K, Shah D, Slager AM, Sylvester AJ, Khan A, Boderick KE, Juba R, Herring TA, Boyer J, Lee J, Sardesai NY, Weiner DB, Bagarazzi ML. Safety, efficacy, and immunogenicity of VGX-3100, a therapeutic synthetic DNA vaccine targeting human papillomavirus 16 and 18 E6 and E7 proteins for cervical intraepithelial neoplasia 2/3: a randomised, double-blind, placebo-controlled phase 2b trial. Lancet. 2015;386(10008):2078–88. https://doi.org/10.1016/S0140-6736(15)00239-1.
17. Stratton SL, Spencer HJ, Greenfield WW, Low G, Hitt WC, Quick CM, Jeffus SK, Blackmon V, Nakagawa M. A novel use of a statewide telecolposcopy network for recruitment of participants in a phase I clinical trial of a human papillomavirus therapeutic vaccine. Clin Trials. 2015;12(3):199–204. https://doi.org/10.1177/1740774514566333.
18. Coleman HN, Greenfield WW, Stratton SL, Vaughn R, Kieber A, Moerman-Herzog AM, Spencer HJ, Hitt WC, Quick CM, Hutchins LF, Mackintosh SG, Edmondson RD, Erickson SW, Nakagawa M. Human papillomavirus type 16 viral load is decreased following a therapeutic vaccination. Cancer Immunol Immunother. 2016;65(5):563–73. https://doi.org/10.1007/s00262-016-1821-x.
19. Ikeda Y, Uemura Y, Asai-Sato M, Nakao T, Nakajima T, Iwata T, Akiyama A, Satoh T, Yahata H, Kato K, Maeda D, Aoki D, Kawana K. Safety and efficacy of mucosal immunotherapy using human papillomavirus (HPV) type 16 E7-expressing lactobacillus-based vaccine for the treatment of high-grade squamous intraepithelial lesion (HSIL): the study protocol of a randomized

placebo-controlled clinical trial (MILACLE study). Jpn J Clin Oncol. 2019;49:877–80. https://doi.org/10.1093/jjco/hyz095.

20. Park YC, Ouh YT, Sung MH, Park HG, Kim TJ, Cho CH, Park JS, Lee JK. A phase 1/2a, dose-escalation, safety and preliminary efficacy study of oral therapeutic vaccine in subjects with cervical intraepithelial neoplasia 3. J Gynecol Oncol. 2019;30(6):e88. https://doi.org/10.3802/jgo.2019.30.e88.
21. Choi YJ, Hur SY, Kim TJ, Hong SR, Lee JK, Cho CH, Park KS, Woo JW, Sung YC, Suh YS, Park JS. A phase II, prospective, randomized, multicenter, open-label study of GX-188E, an HPV DNA vaccine, in patients with cervical intraepithelial neoplasia 3. Clin Cancer Res. 2020;26(7):1616–23. https://doi.org/10.1158/1078-0432.CCR-19-1513.
22. Kojima S, Kawana K, Fujii T, Yokoyama T, Miura S, Tomio K, Tomio A, Yamashita A, Adachi K, Sato H, Nagamatsu T, Schust DJ, Kozuma S, Taketani Y. Characterization of gut-derived intraepithelial lymphocyte (IEL) residing in human papillomavirus (HPV)-infected intraepithelial neoplastic lesions. Am J Reprod Immunol. 2011;66:435–43.
23. Adachi K, Kawana K, Yokoyama T, et al. Oral immunization with lactobacillus casei vaccine expressing human papillomavirus (HPV) type 16 E7 is an effective strategy to induce mucosal cytotoxic lymphocyte against HPV16 E7. Vaccine. 2010;28:2810–7.
24. Komatsu A, Igimi S, Kawana K. Optimization of human papillomavirus (HPV) type 16 E7-expressing lactobacillus-based vaccine for induction of mucosal E7-specific IFNγ-producing cells. Vaccine. 2018;36(24):3423–6.
25. Ikeda Y, Uemura Y, Asai-Sato M, Nakao T, Nakajima T, Iwata T, Akiyama A, Satoh T, Yahata H, Kato K, Maeda D, Aoki D, Kawana K. Safety and efficacy of mucosal immunotherapy using human papillomavirus (HPV) type 16 E7-expressing *lactobacillus*-based vaccine for the treatment of high-grade squamous intraepithelial lesion (HSIL): the study protocol of a randomized placebo-controlled clinical trial (MILACLE study). Jpn J Clin Oncol. 2019;49:877–80.

Part IV

Surgical Treatments of Cervical Cancer

8 Surgical Treatment of Locally Advanced Cervical Cancer

Takahide Arimoto

Abstract

Abdominal radical hysterectomy is the standard surgery for stage IB–IIB cervical cancer in the world. In locally advanced cervical cancer, there is no significant difference in survival rates between surgery and chemoradiotherapy, and there is no clear evidence for treatment strategies based on histological type, but surgery may be a viable option for less radiosensitive adenocarcinomas and special histological types of cancer (gastric-type mucinous and small cell neuroendocrine cancers) under the care of a physician sufficiently skilled in surgical techniques. Recently, the usefulness of nerve-sparing techniques has also been reported. The standard treatment for stage IVA cervical cancer is concurrent chemoradiotherapy, although pelvic exenteration can be chosen in cases where the tumor does not reach the pelvic wall and para-aortic lymph nodes are negative for cancer. On the other hand, less-invasive surgery can be considered for stage IB1 cervical cancer. In 2023, the efficacy and safety of modified radical hysterectomy for stage IB1 cervical cancer has been reported from the Japan Clinical Oncology Group (JCOG).

Keywords
Radical hysterectomy · Nerve-sparing · Radiosensitive · Gastric-type mucinous carcinoma · Pelvic exenteration · Less-invasive surgery

T. Arimoto (✉)
Department of Obstetrics and Gynecology, Toranomon Hospital, Tokyo, Japan
e-mail: arimoto@toranomon.gr.jp

D. Aoki (ed.), *Recent Topics on Prevention, Diagnosis, and Clinical Management of Cervical Cancer*, Comprehensive Gynecology and Obstetrics,
https://doi.org/10.1007/978-981-99-9396-3_8

8.1 Surgical Treatment for T1b-2b Cervical Cancer

The standard surgery for locally advanced cervical cancer (T1b-2b) is a radical hysterectomy (Piver-Rutluge-Smith Class III hysterectomy, Querleu and Morrow type C1 hysterectomy). To control lateral extension from the uterine parametrium to the pelvic wall and regional lymph node metastasis is necessary to ensure curability.

In Japan, radical hysterectomy using the Okabayashi technique, which is considered to have excellent curative properties, has been widely used as a surgical treatment. Advantages of surgical treatment include the assessment of the risk of recurrence based on histopathological findings and the possibility of individualizing subsequent treatment. On the other hand, radical hysterectomy often results in autonomic nerve damage in the pelvic region, which impairs urinary, bowel, and sexual function and reduces post-operative quality of life. In recent years, the effectiveness of pelvic nerve-sparing techniques has been reported not only in stages IB1 and IB2, but also in stages IB3 and IIA2 [1, 2]. The procedure for nerve-sparing radical hysterectomy is given in Table 8.1 [3, 4].

The only interventional study comparing surgery and radiotherapy for stage IB and IIA (FIGO 2008) is the Landoni randomized controlled trial [5]. In that study, there was no significant difference in overall survival with a hazard ratio (HR) of 0.8 (95% CI: 0.5–1.2) for radiotherapy compared to surgery. Five-year survival and 5-year disease-free survival in subgroup analyses with a maximum tumor diameter greater than 4 cm were similar for surgery and radiation (70% vs. 72% and 63% vs. 57%, respectively). On the other hand, a subgroup analysis restricted to adenocarcinoma showed that both survival and disease-free survival were significantly better in the surgery group. However, concurrent chemoradiation (CCRT) was not included

Table 8.1 Procedures of nerve-sparing radical hysterectomy

1. Opening abdomen
2. Ligation and cutting of the round and infundibulopelvic ligaments, followed by incision of broad ligaments
3. Exploration of paravesical space
4. Pelvic lymphadenectomy
5. Exploration of pararectal space (Latzko's space)
6. Treatment of uterine artery
7. Identification of hypogastric nerve
8. Treatment of cardinal ligament
9. Exploration of pararectal space (Okabayashi)
10. Treatment of rectovaginal ligament
11. Mobilization of bladder
12. Treatment of anterior leaf of vesicouterine ligament
13. Lateral mobilization of ureter
14. Isolation and treatment of uterine branch of the inferior hypogastric plexus
15. Treatment of posterior leaf of vesicouterine ligament
16. Treatment of paracolpium
17. Amputation of vagina
18. Closing vaginal vault
19. Closing abdomen

in radiotherapy in this study. There were also significantly more complications with therapeutic intervention in the surgery group.

There have been three observational studies looking at prognosis from a retrospective perspective, all of which analyzed data from the Surveillance, Epidemiology, and End Results (SEER) in the USA. In a study of stage IB, IIA tumors (FIGO2008) > 4 cm in diameter enrolled between 1988–1995, the risk ratio of mortality for radiotherapy to surgery was 1.26 (95%CI: 0.72–2.22), not significantly different [6]. A study of patients registered as stage IB2 (FIGO2008) and node-negative between 2000–2006 found that both overall and disease-specific survival were significantly better in the surgery group ($P < 0.0001$, $P = 0.002$ respectively) [7]. A study examining overall survival in stage IB and stage IIA (FIGO 2008) patients enrolled between 2004 and 2013 and matched by propensity score showed no significant difference in the hazard ratio of radiotherapy compared with surgery at 0.96 (95% CI: 0.76–1.22) [8].

No clear evidence has been presented to support treatment strategies based on histology. A retrospective review of seven RCTs (stage IB-IVA: 1671 cases) of CCRT for cervical cancer conducted by the Gynecologic Oncology Group (GOG) showed that in the radiation alone group, adenocarcinoma had a shorter overall survival than squamous cell carcinoma, whereas in CCRT there was no clear difference in treatment outcome according to histological type [9]. However, multidisciplinary treatment with surgery and chemotherapy may be an option under certain conditions for non-squamous carcinoma of the cervix, which is less radiosensitive. In Japan, a retrospective study of 5964 cases of radical hysterectomy at stage IBI-IIB (FIGO 2008) (JGOG1072s) reported significantly better disease-free survival and control of local recurrence in centers with more experienced operation than in other centers, showing an association between curative surgical treatment and inter-center differences [10]. In Japan, surgery is the treatment of choice for stage IB-II less radiosensitive non-squamous cell carcinoma (including adenocarcinoma) of the cervix [11].

In recent, two RCTs have been reported comparing neo-adjuvant chemotherapy (NAC) followed by radical hysterectomy with CCRT in stage IB3-IIB (FIGO 2018) cervical cancer [12, 13]. Both trials showed no significant difference in overall survival between the two groups, but CCRT was significantly better than NAC plus radical hysterectomy in terms of disease-free survival. In a subgroup analysis by clinical stage, NAC plus radical hysterectomy for stage IIB had a poor outcome compared with CCRT with HR 1.90 (95% CI 1.25–2.89). Therefore, in principle, NAC is not recommended as a treatment strategy for locally advanced cervical cancer. For stage IIB cervical cancer, the NCCN guidelines recommend CCRT rather than surgery [14]. However, in the above-mentioned retrospective study [10], disease-free survival and control of local recurrence were significantly better in high-volume centers, as was the case in other stages in the subgroup analysis at stage IIB. Considering patient characteristics and histology, radical hysterectomy for stage IIB is recommended to be performed by a physician who is well-trained in the surgical technique.

8.2 Surgical Treatment for Special Histological Types (Gastric-Type Mucinous Adenocarcinoma and Small Cell Neuroendocrine Carcinoma)

Gastric-type mucinous carcinomas are reported to have a poor prognosis, account for 20–25% of cervical adenocarcinomas and are often HPV negative [15–17]. A retrospective study with the largest number of cases has been reported from Japan [18]. Ninety-five gastric-type mucinous carcinomas out of 328 stage I, II (FIGO2008) cervical adenocarcinomas were investigated by the Gynecologic Cancer Study Group of the Japan Clinical Oncology Group (JCOG-GCSG). In the study, gastric-type mucinous carcinomas were significantly larger in tumor diameter than usual type adenocarcinomas of the endocervix and were more often associated with deep stromal invasion, vascular invasion, parametrial invasion and ovarian metastasis, positive ascites cytology, and pelvic lymph node metastasis. The response rate to radiotherapy for recurrent foci of gastric-type mucinous carcinoma was 50% compared with 82% for usual type endocervical adenocarcinoma. The median progression-free survival for gastric-type mucinous carcinoma was 42 months and 63 months for usual type endocervical adenocarcinoma, with shorter progression-free survival and overall survival and a poorer prognosis, especially in pT1a-pT1b1 (FIGO 2008) cases. In addition, a multicenter phase II trial of docetaxel and carboplatin as NAC prior to radical hysterectomy for adenocarcinoma including gastric-type mucinous carcinoma at stage IB2-IIB (FIGO 2008) has been reported [19]. The response rate to the chemotherapy in this trial was lower for gastric-type mucinous carcinoma (46%) compared with 85% for usual type endocervical adenocarcinoma, with a 5-year progression-free survival rate of 39% vs. 75% ($P = 0.011$) and overall survival rate of 37% vs. 90% ($P < 0.001$), indicating a significantly worse prognosis for gastric-type mucinous carcinoma. It is considered that radiation and chemotherapy are less effective for gastric-type mucinous carcinoma and surgical removal is necessary.

Small cell neuroendocrine carcinoma (SCNEC) of the cervix is a rare tumor and there is no established treatment. A recent systematic review and meta-analysis of SCNEC of the cervix has been reported that radical surgery combined with NAC or adjuvant chemotherapy was performed most frequently [20]. The NCCN guidelines also recommend radical hysterectomy followed by adjuvant chemotherapy for cases with tumor diameters of 4 cm or less SCNEC. For cases with tumors larger than 4 cm in diameter, hysterectomy after CCRT or NAC with cisplatin and etoposide (PE) therapy has been considered [14]. The prognosis for SCNEC of the cervix is extremely poor, with progression-free survival averaging 16 months and 2- and 5-year survival rates reported to be 50% and 34%, respectively [20]. Therefore, some reports suggest 5–6 cycles of PE therapy after radical hysterectomy, even for early-stage IA cases [21].

In the NCCN Guidelines, radical trachelectomy for gastric-type mucinous carcinoma and small cell neuroendocrine carcinoma is not acceptable due to lack of safety evidence.

8.3 Pelvic Exenteration for Stage IVA Cervical Cancer

The standard treatment for stage IVA cervical cancer is concurrent chemoradiotherapy, although several retrospective studies have reported pelvic exenteration as initial treatment [22–26]. Among stage IVA cervical cancer, pelvic exenteration is indicated in cases where the tumor does not reach the pelvic wall, with reported 5-year overall survival rates as good as 40–53%. However, the prognosis is poor in cases with para-aortic lymph node metastases. In cases of suspicion of para-aortic lymph node metastases preoperatively, the indication for surgery must be carefully determined. For pelvic lymph node metastases, some reports indicate a poor prognosis [24, 25], while others report that they are controllable and do not affect prognosis [27]. Severe post-operative complications of pelvic exenteration, such as rectovaginal fistula, sepsis, intestinal anastomotic leakage, urinary tract infection, bowel obstruction and unknown fever are frequent and require strict post-operative management. A literature review has been reported that double barrel wet colostomy (one stoma) was associated with shorter hospitalization and reduced 30-day morbidity compared with traditional ileal conduit with colostomy (two stomas) as a method of reconstruction for pelvic exenteration [28].

8.4 Less-Invasive Surgery for Stage IB1 Cervical Cancer

In Japan, a multi-institutional non-randomized single-arm confirmatory phase III trial (JCOG1101) was conducted by the Gynecologic Cancer Study Group of the Japan Clinical Oncology Group (JCOG-GCSG) to evaluate the efficacy and safety of modified radical hysterectomy (MRH) in patients with tumor diameter $\leq$ 2 cm FIGO Stage IB1 (FIGO2008) uterine cervical cancer [29]. The results of JCOG1101 trial reported at ASCO2023 are described here [30]. Stage IB1 cervical cancer is generally not considered locally advanced, although JCOG1101 trial includes some cases of locally advanced lymph node metastases (Stage IIIC1, FIGO2018).

The standard surgery for Stage IB1 cervical cancer is radical hysterectomy. The frequency of pathological parametrial invasion and lymph node metastasis is reportedly very low and relapse-free survival is good enough, especially when the tumor diameter is 2 cm or less [31–33]. However, radical hysterectomy causes loss of desire to void because of damage to the pelvic splanchnic nerve due to surgery [34]. Self-catheterization is required in some patients for the rest of their life, which often impairs quality of life, especially for young women. Persistent urination disorder can secondarily cause chronic urinary tract infection and renal failure. Because of such disadvantages for patients, a less-invasive surgery that does not impair the prognosis should be established.

Modified radical hysterectomy (MRH) has been a standard treatment for minimally invasive cancer of the uterine cervix. Compared with radical hysterectomy, pelvic splanchnic nerves can be preserved in MRH and it can prevent urination disorder. MRH can reduce the number of days until self-urination from catheter removal and the number of days until residual urine disappearance compared with radical hysterectomy [35, 36]. It has been reported that MRH shortened mean time to voiding and reduced post-operative voiding difficulty [37]. However, the prognosis of Stage IB1 cervical cancer treated with MRH has yet to be well examined.

Prior to the JCOG1101 trial, from 2008 to 2009, JCOG-GCSG performed an observational study (JCOG0806-A) of surgical procedures and pathological findings for Stage IB1 cervical cancer [38]. Five-year overall survival was 95.8% and the proportion of pathological parametrial involvement was 1.9% in patients with tumor diameter ≤ 2 cm Stage IB1 cervical cancer treated by radical hysterectomy. On the other hand, 5-year overall survival was 97.0% in 31 patients with tumor diameter ≤ 2 cm Stage IB1 cervical cancer treated by MRH. From the results of the study, MRH is considered to be a promising treatment, even in terms of the efficacy, but this should be confirmed in a prospective study.

From January 2013 to August 2017, 240 patients were enrolled in JCOG1101 trial from 40 institutions in Japan. The study design is shown in Fig. 8.1. Eligibility criteria included: (1) FIGO 2008 Stage IB1 cervical cancer; (2) histologically proven squamous cell carcinoma, adenocarcinoma (mucinous or endometrioid) or adenosquamous carcinoma; (3) tumor diameter ≤ 2 cm (measured by MRI or conization specimen); (4) neither distant LN metastasis nor distant metastasis in CT; (5) ECOG PS 0–1; (6) 20–70 years old; and (7) no prior surgery for uterine cervical cancer (except for conization), no prior surgery for lower abdominal or pelvic malignancy, no prior radiation therapy or chemotherapy. In case that the cancer could be microinvasive, conization was required to exclude Stage IA cases. The protocol surgery involved cutting the anterior layer of the vesicouterine ligament of the uterus and dissecting regional lymph nodes. Only laparotomy was permitted: laparoscopy and robotic surgery were not allowed. Post-operative irradiation was administered in cases where pelvic LN or parametrial invasion was positive, depth in the cervical wall invasion was ≥2/3, or surgical margin was <1 cm by pathological findings. The primary endpoint was 5-year overall survival. The secondary endpoints were relapse-free survival, local relapse-free survival, % completion of MRH, % local relapse, % pathological parametrial involvement, days until self-urination and residual urine disappearance, blood loss, operation time, %

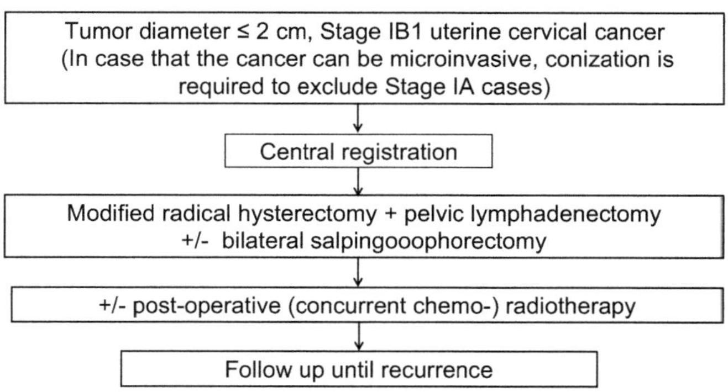

Fig. 8.1 Study design of JCOG1101

post-operative radiotherapy, adverse events (CTCAE ver.4.0), serious adverse events. They set the expected 5-year overall survival of MRH at 95.8% (5-year overall survival of radical hysterectomy in JCOG0806-A) and the threshold 5-year overall survival at 90.8%.

Among 225 eligible patients, 193 (85.8%) were pT1b1 (UICC 7th), and 184 (81.8%) had pathological maximal tumor diameter ≤ 2 cm. Parametrial involvement, lymph node metastasis, ≥ 2/3 stromal invasion and < 1 cm surgical margin were observed in 3 (1.3%), 16 (7.1%), 30 (13.3%) and 11 (4.9%) patients, respectively. Thirty-nine patients (17.3%) underwent adjuvant radiation or chemoradiation. Median follow-up was 77.7 months. Five patients (2.2%) died, and 5-year overall survival was 98.2% (90% CI: 96.0–99.2, > 90.8%). Thirteen patients (5.8%) relapsed (eight local recurrence and five distant recurrence), and 5-year relapse-free survival was 94.7% (95% CI: 90.8–96.9%). Self-urination was observed in all patients, and residual urine disappearance up to 56 days after urethral catheter removal was observed in 213 patients (94.7%). Median time to disappearance of residual urine after urethral catheter removal was 1 day. There was no treatment-related death. Grade 3/4 non-hematological adverse events were observed in 17 patients (7.6%), including eight infection and four hemorrhage.

In conclusion, MRH was as effective as radical hysterectomy and less invasive. MRH can be considered a standard surgery for tumor diameter ≤ 2 cm Stage IB1 uterine cervical cancer.

References

1. Long Y, et al. Clinical efficacy and safety of nerve-sparing radical hysterectomy for cervical cancer: a systematic review and meta-analysis. PLoS One. 2014;9:e94116.
2. Roh JW, et al. Efficacy and oncologic safety of nerve-sparing radical hysterectomy for cervical cancer: a randomized controlled trial. J Gynecol Oncol. 2015;26:90–9.
3. Fujii S, et al. Anatomic identification and functional outcomes of the nerve sparing Okabayashi radical hysterectomy. Gynecol Oncol. 2007;107:4–13.
4. Konishi I. The Okabayashi radical hysterectomy: basic principle and step-by-step procedure. Surg J (N Y). 2021;7(Suppl 2):S57–69.
5. Landoni F, et al. Randomised study of radical surgery versus radiotherapy for stage IB-IIA cervical cancer. Lancet. 1997;350:535–40.
6. Brewster WR, et al. Intent-to-treat analysis of stage Ib and IIa cervical cancer in the United States: radiotherapy or surgery 1988-1995. Obstet Gynecol. 2001;97:248–54.
7. Rungruang B, et al. Surgery versus radiation therapy for stage IB2 cervical carcinoma: a population-based analysis. Int J Gynecol Cancer. 2012;22:484–9.
8. Ross Green W, et al. Revisiting milan cervical cancer study: do the original findings hold in the era of chemotherapy? Gynecol Oncol. 2017;144:299–304.
9. Rose PG, et al. Locally advanced adenocarcinoma and adenosquamous carcinomas or the cervix compared to squamous cell carcinomas of the cervix in gynecologic oncology group trials of cisplatin-based chemoradiation. Gynecol Oncol. 2014;135:208–12.
10. Matsuo K, et al. Association of radical hysterectomy surgical volume and survival for early-stage cervical cancer. Obstet Gynecol. 2019;133:1086–98.
11. Japan Society of Gynecologic Oncology. Guidelines for treatment of uterine cervical cancer: Japan Society of Gynecologic Oncology (JSGO) 2022 edition.

12. Gupta S, et al. Neoadjuvant chemotherapy followed by radical surgery versus concomitant chemotherapy and radiotherapy in patients with stage IB2, IIA, or IIB squamous cervical cancer: a randomized controlled trial. J Clin Oncol. 2018;36:1548–55.
13. Kenter G, et al. Results from neoadjuvant chemotherapy followed by surgery compared to chemoradiation for stage Ib2-IIb cervical cancer, EORTC55994. J Clin Oncol. 2019;37:5503.
14. Cervical Cancer Guideline (Version 1, 2021). NCCN clinical practice guidelines in oncology.
15. International Agency for Research on Cancer. WHO classification of tumors of female reproductive organs. 5th ed. Lyon: IARC Press; 2019.
16. Mikami Y, et al. Gastrointestinal immunophenotype in adenocarcinomas of the uterine cervix and related glandular lesions: a possible link between lobular endocervical glandular hyperplasia/ pyloric gland metaplasia and 'Adenoma malignum'. Mod Pathol. 2004;17:962–72.
17. Kojima A, et al. Gastric morphology and immunophenotype predict poor outcome in mucinous adenocarcinoma of the uterine cervix. Am J Surg Pathol. 2007;31:664–72.
18. Nishio S, et al. Analysis of gastric-type mucinous carcinoma of the uterine cervix- an aggressive tumor with a poor prognosis: a multi-institutional study. Gynecol Oncol. 2019;153:13–9.
19. Kojima A, et al. Chemoresistance of gastric-type mucinous carcinoma of the uterine cervix: a study of the Sankai gynecology study group. Int J Gynecol Cancer. 2018;28:99–106.
20. Temper CB, et al. Neuroendocrine carcinoma of the cervix: a systematic review of the literature. BMC Cancer. 2018;18:530–46.
21. Gadducci A, et al. Neuroendocrine tumors of the uterine cervix: a therapeutic challenge for gynecologic oncologists. Gynecol Oncol. 2017;144:637–46.
22. Tanaka S, et al. Clinical outcome of pelvic exenteration in patients with advanced or recurrent uterine cervical cancer. Int J Clin Oncol. 2014;19:133–8.
23. Marnitz, et al. Indications for primary and secondary exenterations in patients with cervical cancer. Gynecol Oncol. 2006;103:1023–30.
24. Forner DM, et al. Exenteration as a primary treatment for locally advanced cervical cancer: long-term results and prognostic factors. Am J Obstet Gynecol. 2011;205(148):e1–6.
25. Chiantera V, et al. Survival after curative pelvic exenteration for primary or recurrent cervical cancer: a retrospective multicentric study of 167 patients. Int J Gynecol Cancer. 2014;24:916–22.
26. Ungar L, et al. Primary pelvic exenteration in cervical cancer patients. Gynecol Oncol. 2008;111(2 Suppl):S9–12.
27. Schmidt AM, et al. Indications and long-term clinical outcomes in 282 patients with pelvic exenteration for advanced or recurrent cervical cancer. Gynecol Oncol. 2012;125:604–9.
28. Jason G, et al. Literature review: double-Barrelled wet colostomy (one stoma) versus Ileal conduit with colostomy (two stomas). Urol Int. 2017;98:249–54.
29. Kunieda F, et al. Non-randomized confirmatory trial of modified radical hysterectomy for patients with tumor diameter 2 cm or less FIGO stage IB1 uterine cervical cancer: Japan Clinical Oncology Group Study (JCOG1101). Jpn J Clin Oncol. 2015;45:123–6.
30. Arimoto T et al. A confirmatory trial of modified radical hysterectomy for FIGO Stage IB1 cervical cancer patients with tumor diameter preoperatively estimated 2 cm or less: Japan Clinical Oncology Group Study, JCOG1101. ASCO2023.
31. Sartori E, et al. Extended radical hysterectomy in early-stage carcinoma of the uterine cervix: tailoring the radicality. Int J Gynecol Cancer. 1995;5:143–7.
32. Kinney WK, et al. Identification of a low-risk subset of patients with stage IB invasive squamous cancer of the cervix possibly suited to less radical surgical treatment. Gynecol Oncol. 1995;57:3–6.
33. Kristensen GB, et al. Tumor size, depth of invasion, and grading of the invasive tumor front are the main prognostic factors in early squamous cell cervical carcinoma. Gynecol Oncol. 1999;74:245–51.
34. Noda K, et al. Keeping of vesical and rectal functions after radical operation of uterine cervical cancer. Acta Obstet Gynaecol Jpn. 1972;24:99–106.
35. Matuzawa M. Urination disorder and function preserving surgery in gynecology. In: Kotsuban Geka. Tokyo: Ishiyaku Publishers; 1982; (in Japanese).

36. Yamabe T. Hysterectomy for primary uterine cervical cancer (modified radical hysterectomy—provisional title). Sanfujinka Chiryou. 1974;28:599–606; (in Japanese).
37. Yang YC, et al. Modified radical hysterectomy for early Ib cervical cancer. Gynecol Oncol. 1999;74:241–4.
38. Kato T, et al. Clinical tumor diameter and prognosis of patients with FIGO stage IB1 cervical cancer (JCOG0806-A). Gynecol Oncol. 2015;137:34–9.

Minimally Invasive Surgery for Cervical Cancer

9

Hiroshi Nishio

Abstract

Surgery is the standard treatment for early stage cervical cancer. Over the last few decades, growing evidence has supported the adoption of minimally invasive radical hysterectomy for the treatment of patients with surgical indications. Retrospective data suggested that minimally invasive surgery (MIS) improved perioperative outcomes without affecting oncologic outcomes until the unexpected results of the phase III randomized Laparoscopic Approach to Cervical Cancer (LACC) trial revealed that, compared with the open abdominal approach, MIS correlated with worse disease-free and cancer-specific survival. Other retrospective studies corroborated this result. In this chapter, we assess the current status and unresolved issues around MIS in patients with early stage cervical cancer. We conclude that minimally invasive surgery should be offered in the context of clinical trials with detailed informed consent, and that ongoing trials with well-designed protocols may improve the status of early stage cervical cancer treatment.

Keyword

Radical hysterectomy · Minimally invasive surgery · LACC trial

H. Nishio (✉)
Department of Obstetrics and Gynecology, Keio University School of Medicine, Tokyo, Japan
e-mail: nishio@z3.keio.jp

D. Aoki (ed.), *Recent Topics on Prevention, Diagnosis, and Clinical Management of Cervical Cancer*, Comprehensive Gynecology and Obstetrics,
https://doi.org/10.1007/978-981-99-9396-3_9

9.1 Introduction

Surgery is the primary treatment for early stage cervical cancer [1, 2]. Radical hysterectomy allows complete tumor removal and the identification of risk factors for adjuvant treatments [3]. During the past decades, there has been robust evidence of the safety and effectiveness of radical hysterectomy plus pelvic lymphadenectomy in early stage cervical cancer, initially using an open or vaginal approach, and recently using minimally invasive surgery (MIS) by either laparoscopic or robotic surgery [4–6]. The International Federation of Gynecology and Obstetrics (FIGO) recommended the utilization of radical hysterectomy, and the National Comprehensive Cancer Network (NCCN) in 2017 and European Society of Gynecology Oncology (ESGO) in 2018 recommended the application of radical hysterectomy via open or MIS [7]. Retrospective evidence has supported the safety and usefulness of minimally invasive radical hysterectomy [8–10] and has validated that the disease-free and overall survival of MIS are comparable to those of the open approach. A retrospective propensity score-matched analysis conducted by Ditto et al. with 60 cervical cancer patients who underwent type B radical hysterectomy with either open surgery or MIS showed comparable survival outcomes in terms of 5-year disease-free survival between these groups [11]. They selected 157 consecutive women with FIGO 2009 stage IA2 and IB1 < 2 cm cervical cancer. Patients undergoing laparoscopic surgery experienced a longer operative time than those undergoing abdominal surgery. MIS did not influence the site of recurrence or survival outcomes in terms of 5-year disease-free survival and overall survival. Another meta-analysis conducted by Wang et al. evaluated 12 studies comparing laparoscopic radical hysterectomy (754 patients) with open radical hysterectomy (785 patients). Their findings revealed no significant differences in the 5-year overall survival rate (hazard ratio [HR] 0.91; 95% confidence interval [CI], 0.48–1.71) or 5-year rate of disease-free survival (HR 0.97; 95% CI, 0.56–1.68) [10]. However, because we still have not been convinced by the prospective phase III setting, the Laparoscopic Approach to Cervical Cancer (LACC) trial was conducted to verify the effectiveness of minimally invasive radical hysterectomy compared with the open approach for cervical cancer of stage IA1 (with lymphovascular invasion), IA2, and IB1 and for the histological subtypes squamous cell carcinoma, adenocarcinoma, and adenosquamous carcinoma in a prospective randomized trial [12]. The results of this phase III multicenter randomized trial results regarding the oncological outcomes of open surgery compared to those of MIS showed that the prognosis following MIS (laparoscopic or robot-assisted radical hysterectomy) for early stage cervical cancer was not comparable to that of open surgery, and included increased risks of recurrence and death. The aim of this review is to assess the current evidence and unresolved issues around the use of MIS in patients with early stage cervical cancer.

9.2 The Laparoscopic Approach to Cervical Cancer (LACC) Trial

Until the unprecedented results of the LACC trial published by Ramirez et al. in 2018 [12], minimally invasive radical hysterectomy was the recommended approach for treating patients with early stage cervical cancer [11]. The LACC trial is the only open-label, randomized trial to compare the oncologic outcomes between open abdominal hysterectomy and minimally invasive radical hysterectomy. Owing to the prospective, randomized study design, each group contained a homogenous population. Among the patients with MIS, 84.4% and 15.6% underwent laparoscopic and robot-assisted surgery, respectively. Most patients had stage IB1 disease (91.9%), and the protocol included either type II or III radical hysterectomy. Surprisingly, the study was discontinued early by the data and safety monitoring committee following evaluation of 631 of the planned 740 patients owing to an imbalance in deaths between these two groups. The authors reported that patients who underwent MIS had worse 4.5-year survival outcomes than those who underwent open radical hysterectomy. In particular, the rate of disease-free survival was 86% after MIS and 96.5% after the open approach. The risks of recurrence, locoregional recurrence, and all-cause mortality were 3.74-, 4.26- and 6.00-times higher, respectively, with MIS than with open surgery. These differences remained even after adjusting for age, body mass index, disease stage, lymphovascular invasion, and lymph node involvement.

The results of the LACC trial dramatically shifted the surgical approach toward cervical cancer [13, 14]. Following this evidence, several multi-institutional observational studies designed based on the results of the LACC trial have confirmed inferior treatment or survival outcomes in patients with MIS. In the same issue of the NEJM that published the LACC trial result, Melamed et al. reported a nationwide observational study in the USA that demonstrated inferior surgical outcomes among patients with stage IA2 or IB1 cervical cancer treated with MIS compared to those patients who underwent open surgery [15]. In their report, the authors performed two different analyses using data from the Commission on Cancer-accredited Hospitals in the USA (2010–2013) and from the Surveillance, Epidemiology, and End Results (SEER) program database (2000–2010). The primary analysis included 2461 cervical cancer patients with who underwent 1225 MIS procedures. Patients who underwent MIS were more likely to have smaller, lower-grade tumors. The authors adopted inverse probability weighting analysis to correct for confounding factors. As a result, the 4-year mortality was 9.1% and 5.3% for patients having MIS and open radical hysterectomy respectively (HR 1.65; 95% CI 1.22–2.22). In the second analysis, the authors observed that MIS adoption coincided with a decrease in the survival rate of 0.8% per year. In contrast, the 4-year relative survival rate among women who underwent radical hysterectomy for cervical cancer remained stable before the adoption of MIS during 2000–2006 period. They concluded that MIS was associated with a higher risk of death than was open surgery among women who underwent radical hysterectomy for early stage cervical cancer, irrespective of the approach (laparoscopic or robotic), tumor size, or histological type.

A meta-analysis conducted by Nitecki et al. involving 9499 patients and including 15 studies was consistent with the LACC trial result in that the pooled HR was 71% higher for patients with MIS compared with the open approach (HR 1.71; 95% CI, 1.36–2.15) [16]. Among the MIS patients, 49% ($n = 4684$) received MIS, and of those patients, 57% ($n = 2675$) received robot-assisted laparoscopy with low to moderate heterogeneity. They found no association between the prevalence of robot-assisted surgery and the magnitude of the association between MIS and the risk of recurrence, death, or all-cause mortality. A European cohort study (SUCCOR, the Surgery in Cervical Cancer, Observational, Retrospective study) reviewed 1272 patients with FIGO 2009 stage IB1 during 2013 and 2014 to determine disease-free survival after radical hysterectomy for the two modalities. They investigated the risk of relapse for the two approaches with a particular focus on surgical maneuvers, namely, the use of a uterine manipulator and protective closure of the colpotomy over the tumor. They selected 1116 patients and excluded 423 patients with a previous history of cone resection and analyzed the remaining 693 patients (402 patients who underwent open surgery and 291 patients who underwent MIS) with inverse probability weighting using propensity scores. They found that the risk of recurrence for MIS treated patients was twice as high as for those receiving open surgery (HR; 2.07, 95% CI, 1.35–3.15) and that MIS was also associated with a lower rate of overall survival than was open surgery [17]. Twenty-eight patients among 291 patients died from MIS, while 21 of the 402 patients who underwent open surgery died. They confirmed those differences in the subgroup of patients with tumors greater than 2 cm (HR, 2.31, 95% CI, 0.37–3.90, $P = 0.002$) while for the group of patients with tumors smaller or equal than 2 cm, those differences were not significant (HR, 1.63, 95% CI, 0.79–3.40, $P = 0.19$). Paik et al. reviewed 738 women who underwent radical hysterectomy for FIGO stage IB-IIA cervical cancer and selected 119 patients who underwent laparoscopic radical hysterectomy and 357 patients who underwent abdominal radical hysterectomy. They demonstrated that patients treated with MIS had inferior disease-free survival compared with those who had open surgery (HR, 2.74, 95% CI 1.3–5.7), with a significant difference in pelvic and hematogenous recurrence [18]. A population-based cancer registry study from Canada found a statistically significant interaction between tumor stage and MIS; increased risk of recurrence and death may be limited to patients with macroscopic disease [19], but they concluded that open radical hysterectomy should be the recommended approach for early stage cervical cancer. Based on this evidence, the NCCN suggested that open surgery should be "the standard and recommended approach to radical hysterectomy" [20]. The Society of Gynecologic Oncology (SGO) encouraged surgeons to discuss the data from the LACC trial with patients, thus providing adequate counseling. ESGO and the European Society for Medical Oncology also modified their guidelines.

After the LACC trial, the number of laparoscopic and robot-assisted surgical procedures decreased dramatically. Lewicki reported the effects of the publication of the LACC trial results on clinical practice in the USA. They observed a decrease in the adoption of MIS from 58.0% to 42.9% ($P < 0.0001$) involving 2437 patients who received care at 283 centers between November 2015 and March 2020, especially in academic centers [13]. At academic centers, the odds ratio for MIS after publication of LACC trial was 0.27 (95% CI, 0.17–0.43, $P < 0.0001$), as compared with 0.81 (95% CI, 0.45–1.47, $P = 0.49$) at non-academic centers. They also compared the trend in the use of a minimally invasive approach for hysterectomy for uterine fibroids as a negative control. No change was observed in the percentage of patients in these populations who underwent MIS. Table 9.1 lists previous meta-analyses that evaluated open radical hysterectomy versus MIS.

However, several studies have disagreed on the implications of this paradigm shift. Some investigators have suggested that the increased adoption of open radical hysterectomy correlates with an increased risk of postoperative events [14, 21]. An analysis of the National Inpatient Sample from 2015 to 2018 suggested that after

Table 9.1 Meta-analyses of oncologic outcomes of laparoscopic or robotic-assisted radical hysterectomy

Authors	Study year	Number of studies	Stage (FIGO 2008)	Control (n)	Experimental (n)	HR(95% CI)	Result
Cao et al.	2007–2014	22	IA1-IIB	ARH ($n = 1692$)	LRH ($n = 1230$)	1.01 (0.90–1.11)	DFS and OS showed no difference between two arms
Wang et al.	2007–2014	12	IA1-IIA2	ARH ($n = 785$)	LRH ($n = 754$)	0.97 (0.56–1.68)	5-year DFS and OS showed no difference between two arms
Nitecki et al.	2012–2020	15	IA1-IIA	ARH ($n = 4815$)	LRH ($n = 2009$), RRH ($n = 2675$)	1.71 (1.76–2.15)	MIS is associated with elevated risk of recurrence and death compared with ARH
Kampers et al.	2007–2020	30	IA1-IIA	ARH ($n = 7701$)	LRH ($n = 7058$)	0.95 (0.93–0.98)	Inferiority of MIS compared with ARH Higher DFS in ARH compared with MIS
Marchand et al.	2003–2017	60	IA1-IIB	ARH ($n = 4834$)	LRH ($n = 5062$)	1.00 (0.80–1.26)	Increased DFS and OS is not seen in LRH when excluding RRH

ARH abdominal radical hysterectomy, *CI* confidence interval, *DFS* disease-free survival, *HR* hazard ratio, *LRH* laparoscopic radical hysterectomy, *MIS* minimally invasive surgery, *OS* overall survival, *RRH* robotic radical hysterectomy publication of the LACC trial, cervical cancer patients were less likely to undergo MIS (−63%) but more likely to develop perioperative complications (+23%) and have a longer length of hospital stay (3 vs. 2 days) [21]. Another intriguing report published by the Italian Gynecological Cancer Study Group observed that the adoption of MIS for cervical cancer decreased following the publication of the LACC trial from 64.9% to 30.4% ($P < 0.001$) [22]. However, the morbidity rate was not affected. Overall, 90-day complications occurred in 110 (18.9%) and 119 (16.6%) patients before and after the publication of the LACC trial, respectively ($P = 0.795$). Similarly, the number of severe complications (grade 3 or worse) did not differ between the two periods (6.5% and 5.1%, respectively). Overall and severe 90-day complications were consistent between periods, even for stages IA ($P = 0.471$), IB1 ($P = 0.929$), and IB2 ($P = 0.929$). These data highlight that the shift from MIS to the open approach does not influence the 90-day surgery-related morbidity, irrespective of disease stage.

9.3 Reasons for Worse Outcome in MIS

The exact reasons and poor prognostic factors explaining why MIS correlates with worse disease-free and overall survival while previous retrospective studies of minimally invasive radical hysterectomy showed promising results are still unknown and controversial. Ramiez et al. mentioned several issues regarding their unexpected results. One is the different clinical trial settings between their prospective, randomized trial and the previously reported retrospective studies. Most retrospective studies involved sequential comparisons rather than concurrent analyses. Other reasons for the inferior oncological outcomes in the MIS group included the routine use of a uterine manipulator, which might cause tumor cells to disseminate to both salpinges and increase the probability of tumor spillage. In addition, consideration of the effect of gas insufflation on tumor cell growth or spread is warranted [12]. Carbon dioxide is supplied during laparoscopic operations to maintain the pneumoperitoneum, which can cause implantation and proliferation of tumor cells exposed to the peritoneal cavity. Although the LACC trial was not sufficiently powered to enable analysis based on the stage of cervical cancer, the authors observed that the surgical approach influenced the risk of recurrence in patients with tumors larger than 2 cm [12].

Some experts have mentioned possible reasons for the inferiority of MIS compared to the abdominal approach, including (1) lack of radicality, (2) cancer spillage during surgery, and (3) the surgeon's learning curve [23]. In terms of radicality, the rate of tumor-free surgical margin status was comparable between the MIS and open surgery groups in the LACC trial [12]; however, closed surgical margins may have been more common in the MIS group, which could impact oncologic outcome [24]. One thing we need to be aware of is that the subgroup analysis of this trial showed a detrimental effect on patients with a tumor size >2 cm. Open surgery may allow for greater anterior traction of the uterus, thereby facilitating greater resection of the uterosacral ligaments and parametria, especially in patients with larger tumors.

While this association was not demonstrated in patients with tumors <2 cm, the level of radicality did not influence the outcomes of patients with tumors <2 cm. In those patient population with tumor size <2 cm, in the prospective, single arm, multicenter study ConCerv trial patients with grade 1 and 2 cervical cancer with tumor <2 cm, stromal invasion <10 mm, and no lymphovascular space involvement were offered to have conserve surgery and/or simple hysterectomy with lymphadenectomy [25]. They reported three cases of recurrent disease within 2 years of surgery and a cumulative incidence of 3.5% (95% CI, 0.9–9.0%). Most patients included in the LACC trial had stage IB1 disease, whereas only 51 had stage IA disease. In a previously reported population-based study, the authors evaluated the impact of surgical approach on patients with cervical cancer (stage IA ($n = 244$), IB ($n = 543$), II ($n = 124$), and unknown ($n = 56$)). In this study, the surgical approach did not affect the survival outcomes of patients with stage IA disease. However, we need to consider that a larger size fulfills the statistical number to show any difference learned by the LACC trial. Therefore, even in the setting of stage IA cervical cancer, we be adopted with caution by counseling patients about the available evidence.

Regarding the second issue of cancer spillage, whether the use of manipulators contributed to an increased recurrence rate has been debated [25]. In addition to the use of manipulators, several possibilities should be considered. One is that tumor cells can be exposed to the peritoneal cavity when the cervix is exposed during intracorporeal colpotomy and tumor cells exposed to the peritoneal cavity can travel upwards when the patient's position is maintained in the Trendelenburg position during minimally invasive operations, leading to distant metastasis. One study with 2661 early stage endometrial cancer retrospectively assessed the oncologic outcomes of uterine manipulator use. The study population consisted of 1756 patients who underwent hysterectomy with a uterine manipulator and 905 who did not. Each group was balanced with respect to histology, tumor grade, myometrial invasion, FIGO stage, and adjuvant therapy. The recurrence rates were 11.69% and 7.4% in the uterine manipulator group and group without manipulator, respectively ($P < 0.001$). The use of a manipulator was associated with a higher risk of recurrence (HR, 2.31; 95% CI 1.27–4.20). A European cohort observational study comparing MIS with open radical hysterectomy in patients with stage IB1 cervical cancer (SUCCOR) suggested that patients undergoing minimally invasive radical hysterectomy experienced a 2–2.4-fold increase in the risk of recurrence and death and demonstrated a negative impact of uterine manipulators on disease-free survival. Disease-free survival at 4.5 years was 73% in the manipulator group and 83% in the non-manipulator group ($P = 0.0001$). However, avoiding the uterine manipulator and using maneuvers to avoid tumor spread during colpotomy in MIS were associated with outcomes similar to open surgery [17]. They found that the disease-free survival at 4.5 years was 93% with protective vaginal closure and 74% without it ($P < 0.001$). Those who underwent MIS with vaginal closure had similar rates of relapse to those who underwent open surgery (HR 0.63, 95% CI, 0.91–4.27). These differences remained in patients with tumors >2 cm (HR 2.99, 95% CI, 1.59–5.15), but were not found in those with tumor <2 cm (HR, 1.96, 95% CI 0.91–4.27). Li et al. reported conflicting systematic reviews and meta-analyses on manipulator use during minimally invasive radical hysterectomies. They selected six observational studies involving 2150 women treated with MIS without a manipulator or open surgery. The MIS group without manipulator usage had a significantly higher risk of cancer relapse comparing with open surgery group (HR 1.55; 95% CI 1.15–2.10) [26]. An ongoing trial evaluating MIS for early stage cervical cancer, which prohibits the use of manipulators, could address these issues.

The pattern of recurrence is another proof of possible tumor dissemination at the time of colpotomy. Kong et al. assessed whether colpotomy (intracorporeal vs. vaginal) influenced the oncological outcomes of MIS (laparoscopic or robot-assisted) in 128 patients with cervical cancer FIGO stages IB to IIA, indicating that intracorporeal colpotomy provided poorer oncological outcomes than vaginal colpotomy [27]. In addition to those evidence, growing evidence showed that tumor removal with preoperative conization is associated with similar outcomes to open surgery, indicating removing the primary tumor before surgery avoids any source of spillover [28]. Another study suggested that patients undergoing laparoscopy-associated vaginal hysterectomy experienced similar outcomes to those undergoing open surgery by avoiding contact between the cervical tumor the peritoneal cavity [29]. In several ongoing trials verifying MIS for cervical cancer, protective maneuvers are required for registration.

Regarding open surgery for cervical cancer, it has been reported that institutions that are highly experienced in surgery have better oncologic outcomes than those with little experience [30]. However, the LACC trial did not find any differences in complication rates between MIS and open surgery. However, it is difficult to assess a surgeon's experience and skills in all patients. Recurrent cases were limited to only fourteen of the 31 centers enrolled in this trial, suggesting that the quality of surgery may have differed among the centers. Cancer control after radical prostatectomy appears to be sensitive to surgeon's experience [31], and several studies have demonstrated that the learning curve in minimally invasive radical hysterectomy might be associated with cervical cancer recurrence, requiring more surgical cases than open surgery to achieve acceptable oncologic outcomes [16, 32–34]. Li et al. retrospectively selected 282 patients with cervical cancer and reported that the number of surgeries during the learning period was 30 and 60 in the open surgery and MIS groups, respectively. All patients with tumors <2 cm had similar 5-year disease-free survival rates, regardless of the operation mode or learning curve. The MIS group had lower survival rates than the open surgery group when the tumors were > 2 cm in the skilled phase.

9.4 Ongoing Trials

Prospective randomized trials have not been completed since the LACC trial. One issue with the LACC trial was the low rate of robot-assisted radical hysterectomies. A recently published meta-analysis of 1244 studies by Marchard et al. mentioned that laparoscopic radical hysterectomy, excluding the robotic approach, had no significant difference in 5-year overall survival, and they concluded that the laparoscopic approach, excluding the robotic approach, could be comparable to the abdominal approach, with a significantly lower incidence of blood loss and postoperative complications [35]. Table 9.2 summarizes ongoing trials comparing MIS and open surgery for early stage cervical cancer. The Robot-assisted Approach to Cervical Cancer (RACC) trial focused on the role of robot-assisted surgery in stage IB1–IIA1 patients. This trial enrolled 800 patients who were randomized to undergo robot-assisted radical hysterectomy or open radical hysterectomy. The primary endpoint is progression-free survival. The Randomized Controlled Trial of Robotic Versus Open Radical Hysterectomy for Cervical Cancer (ROCC) was a multicenter, open level, randomized, noninferiority trial. The primary endpoint of this study was disease-free survival, which was aimed at 840 patients with stage IA2-IB1 (FIGO 2018). The third study, Minimally Invasive Therapy Versus Open Radical Hysterectomy (MITOR) for the management of early stage cervical cancer (stages IA1 to IIA1), aimed to compare laparoscopic and open radical hysterectomy with

Table 9.2 Ongoing trials evaluating roles of MIS in early stage cervical cancer

Study	Study design	Participants	Procedures	Stage	Protective methods
NCT03955185, RWS-01	Prospective, non-randomized	2000	LRH/RRH vs. ARH	IA1 with LVSI-IIA1 (FIGO 2018)	1. Cup-shaped uterine manipulator is prohibited; uterus hanging wire is allowed. 2. Avoid tumor cells shedding into the pelvis: (a) Cut the vagina with the transvaginal method. (b) Cut the vagina after closed loop ligation of the vagina
NCT04934982	Prospective randomized	690	LRH/RRH vs. ARH	IA1 with LVSI-IA2	Not specified
NCT04831580 ROCC	Prospective randomized	840	RRH vs. ARH	IA2-IB1 (FIGO 2018)	Vagina must be closed prior to intracorporeal colpotomy
NCT03719547 RACC	Prospective randomized	800	RRH vs. ARH	IB1-IIA1 (FIGO 2018)	Not specified
NCT04999696 MITOR	Prospective randomized	820	LRH vs. ARH	IA1 with LVSI-IIA1	Not specified
NCT04370496 SOLUTION	Prospective, single arm	124	LRH and RRH	IB1 (FIGO 2018)	Endoscopic stapler
JGOG1087	Prospective, single arm	440	LRH	IA2-IIA1(FIGO 2018)	Manipulator is prohibited. Vagina must be closed prior to intracorporeal colpotomy

ARH abdominal radical hysterectomy, *LRH* laparoscopic radical hysterectomy, *LVSI* lymphovascular space invasion, *MIS* minimally invasive surgery, *RRH* robotic radical hysterectomy

820 included patients, which is not currently recruiting. The RWS-01 trial (NCT03955185) is a multicenter, prospective, non-randomized study aimed at enrolling 2000 patients with IA1 to IIA1 (FIGO 2018) having MIS and open radical hysterectomy. Several other phase II trials including JGOG1087, a non-randomized controlled laparoscopic radical hysterectomy in Japan, aims to enroll 440 patients with stage IA2–IIA1. Another phase 2 study, SOLUTION, is a noninferiority trial evaluating the oncologic outcomes of MIS using an endoscopic stapler as a tool to prevent cancer spillage [36].

9.5 Conclusion

We reviewed the current evidence regarding use of MIS in early stage cervical cancer. The LACC trial has clearly shown that minimally invasive radical hysterectomy is associated with worse survival in patients with early stage cervical cancer. Based on this level A evidence, MIS should be offered in the context of clinical trials with detailed informed consent. Ongoing trials with well-designed protocols may improve the status of early stage cervical cancer treatment.

Acknowledgments The authors thank Ms. Keiko Abe and Ms. Hitomi Nishino for their help in revising the manuscript.

References

1. Raspagliesi F, Ditto A, Fontanelli R, Zanaboni F, Solima E, Spatti G, et al. Type II versus type III nerve-sparing radical hysterectomy: comparison of lower urinary tract dysfunctions. Gynecol Oncol. 2006;102(2):256–62. https://doi.org/10.1016/j.ygyno.2005.12.014; Epub 2006 Jan 30.
2. Ditto A, Martinelli F, Mattana F, Reato C, Solima E, Carcangiu M, et al. Class III nerve-sparing radical hysterectomy versus standard class III radical hysterectomy: an observational study. Ann Surg Oncol. 2011;18(12):3469–78. https://doi.org/10.1245/s10434-011-1767-3; Epub 2011 May 10.
3. Cohen PA, Jhingran A, Oaknin A, Denny L. Cervical cancer. Lancet. 2019;393(10167):169–82. https://doi.org/10.1016/S0140-6736(18)32470-X.
4. Nam JH, Park JY, Kim DY, Kim JH, Kim YM, Kim YT. Laparoscopic versus open radical hysterectomy in early-stage cervical cancer: long-term survival outcomes in a matched cohort study. Ann Oncol. 2012;23(4):903–11. https://doi.org/10.1093/annonc/mdr360; Epub 2011 Aug 12.
5. Bogani G, Cromi A, Uccella S, Serati M, Casarin J, Pinelli C, et al. Laparoscopic versus open abdominal management of cervical cancer: long-term results from a propensity-matched analysis. J Minim Invasive Gynecol. 2014;21(5):857–62. https://doi.org/10.1016/j.jmig.2014.03.018; Epub 2014 Mar 31.
6. Sert BM, Boggess JF, Ahmad S, Jackson AL, Stavitzski NM, Dahl AA, et al. Robot-assisted versus open radical hysterectomy: a multi-institutional experience for early-stage cervical cancer. Eur J Surg Oncol. 2016;42(4):513–22. https://doi.org/10.1016/j.ejso.2015.12.014; Epub 2016 Jan 21.
7. Cibula D, Pötter R, Planchamp F, Avall-Lundqvist E, Fischerova D, Haie Meder C, et al. The European Society of Gynaecological Oncology/European Society for Radiotherapy

and Oncology/European Society of Pathology Guidelines for the management of patients with cervical cancer. Int J Gynecol Cancer. 2018;28(4):641–55. https://doi.org/10.1097/IGC.0000000000001216.
8. Geetha P, Nair MK. Laparoscopic, robotic and open method of radical hysterectomy for cervical cancer: a systematic review. J Minim Access Surg. 2012;8(3):67–73. https://doi.org/10.4103/0972-9941.97584.
9. Cao T, Feng Y, Huang Q, Wan T, Liu J. Prognostic and safety roles in laparoscopic versus abdominal radical hysterectomy in cervical cancer: a meta-analysis. J Laparoendosc Adv Surg Tech A. 2015;25(12):990–8. https://doi.org/10.1089/lap.2015.0390; Epub 2015 Nov 19.
10. Wang YZ, Deng L, Xu HC, Zhang Y, Liang ZQ. Laparoscopy versus laparotomy for the management of early stage cervical cancer. BMC Cancer. 2015;15:928. https://doi.org/10.1186/s12885-015-1818-4.
11. Ditto A, Martinelli F, Bogani G, Gasparri ML, Di Donato V, Zanaboni F, et al. Implementation of laparoscopic approach for type B radical hysterectomy: a comparison with open surgical operations. Eur J Surg Oncol. 2015;41(1):34–9. https://doi.org/10.1016/j.ejso.2014.10.058; Epub 2014 Nov 6.
12. Ramirez PT, Frumovitz M, Pareja R, Lopez A, Vieira M, Ribeiro R, et al. Minimally invasive versus abdominal radical hysterectomy for cervical cancer. N Engl J Med. 2018;379(20):1895–904. https://doi.org/10.1056/NEJMoa1806395; Epub 2018 Oct 31.
13. Lewicki PJ, Basourakos SP, Qiu Y, Hu JC, Sheyn D, Hijaz A, Shoag JE. Effect of a randomized, controlled trial on surgery for cervical cancer. N Engl J Med. 2021;384(17):1669–71. https://doi.org/10.1056/NEJMc2035819.
14. Bogani G, Di Donato V, Muzii L, Casarin J, Ghezzi F, Malzoni M, et al. Assessing the role of minimally invasive radical hysterectomy for early-stage cervical cancer. Eur J Obstet Gynecol Reprod Biol. 2022;275:64–9. https://doi.org/10.1016/j.ejogrb.2022.06.004; Epub 2022 Jun 8.
15. Melamed A, Margul DJ, Chen L, Keating NL, Del Carmen MG, Yang J, et al. Survival after minimally invasive radical hysterectomy for early-stage cervical cancer. N Engl J Med. 2018;379(20):1905–14. https://doi.org/10.1056/NEJMoa1804923; Epub 2018 Oct 31.
16. Nitecki R, Ramirez PT, Frumovitz M, Krause KJ, Tergas AI, Wright JD, et al. Survival after minimally invasive vs open radical hysterectomy for early-stage cervical cancer: a systematic review and meta-analysis. JAMA Oncol. 2020;6(7):1019–27. https://doi.org/10.1001/jamaoncol.2020.1694.
17. Chiva L, Zanagnolo V, Querleu D, Martin-Calvo N, Arévalo-Serrano J, Căpîlna ME, SUCCOR Study Group, et al. SUCCOR study: an International European cohort observational study comparing minimally invasive surgery versus open abdominal radical hysterectomy in patients with stage IB1 cervical cancer. Int J Gynecol Cancer. 2020;30(9):1269–77. https://doi.org/10.1136/ijgc-2020-001506; Epub 2020 Aug 11.
18. Paik ES, Lim MC, Kim MH, Kim YH, Song ES, Seong SJ, et al. Comparison of laparoscopic and abdominal radical hysterectomy in early stage cervical cancer patients without adjuvant treatment: ancillary analysis of a Korean gynecologic oncology group study (KGOG 1028). Gynecol Oncol. 2019;154(3):547–53. https://doi.org/10.1016/j.ygyno.2019.06.023; Epub 2019 Jul 1.
19. Cusimano MC, Baxter NN, Gien LT, Moineddin R, Liu N, Dossa F, et al. Impact of surgical approach on oncologic outcomes in women undergoing radical hysterectomy for cervical cancer. Am J Obstet Gynecol. 2019;221(6):619.e1–619.e24. https://doi.org/10.1016/j.ajog.2019.07.009; Epub 2019 Jul 6.
20. Abu-Rustum NR, Yashar CM, Bean S, Bradley K, Campos SM, Chon HS, et al. NCCN guidelines insights: cervical cancer, version 1.2020. J Natl Compr Cancer Netw. 2020;18(6):660–6. https://doi.org/10.6004/jnccn.2020.0027.
21. Kohut AY, Kuhn T, Conrad LB, Chua KJ, Abuelafiya M, Gordon AN, et al. Thirty-day postoperative adverse events in minimally invasive versus open abdominal radical hysterectomy for early-stage cervical cancer. J Minim Invasive Gynecol. 2022;29(7):840–7. https://doi.org/10.1016/j.jmig.2022.03.014; Epub 2022 Apr 9.

22. Bogani G, Donato VD, Scambia G, Landoni F, Ghezzi F, Muzii L, Investigator of the Italian Gynecological Cancer Study Group, et al. Practice patterns and 90-day treatment-related morbidity in early-stage cervical cancer. Gynecol Oncol. 2022;166(3):561–5. https://doi.org/10.1016/j.ygyno.2022.07.022; Epub 2022 Jul 29.
23. Klapdor R, Hertel H, Hillemanns P, Röttger M, Soergel P, Kuehnle E, et al. Peritoneal contamination with ICG-stained cervical secretion as surrogate for potential cervical cancer tumor cell dissemination: a proof-of-principle study for laparoscopic hysterectomy. Acta Obstet Gynecol Scand. 2019;98(11):1398–403. https://doi.org/10.1111/aogs.13681; Epub 2019 Jul 23.
24. McCann GA, Taege SK, Boutsicaris CE, Phillips GS, Eisenhauer EL, Fowler JM, et al. The impact of close surgical margins after radical hysterectomy for early-stage cervical cancer. Gynecol Oncol. 2013;128(1):44–8. https://doi.org/10.1016/j.ygyno.2012.10.028; Epub 2012 Nov 5.
25. Schmeler KM, Pareja R, Lopez Blanco A, Humberto Fregnani J, Lopes A, Perrotta M, et al. ConCerv: a prospective trial of conservative surgery for low-risk early-stage cervical cancer. Int J Gynecol Cancer. 2021;31(10):1317–25. https://doi.org/10.1136/ijgc-2021-002921; Epub 2021 Sep 7.
26. Li RZ, Sun LF, Li R, Wang HJ. Survival after minimally invasive radical hysterectomy without using uterine manipulator for early-stage cervical cancer: a systematic review and meta-analysis. BJOG. 2023;130(2):176–83. https://doi.org/10.1111/1471-0528.17339; Epub 2022 Nov 13.
27. Kong TW, Chang SJ, Piao X, Paek J, Lee Y, Lee EJ, et al. Patterns of recurrence and survival after abdominal versus laparoscopic/robotic radical hysterectomy in patients with early cervical cancer. J Obstet Gynaecol Res. 2016;42(1):77–86. https://doi.org/10.1111/jog.12840; Epub 2015 Nov 10.
28. Bogani G, Ditto A, Chiappa V, Pinelli C, Sonetto C, Raspagliesi F. Primary conization overcomes the risk of developing local recurrence following laparoscopic radical hysterectomy in early stage cervical cancer. Int J Gynaecol Obstet. 2020;151(1):43–8. https://doi.org/10.1002/ijgo.13260; Epub 2020 Jul 9.
29. Kwon BS, Roh HJ, Lee S, Yang J, Song YJ, Lee SH, et al. Comparison of long-term survival of total abdominal radical hysterectomy and laparoscopy-assisted radical vaginal hysterectomy in patients with early cervical cancer: Korean multicenter, retrospective analysis. Gynecol Oncol. 2020;159(3):642–8. https://doi.org/10.1016/j.ygyno.2020.09.035; Epub 2020 Oct 9.
30. Matsuo K, Shimada M, Yamaguchi S, Matoda M, Nakanishi T, Kikkawa F, et al. Association of radical hysterectomy surgical volume and survival for early-stage cervical cancer. Obstet Gynecol. 2019;133(6):1086–98. https://doi.org/10.1097/AOG.0000000000003280.
31. Vickers AJ, Bianco FJ, Serio AM, Eastham JA, Schrag D, Klein EA, et al. The surgical learning curve for prostate cancer control after radical prostatectomy. J Natl Cancer Inst. 2007;99(15):1171–7. https://doi.org/10.1093/jnci/djm060; Epub 2007 Jul 24.
32. Fusegi A, Kanao H, Tsumura S, Murakami A, Abe A, Aoki Y, et al. Minimally invasive radical hysterectomy and the importance of avoiding cancer cell spillage for early-stage cervical cancer: a narrative review. J Gynecol Oncol. 2023;34(1):e5. https://doi.org/10.3802/jgo.2023.34.e5; Epub 2022 Nov 10.
33. Paek J, Lim PC. The early surgical period in robotic radical hysterectomy is related to the recurrence after surgery in stage IB cervical cancer. Int J Med Sci. 2021;18(12):2697–704. https://doi.org/10.7150/ijms.59267.
34. Li LY, Wen LY, Park SH, Nam EJ, Lee JY, Kim S, et al. Impact of the learning curve on the survival of abdominal or minimally invasive radical hysterectomy for early-stage cervical cancer. Cancer Res Treat. 2021;53(1):243–51. https://doi.org/10.4143/crt.2020.063; Epub 2020 Oct 12.
35. Marchand G, Masoud AT, Abdelsattar A, King A, Ulibarri H, Parise J, et al. Meta-analysis of laparoscopic radical hysterectomy, excluding robotic assisted versus open radical hysterectomy for early stage cervical cancer. Sci Rep. 2023;13(1):273. https://doi.org/10.1038/s41598-023-27430-9.

36. Park SJ, Kong TW, Kim T, Lee M, Choi CH, Shim SH, et al. Safety and efficacy study of laparoscopic or robotic radical surgery using an endoscopic stapler for inhibiting tumour spillage of cervical malignant neoplasms evaluating survival (SOLUTION): a multi-centre, open-label, single-arm, phase II trial protocol. BMC Cancer. 2022;22(1):331. https://doi.org/10.1186/s12885-022-09429-z.

Fertility-Sparing Treatment of Early and Locally Advanced Cervical Cancer

10

Isao Murakami and Kyoko Tanaka

Abstract

With the advent of improved widespread screening for cervical cancer, the number of patients diagnosed with early stage disease, and with that, the proportion of those of child-bearing age who wish to preserve their fertility, is increasing. The prognosis of these patients is considerably more positive than patients with advanced disease, and fertility-sparing options should be carefully considered. In this chapter, we discuss the treatment approaches that could achieve such an outcome, including radical trachelectomy (RT), and compare RT with the effects of radical hysterectomy. We describe the criteria for patient selection to achieve the best oncological outcome and the importance of pre-operative assessment, such as imaging, to determine patient suitability for RT. The advantages and disadvantages of various surgical methods for RT are considered, including abdominal and vaginal approaches and laparoscopic and robotic techniques, as well as the impact of frozen section analysis, uterine artery preservation, and cervical cerclage on successful treatment. Complications associated with these approaches are also explored, including the risk of miscarriage in women who have undergone RT. The chapter concludes with an overview of the impact of RT on oncological and obstetric outcomes, including patient survival and successful full-term delivery following appropriate perinatal management.

Keywords

Cervical cancer · Early stage · Fertility preservation · Surgical techniques · Radical trachelectomy · Patient outcomes

I. Murakami · K. Tanaka (✉)
Department of Obstetrics and Gynecology, Toho University Ohashi Medical Center, Tokyo, Japan
e-mail: kyoko.tanaka@med.toho-u.ac.jp

D. Aoki (ed.), *Recent Topics on Prevention, Diagnosis, and Clinical Management of Cervical Cancer*, Comprehensive Gynecology and Obstetrics,
https://doi.org/10.1007/978-981-99-9396-3_10

10.1 Introduction

Cervical cancer ranks fourth in incidence and mortality, accounting for an estimated 570,000 cases and more than 311,000 deaths in women worldwide [1–3]. Moreover, it is one of the most common causes of mortality in women younger than 40 years who have a strong desire to retain their fertility. With the widespread implementation of cervical cancer screening programs, the proportion of people diagnosed with early stage disease is increasing. Cases with localized disease have a considerably more favorable prognosis. Therefore, fertility-sparing options could be cervical conization, cone biopsy with pelvic lymph node assessment, or radical trachelectomy (RT) for cases with localized disease who have a strong desire to retain their fertility.

RT was developed in 1994 by Daniel Dargent for the treatment of early invasive cervical cancer to preserve fertility. He reported on the first vaginal RT (VRT), which comprised excision of the cervix with the parametria accompanied by laparoscopic pelvic lymphadenectomy. Abdominal RT (ART) was subsequently described in 1997 by Smith et al. [4, 5] and its use has become worldwide in recent years. Therefore, RT has become the standard treatment for early stage cervical cancer. RT consists of en bloc removal of the cervix, vaginal margins, and parametrial while leaving the uterine body and fundus in situ. RT surgical methods comprise multiple approaches including vaginal, abdominal, laparoscopic, and robotic techniques. Gizzo et al. reported nearly 300 pregnancies with 173 live births in their recent systematic review that analyzed 1300 RTs [6] and found a 3% risk of cancer recurrence, with the most reported complications being miscarriage and chorioamnionitis.

Compared with radical hysterectomy (RH), there is increased surgery time in patients undergoing RT. Blood loss, complication rates, recurrence rates, 5-year overall survival, and recurrence-free survival were similar between RT and RH. Moreover, patients undergoing RT had a shorter post-operative hospital stay [7].

In this chapter, we will review patient selection, pre-operative assessment, surgical techniques, common post-operative complications, and oncological and obstetric outcomes.

10.2 Applicable Patients and Pre-Operative Assessment

Strict indication criteria should be followed to achieve the best oncological results while preserving fertility. Criteria to determine appropriate candidates for RT have remained similar to when RT was first described (Table 10.1). Some of the most important criteria is the patient's strong desire to retain her fertility and that the patient is of reproductive age, typically <40–45 years of age. As a pathological factor, RT should be oncologically safe for stage IA1 with lymphovascular space invasion, stage IA2, or stage IB1, especially those with tumors smaller than 2 cm and an indication of negative pelvic lymph nodes. Moreover, other than squamous cell carcinoma and adenocarcinoma, histology approaches—such as small cell carcinoma,

Table 10.1 Criteria to determine appropriate candidates for RT

Reproductive age, typically <40–45 years old
Squamous cell or adenocarcinoma pathology
Stage IA1 with lymphovascular space invasion, IA2, or IB1
Tumor size <2 cm
No extra-uterine lesions on PET-CT or MRI
Adequate remaining cervical length
Strong desire to preserve fertility

neuroendocrine carcinoma, gastric type adenocarcinoma, clear cell carcinoma, and adenoma malignum—are not considered suitable for RT because they are often associated with a poor prognosis and a high risk of distant metastasis.

Using the above criteria, Sonoda et al. investigated 186 patients who had undergone RH and determined that 48% could have been eligible for RT. However, RT needed to be abandoned because of unexpected disease spread [8]. Therefore, pre-operative assessment is particularly important for RT. Colposcopy and clinical examinations such as ultrasound examination are integral features of pre-operative assessment. Moreover, cone biopsy is essential for precise diagnosis of clinically undetectable cervical cancer. Recently, pre-operative imaging techniques for the evaluation of disease spread have been employed. Pre-operative imaging is crucial in the assessment of tumor dimensions, the amount of healthy cervical stroma, and the involvement of the parametrium and lymph node metastasis. Magnetic resonance imaging (MRI) plays a vital role in the pre-operative assessment of potential candidates for RT because it can be used to determine the tumor dimensions, the amount of healthy cervical stroma, the involvement of the parametrium, and the length of the canal. In patients with early cervical cancer, computed tomography, positron emission tomography, and MRI have shown low detection of lymph node metastasis [9, 10]. Hence, the most precise method identified to date is rapid pathological examination during surgery.

10.3 Surgical Techniques

Multiple approaches in RT have been reported, including vaginal, abdominal, laparoscopic, and robotic. However, determination of the most optimal approach is still under study and is influenced by the preferences and skills of the gynecological surgeon. Therefore, we cannot declare that a specific method of RT is more favorable than another. However, ART could be considered more familiar to gynecological oncologists, and potentially allows more efficient parametrial and paracervical resection compared with VRT. Several investigators reported that the median surgery time was less for VRT than for ART and laparoscopic RT (LRT). However, estimated blood loss was lowest for LRT. The conversion to RH for VRT was lower

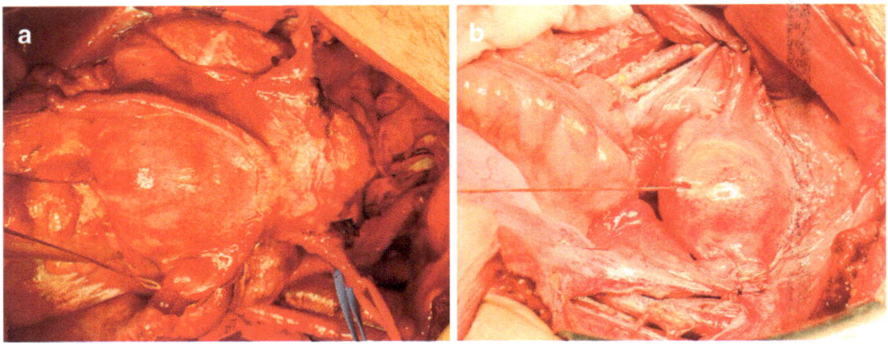

Fig. 10.1 Opening of the vagina and partial resection of the cervix (**a**). Anastomosis of the round ligament and partial closure of the retroperitoneum (**b**)

than ART and LRT by more than twofold, and outcomes such as recurrence rate and recurrence-free and overall survival were favorable [11]. Further trials are warranted to optimize the best approach that could combine oncological safety with improved fertility outcomes in patients with early stage cervical cancer.

10.3.1 Abdominal Approach

The abdominal approach for RT is more radical in terms of parametrical and paracervical resection compared with the vaginal approach. ART is a modification of RH, which brings the advantage of minimal required special surgical experience except for the RH technique.

10.3.1.1 Surgical Steps

1. Laparotomy—resection of the round ligament and uterine traction—development of pararectal/paravesical cavity.
2. Pelvic lymphadenectomy.
3. Identification of the uterine artery.
4. Resection of the cardinal ligament, vesicouterine ligament (anterior/posterior), sacrouterine ligament, rectovaginal ligament, and paracolpium tissues.
5. Opening of the vagina and partial resection of the cervix (Fig. 10.1a).
6. Neocervix plasty and anastomosis of the neocervix to the vagina.
7. Anastomosis of the round ligament and partial closure of the retroperitoneum (Fig. 10.1b).
8. Closure of the abdomen (insertion of drain, use of anti-adhesive agents).

Laparotomy: Resection of the Round Ligament and Uterine Traction: Development of the Pararectal/Paravesical Cavity

A vertical incision is made below the navel and the round uterine ligament is cut. Z suture is performed at the bottom of the uterus. The uterus is pulled by three threads.

Then the retroperitoneal incision is extended, and the pararectal and paravesical cavity are developed.

Pelvic Lymphadenectomy

Lymphadenectomy is performed in a similar manner to standard abdominal radical hysterectomy. Lymphadenectomy is performed up to the level of the bifurcation of the common iliac artery and includes the common iliac, internal iliac, external iliac, cardinal, obturator, supra-inguinal, and presacral nodes. Intraoperative frozen sections of some enlarged lymph nodes are taken for histopathological examination. If a positive lymph node is diagnosed, trachelectomy is converted to conventional radical hysterectomy.

Identification of Uterine Artery

The umbilical ligament is identified in the connective tissue of the paravesical cavity. The uterine artery from the internal iliac artery can be seen and its main stem and ascending branches are preserved. The ureter is separated from the posterior broad ligament to near the entrance of the so-called ureteral tunnel with scissors. The ureteral branch of the uterine artery is then clamped, cut, and ligated or resected.

Resection of the Cardinal Ligament, Vesicouterine Ligament (Anterior/Posterior), Sacrouterine Ligament, Rectovaginal Ligament, and Paracolpium Tissues

Thorough dissection of the lymph nodes surrounding the cardinal ligament is performed to identify the cardinal ligament vessels. The cardinal ligament vessels are treated on the pelvic side in the same way as conventional radical hysterectomy (level III of the Piver classification). The anterior layer of the vesicouterine ligament is resected. The ureter is mobilized outside and then the posterior layer of the vesicouterine ligament is resected. The sacrouterine ligament and rectovaginal ligament are dissected to separate the vagina and the rectum. The paracolpium is resected.

Opening of the Vagina and Partial Resection of the Cervix

Both ends of the vaginal canal are pinched with curved serrated multipurpose forceps, and the upper level of the vaginal wall is clamped by vaginal clamp forceps to prevent cancer spillage. The vaginal canal is resected with a cuff of approximately 2 cm from the cervical edge. The vaginal wall is then opened and the paracolpium and the stump of the vaginal edge are sutured to fit the size of the neocervix. The descending branch of the uterine artery is sacrificed. The partial cervix is resected 5–10 mm underneath the isthmus using an electric scalpel. Additional cervical tissue is resected by cold scalpel for intraoperative histopathological examination. If the stump is positive, trachelectomy is converted to conventional radical hysterectomy.

Neocervix Plasty and Anastomosis of the Neocervix to the Vagina

The serosa of the uterine body is separated from the stroma. Cerclage to prevent premature delivery is placed in the stroma of the neocervix with non-absorbable sutures. The neocervix is then anastomosed to the vaginal wall with absorbable sutures.

Anastomosis of the Round Ligament and Partial Closure of the Retroperitoneum
The dorsal portion of the retroperitoneum and the bladder peritoneum is closed between the right and left edge of the round ligaments. The lateral portion of the retroperitoneum is open to prevent lymphocyst formation.

Closure of the Abdomen (Insertion of Drain, Use of Anti-Adhesive Agents)
After washing the pelvic cavity with saline, a drain is inserted into the retroperitoneal space. The anti-adhesion agents are used in the retroperitoneal opening space around the uterus and adnexas.

10.3.2 Vaginal Approach

VRT has been well documented and is a modification of the original Schauta–Stockel procedure. At first, retroperitoneal or laparoscopic pelvic lymphadenectomy is performed, consisting of the removal of the lymph node-bearing tissue between each distal common iliac artery, the anterior and medial aspect of the proximal half of the external iliac artery and vein, and the distal half of the obturator fat pad anterior to the obturator nerve. The other part of the procedure consists of VRT with resection of the parametria at the level of RH type B.

10.3.3 Laparoscopic or Robotic Approach

At present, laparoscopic and robotic RT represent a noteworthy alternative approach to performing RT. The steps with either laparoscopic and robotic RT are the same with regards to ART. However, advances in these approaches have allowed the undertaking of many procedures with advantages such as reduced hospital stay and blood loss, decreased blood transfusion rates and complication rates, and improved esthetic outcomes. Burnett et al. proposed the first patient for robotic RT with the intent to demonstrate that robotic RT might circumvent some of the disadvantages related to either VRT or ART [12]. Moreover, Persson et al. confirmed that robotic RT could improve visualization because of its three-dimensional optics, improve tissue manipulation because of the flexibility of the instruments, decrease adjacent tissue trauma and adhesions, and diminish post-operative pain and hospitalization [13].

10.3.4 Frozen Sections

Frozen sections for RT can be advocated to ensure that an acceptable tumor-free margin has been obtained [14–16]. The recommended tumor clearance is at least 5 mm, and where possible, 1 cm [17]. If this is not possible, RH would need to be performed. Frozen sections of any suspicious pelvic nodes should be analyzed prior to RT to ensure that there is no metastatic disease because this would be an indication to abort a fertility-sparing procedure.

10.3.5 Uterine Artery Preservation

One of the most frequently discussed issues is whether uterine artery preservation should be performed. Several authors have addressed uterine perfusion after RT. The first report, by Tang et al., and the most recent report, by Escobar et al., investigated uterine perfusion utilizing laser angiography with indocyanine green in both uterine artery-sparing and -non-sparing RT [18, 19]. The authors concluded that there was no need to preserve the uterine artery during RT to maintain uterine viability. However, this remains controversial, and further consideration and discussion is warranted in respect of preservation of fertility.

10.3.6 Cervical Cerclage

Cervical cerclage following RT is not a standard procedure [20]. Placement of a cervical cerclage at the time of RT plays an important role in preventing premature dilatation of the residual uterine cervical canal and the subsequent occurrence of preterm premature rupture of membranes [21]. We use non-absorbable thread; moreover, the type of suture used to perform the cerclage differs among reports and includes braided and non-braided sutures. Braided sutures are easy to remove, but they provide an environment for bacterial incorporation, which is a known contributor to preterm birth [22]. In contrast, non-braided sutures exhibit less tissue reactivity. However, it is still controversial as to which type is better. Moreover, we tie the knot of the cerclage posteriorly to avoid the theoretical risk of erosion into the bladder. Neither the thread nor the position of the knot has been evaluated in a randomized trial.

10.4 Complications

The general complication rate for RT has been reported to be similar to that of RH. The meta-analysis revealed that no difference was detected with regards to intraoperative and post-operative complications between RT and RH [7, 23]. The only significant difference was in the median operative time (155 min in RT versus 115 min in RH) [24]. The most common intraoperative complication was injury to the urinary tract. Specific complications for RT include amenorrhoea, cervical stenosis, which occurs in approximately 10% of patients, cervical cerclage expulsion, and an increased risk of pregnancy-related complications, such as spontaneous abortion and premature delivery [25]. These issues will be discussed later. Regarding cervical stenosis, in a review of 1547 patients who underwent RT, in whom 424 (27%) used anti-stenosis tools, the incidence of cervical stenosis was 4.6% with the tools and 12.7% without the tools, which was a significant difference [26]. The most commonly used tool to prevent cervical stenosis was a catheter, and the duration of the catheter placement was 3–5 days to 8 weeks [26].

10.5 Oncological Outcomes

Oncological outcomes such as 5-year overall survival and recurrence-free survival following RT were similar with RH for tumors of similar sizes. Some studies investigated that RT could obtain a similar death rate compared with RH and should be a safe alternative for fertility preservation. Zhang et al. identified recurrence rates of 2.3% and mortality rates of 0.7% in their meta-analysis, which included 2479 patients [27]. Follow-up ranged from 9 to 96 months, and 81.4% of the patients had follow-up durations greater than 2 years. A sample of the literature used to compile these numbers is incorporated in Table 10.2 [28–39]. However, the most important issue could be maintaining the strict criteria for patient selection to obtain similar oncological outcomes following RT with RH. Neoadjuvant chemotherapy is proposed to remove possible ovarian micro-metastasis and/or downstage bulky cervical cancer. However, large multicenter studies on these novel approaches are required to obtain a good prognosis.

Table 10.2 Oncologic outcomes following RT

Authors	Case numbers	Disease recurrent No. patients	Disease death
Plante et al. and Roy et al.	100	2	1
Dargent et al. and Mathevet et al.	95	4	3
Burnett et al.	19	0	0
Covens and steed	121	7	4
Schlaerth et al.	10	0	0
Hertel et al.	100	4	2
Shepherd et al.	123	5	2
Ungar et al.	91	2	0
Diaz et al.	40	1	1
Wethington et al.	101	4	0
Total	800	29	13

10.6 Fertility and Obstetric Outcomes

Hundreds of post-operative pregnancies have been reported, mostly with the vaginal approach, but increasingly with the abdominal approach recently (Table 10.3) [28, 30, 31, 34–38, 40–43]. Vaginal delivery is absolutely contraindicated for RT. Therefore, pregnancies must be delivered by cesarean section in these patients. Moreover, the preterm delivery rates in laparoscopic RT were reported to be higher than in the vaginal and abdominal approaches [44]. Interestingly, the post-RT pregnancy rate was highest for the vaginal approach. However, despite differences in pregnancy rates by the vaginal or abdominal approach, live birth rates remain roughly similar across interventions. Rob et al. reported that pregnancy loss rates were 22% and preterm birth rates were 35% among the total number of conceptions and deliveries [25]. In a large systematic review reporting on obstetric outcomes in patients undergoing RT, aggregated rates of miscarriage and preterm labor were 24% and 26.6%, respectively, with a pooled pregnancy rate of 20.5% [27]. Furthermore, there are several complications specific to post-RT pregnancies, such as abnormal bleeding from varices and complications due to the presence of a prophylactic cerclage during pregnancy. However, the guidelines for perinatal management after RT have not been determined. In post-RT pregnancies, one of the most important reasons for preterm delivery was preterm premature rupture of the membranes (PROM), and it is believed that mechanical and/or infectious causes may be responsible. Nishio et al. reported that the relatively lower pregnancy rate among these patients may be due to cervical factors, chronic endometritis, and the larger volume of cervix being resected by RT [45]. Moreover, another theory pertained to the possibility that these complications could be the result of a lack of adequate blood flow to the uterus following transection of the uterine artery.

Table 10.3 Obstetrical outcomes following RT

Authors	Pregnant No.	1st trimester miscarriage	2nd trimester miscarriage	3rd trimester miscarriage	Delivery <32 weeks	Delivery ≥32 weeks
Plante et al.	59	10	2	44	3	41
Dargent et al. and Mathevet	56	11	8	34	5	29
Covents et al. and Bernardini	45	8	3	34	6	28
Schlaerth et al.	4	0	2	0	0	2
Hertel et al.	14	1	0	11	3	8
Shepherd et al.	52	15	7	28	7	21
Ungar et al.	10	4	0	6	1	5
Sonoda et al.	11	1	2	0	0	8
Diaz et al.	9	0	3	0	0	6
Kim et al.	27	1	3	20	0	20
Total	287	51	30	177	25	168

In previous reviews, the incidence of miscarriage in the first trimester (before 12 weeks of gestation) was reported to be 14% [34]. Typically, dilatation and curettage (D&C) is often performed in patients with miscarriage in the first trimester. However, D&C is of concern because of the risk of prophylactic cerclage removal and the development of endometritis in patients after RT. Lavie et al., Bernardini et al., and Planre et al. recommended that expectant management without D&C could be indicated for miscarriage in the first trimester [40, 41, 46]. Therefore, it is suggested that expectant management could be useful and appropriate for first trimester miscarriages after RT.

In previous reviews, the incidence of miscarriage in the second trimester (from 13 to 27 weeks of gestation) was 5.8%–10%, which was higher than in the general population [34]. Of these, 85% could result in delivery after 32 weeks of gestation, with the majority reaching full term (>37 weeks gestation). A major etiology of miscarriage in the second trimester and preterm deliveries could be likely due to mechanical changes to the remaining cervix and support of the growing lower uterine segment. Therefore, although it is hard to predict miscarriage in the second trimester, Kim et al. reported that residual cervical shortening was associated with miscarriage after the second trimester in post- RT pregnancies [21].

There is a concern about how to deliver when patients who have undergone RT have a miscarriage in the second trimester. Plante et al. recommended that with the selection of an expectant treatment, most patients could deliver a miscarriage vaginally without removal of the prophylactic cerclage in the second trimester [47]. However, Kasuga et al. concluded that when patients who have undergone RT undergo vaginal delivery of a miscarriage in the second trimester, they might experience laceration of the residual cervix [48]. In another report, the prophylactic cerclage should be removed when the fetus is delive

red vaginally at 17 weeks of gestation [49]. Therefore, cesarean section could be recommended for patients who have undergone RT and who then suffer a miscarriage in the second trimester. Doing so would allow delivery without lacerating the residual cervix and/or removing the cerclage.

Maternal fetal medicine consultation is critical for patients after RT to ensure they are receiving adequate perinatal care according to the most up-to-date guidelines for the management of a short cervix. Additionally, if patients after RT have recurrent miscarriages in the second trimester, there is evidence to suggest that an abdominal cerclage might be preventative [50].

Despite an increasing number of post-RT pregnancies, there are still insufficient cases on which to formulate an established method of perinatal management. Large multicenter studies on post-RT pregnancies are therefore required to obtain a good prognosis.

References

1. Schlaerth JB, Spirtos NM, Schlaerth AC. Radical trachelectomy and pelvic lymphadenectomy with uterine preservation in the treatment of cervical cancer. Am J Obstet Gynecol. 2003;188:29–34.
2. Costales A, Michener C, Escobar-Rodriguez PF. Radical trachelectomy for early stage cervical cancer. Curr Treat Options Oncol. 2018;19:75.
3. Nishio H, Fujii T, Kameyama K, Susumu N, Nakamura M, Iwata T, Aoki D. Abdominal radical trachelectomy as a fertility-sparing procedure in women with early-stage cervical cancer in a series of 61 women. Gynecol Oncol. 2009;115:51–5.
4. Bernardini M, Barrett J, Seaward G, Covens A. Pregnancy outcomes in patients after radical trachelectomy. Am J Obstet Gynecol. 2003;189:1378–82.
5. Ungár L, Smith JR, Pálfalvi L, Del Priore G. Abdominal radical trachelectomy during pregnancy to preserve pregnancy and fertility. Obstet Gynecol. 2006;108:811–4.
6. Roy M, Plante M. Pregnancies after radical vaginal trachelectomy for early-stage cervical cancer. Am J Obstet Gynecol. 1998;179:1491–6.
7. Israfil-Bayli F, Toozs-Hobson P, Lees C, Slack M, Ismail KMK. Pregnancy outcome after elective cervical cerclage in relation to type of suture material used. Med Hypotheses. 2013;81:119–21.
8. Sonoda Y, Chi DS, Carter J, Barakat RR, Abu-Rustum NR. Initial experience with Dargent's operation: the radical vaginal trachelectomy. Gynecol Oncol. 2008;108:214–9.
9. Dargent D, Martin X, Sacchetoni A, Mathevet P. Laparoscopic vaginal radical trachelectomy: a treatment to preserve the fertility of cervical carcinoma patients. Cancer. 2000;88:1877–82.
10. Escobar PF, Ramirez PT, Garcia Ocasio RE, Pareja R, Zimberg S, Sprague M, Frumovitz M. Utility of indocyanine green (ICG) intra-operative angiography to determine uterine vascular perfusion at the time of radical trachelectomy. Gynecol Oncol. 2016;143:357–61.
11. Ismiil N, Ghorab Z, Covens A, Nofech-Mozes S, Saad R, Dubé V, Khalifa MA. Intraoperative margin assessment of the radical trachelectomy specimen. Gynecol Oncol. 2009;113:42–6.
12. Rob L, Skapa P, Robova H. Fertility-sparing surgery in patients with cervical cancer. Lancet Oncol. 2011;12:192–200.
13. Lavie O, Peer G, Sagi S, Ben Arie A, Auslender R. The management of an early-missed abortion after radical trachelectomy—a case report and a review of the literature. Int J Gynecol Cancer. 2006;16:1688–90.
14. Gizzo S, Ancona E, Saccardi C, et al. Radical trachelectomy: the first step of fertility preservation in young women with cervical cancer (Review). Oncol Rep. 2013;30:2545–54.
15. Shepherd JH, Spencer C, Herod J, Ind TEJ. Radical vaginal trachelectomy as a fertility-sparing procedure in women with early-stage cervical cancer-cumulative pregnancy rate in a series of 123 women. BJOG. 2006;113:719–24.
16. Burnett AF, Roman LD, O'Meara AT, Morrow CP. Radical vaginal trachelectomy and pelvic lymphadenectomy for preservation of fertility in early cervical carcinoma. Gynecol Oncol. 2003;88:419–23.
17. Selman TJ, Mann C, Zamora J, Appleyard T-L, Khan K. Diagnostic accuracy of tests for lymph node status in primary cervical cancer: a systematic review and meta-analysis. CMAJ. 2008;178:855–62.
18. Mathevet P, Laszlo de Kaszon E, Dargent D. Fertility preservation in early cervical cancer. Gynecol Obstet Fertil. 2003;31:706–12.
19. Zhang S, Xu H, Zhang L, Qiao Y. Cervical cancer: epidemiology, risk factors and screening. Chin J Cancer Res. 2020;32:720–8.
20. Steed H, Rosen B, Murphy J, Laframboise S, De Petrillo D, Covens A. A comparison of laparascopic-assisted radical vaginal hysterectomy and radical abdominal hysterectomy in the treatment of cervical cancer. Gynecol Oncol. 2004;93:588–93.

21. Ungár L, Pálfalvi L, Hogg R, Siklós P, Boyle DCM, Del Priore G, Smith JR. Abdominal radical trachelectomy: a fertility-preserving option for women with early cervical cancer. BJOG. 2005;112:366–9.
22. Prodromidou A, Iavazzo C, Fotiou A, Psomiadou V, Douligeris A, Vorgias G, Kalinoglou N. Short- and long term outcomes after abdominal radical trachelectomy versus radical hysterectomy for early stage cervical cancer: a systematic review of the literature and meta-analysis. Arch Gynecol Obstet. 2019;300:25–31.
23. Kim CH, Abu-Rustum NR, Chi DS, Gardner GJ, Leitao MMJ, Carter J, Barakat RR, Sonoda Y. Reproductive outcomes of patients undergoing radical trachelectomy for early-stage cervical cancer. Gynecol Oncol. 2012;125:585–8.
24. Plante M, Renaud M-C, Hoskins IA, Roy M. Vaginal radical trachelectomy: a valuable fertility-preserving option in the management of early-stage cervical cancer A series of 50 pregnancies and review of the literature. Gynecol Oncol. 2005;98:3–10.
25. Plante M. Vaginal radical trachelectomy: an update. Gynecol Oncol. 2008;111:S105–10.
26. Signorelli M, Guerra L, Montanelli L, Crivellaro C, Buda A, Dell'Anna T, Picchio M, Milani R, Fruscio R, Messa C. Preoperative staging of cervical cancer: is 18-FDG-PET/CT really effective in patients with early stage disease? Gynecol Oncol. 2011;123:236–40.
27. Diaz JP, Sonoda Y, Leitao MM, Zivanovic O, Brown CL, Chi DS, Barakat RR, Abu-Rustum NR. Oncologic outcome of fertility-sparing radical trachelectomy versus radical hysterectomy for stage IB1 cervical carcinoma. Gynecol Oncol. 2008;111:255–60.
28. Smith ES, Moon AS, O'Hanlon R, Leitao MMJ, Sonoda Y, Abu-Rustum NR, Mueller JJ. Radical trachelectomy for the treatment of early-stage cervical cancer: a systematic review. Obstet Gynecol. 2020;136:533–42.
29. Li X, Li J, Wu X. Incidence, risk factors and treatment of cervical stenosis after radical trachelectomy: a systematic review. Eur J Cancer. 2015;51:1751–9.
30. Ishioka S, Endo T, Baba T, Akashi Y, Morishita M, Sugio A, Kanayama N, Saito T. Successful delivery after transabdominal cerclage of uterine cervix for cervical incompetence after radical trachelectomy. J Obstet Gynaecol Res. 2015;41:1295–9.
31. Lim YK, Lek SM, Yeo SH. Obstetric care after radical abdominal trachelectomy in a patient with stage IB1 cervical cancer: a case report and a review of medical literature. Gynecol Oncol Rep. 2016;17:86–8.
32. Guo J, Hu Q, Deng Z, Jin X. Outcomes of trachelectomy vs. hysterectomy for early-stage cervical cancer: a systematic review and meta-analysis. Front Surg. 2021;8:735944.
33. Kim M, Ishioka S, Endo T, Baba T, Akashi Y, Morishita M, Adachi H, Saito T. Importance of uterine cervical cerclage to maintain a successful pregnancy for patients who undergo vaginal radical trachelectomy. Int J Clin Oncol. 2014;19:906–11.
34. Bray F, Ferlay J, Soerjomataram I, Siegel RL, Torre LA, Jemal A. Global cancer statistics 2018: GLOBOCAN estimates of incidence and mortality worldwide for 36 cancers in 185 countries. CA Cancer J Clin. 2018;68:394–424.
35. Kasuga Y, Miyakoshi K, Endo T, Takeda T, Nakamura M, Ochiai D, Tanaka M. Sonographic findings of cervical laceration caused by vaginal delivery in pregnancy after radical trachelectomy. J Med Ultrason (2001). 2020;47:655–7.
36. Zhang Q, Li W, Kanis MJ, Qi G, Li M, Yang X, Kong B. Oncologic and obstetrical outcomes with fertility-sparing treatment of cervical cancer: a systematic review and meta-analysis. Oncotarget. 2017;8:46580–92.
37. Zhang D, Ge H, Li J, Wu X. A new method of surgical margin assuring for abdominal radical trachelectomy in frozen section. Eur J Cancer. 2015;51:734–41.
38. Plante M, Renaud M-C, François H, Roy M. Vaginal radical trachelectomy: an oncologically safe fertility-preserving surgery. An updated series of 72 cases and review of the literature. Gynecol Oncol. 2004;94:614–23.
39. Tang J, Li J, Wang S, Zhang D, Wu X. On what scale does it benefit the patients if uterine arteries were preserved during ART? Gynecol Oncol. 2014;134:154–9.
40. Small WJ, Bacon MA, Bajaj A, et al. Cervical cancer: a global health crisis. Cancer. 2017;123:2404–12.

41. Wethington SL, Cibula D, Duska LR, Garrett L, Kim CH, Chi DS, Sonoda Y, Abu-Rustum NR. An international series on abdominal radical trachelectomy: 101 patients and 28 pregnancies. Int J Gynecol Cancer. 2012;22:1251–7.
42. Abu-Rustum NR, Sonoda Y, Black D, Levine DA, Chi DS, Barakat RR. Fertility-sparing radical abdominal trachelectomy for cervical carcinoma: technique and review of the literature. Gynecol Oncol. 2006;103:807–13.
43. Burnett AF, Stone PJ, Duckworth LA, Roman JJ. Robotic radical trachelectomy for preservation of fertility in early cervical cancer: case series and description of technique. J Minim Invasive Gynecol. 2009;16:569–72.
44. Bentivegna E, Maulard A, Pautier P, Chargari C, Gouy S, Morice P. Fertility results and pregnancy outcomes after conservative treatment of cervical cancer: a systematic review of the literature. Fertil Steril. 2016;106:1195–1211.e5.
45. Persson J, Imboden S, Reynisson P, Andersson B, Borgfeldt C, Bossmar T. Reproducibility and accuracy of robot-assisted laparoscopic fertility sparing radical trachelectomy. Gynecol Oncol. 2012;127:484–8.
46. Tanguay C, Plante M, Renaud M-C, Roy M, Têtu B. Vaginal radical trachelectomy in the treatment of cervical cancer: the role of frozen section. Int J Gynecol Pathol. 2004;23:170–5.
47. Sonoda Y, Abu-Rustum NR, Gemignani ML, Chi DS, Brown CL, Poynor EA, Barakat RR. A fertility-sparing alternative to radical hysterectomy: how many patients may be eligible? Gynecol Oncol. 2004;95:534–8.
48. Smith JR, Boyle DC, Corless DJ, Ungar L, Lawson AD, Del Priore G, McCall JM, Lindsay I, Bridges JE. Abdominal radical trachelectomy: a new surgical technique for the conservative management of cervical carcinoma. Br J Obstet Gynaecol. 1997;104:1196–200.
49. Park KJ, Soslow RA, Sonoda Y, Barakat RR, Abu-Rustum NR. Frozen-section evaluation of cervical adenocarcinoma at time of radical trachelectomy: pathologic pitfalls and the application of an objective scoring system. Gynecol Oncol. 2008;110:316–23.
50. Hertel H, Köhler C, Grund D, Hillemanns P, Possover M, Michels W, Schneider A, German Association of Gynecologic Oncologists (AGO). Radical vaginal trachelectomy (RVT) combined with laparoscopic pelvic lymphadenectomy: prospective multicenter study of 100 patients with early cervical cancer. Gynecol Oncol. 2006;103:506–11.

Sentinel Navigation Surgery for Local Advanced Cervical Cancer

11

Yoshito Terai

Abstract

Cervical cancer is the fourth most frequent cancer in women and the fourth leading cause of cancer related deaths in females. Primary surgical treatment, including radical hysterectomy and pelvic lymph node dissection (PLND), is considered the standard of care. However, lymphedema has been observed in 35% of patients who undergo surgery, including lymphadenectomy for cervical cancer. The sentinel lymph nodes (SLN) are the first lymph nodes to receive drainage from their tumor. An SLN biopsy for patients with cervical cancer was first reported in 1995. SLN biopsy appears to be feasible for detecting lymph node metastasis in patients with early-stage cervical cancer. The SLN biopsy can reduce surgical morbidities such as intraoperative blood loss and lower the risk of postoperative complications of lymphedema and lymphocyst for the patients with radical hysterectomy of cervical cancer. Recently, several reports have shown that indocyanine green (ICG) has a feasible detection rate in patients with uterine cervical cancer. Several studies suggest that SLN biopsy without a systematic lymphadenectomy is a safe treatment modality for early-stage cervical cancer and a tumor size ≤2 cm, and there was no significant difference between SLN biopsy and lymphadenectomy in the oncologic outcomes for the patients with cervical cancer. However, SLN biopsy and/or SLN mapping for the patients with cervical cancer has not been yet covered by public health insurance at the present time in Japan, and only 22% facilities have experience in SLN biopsy for gynecological cancers in Japan.

Y. Terai (✉)
Department of Obstetrics and Gynecology, Kobe University Graduate School of Medicine, Kobe, Hyogo, Japan
e-mail: yterai@med.kobe-u.ac.jp

D. Aoki (ed.), *Recent Topics on Prevention, Diagnosis, and Clinical Management of Cervical Cancer*, Comprehensive Gynecology and Obstetrics,
https://doi.org/10.1007/978-981-99-9396-3_11

Keywords
Cervical cancer · Sentinel lymph nodes · SLN biopsy · Pelvic lymph node dissection · OSNA assay

11.1 Principle and History

With nearly 600,000 new cases per year and 340,000 deaths per year in the world, cervical cancer is the fourth most frequent cancer in women and the fourth leading cause of cancer related deaths in females [1]. Primary surgical treatment, including radical hysterectomy and pelvic lymph node dissection (PLND), is considered the standard of care. The most important prognostic factor in locally advanced cervical cancer is lymph node status. The 5-year survival rate decreases from 88–92% to 55–64% in cases with positive nodes [2], and the incidence of lymph node metastasis in patients with locally advanced cervical cancer is approximately 10–27% [3]. Therefore, an accurate assessment of lymph node metastasis is necessary. However, lymphadenectomy is frequently associated with sequelae, including lymphocele, lymphedema, and cellulitis, and lymphedema has the most notable effect upon patient quality of life [4]. Lymphedema has been observed in 35% of patients who undergo surgery, including lymphadenectomy for cervical cancer [5].

The sentinel lymph nodes (SLN) are the first lymph nodes to receive drainage from their tumor; when cancer cells begin their spread through the lymphatic system, the cells are initially trapped in the sentinel lymph nodes. The use of SLN biopsy was initially reported in patients with penile cancer in 1977 by Cabanas [6] and subsequently applied and further developed in the treatment of other human cancers such as melanoma, breast, and vulvar cancers [7–9]. An SLN biopsy using the blue dye lymphazurin for patients with cervical cancer was first reported in 1995 [10]. When an SLN can be intraoperatively diagnosed using frozen sections, a systematic pelvic lymphadenectomy may be omitted, and an SLN biopsy can avoid complications such as bleeding, nerve damage, lymphocysts, and lymphedema caused by a systematic lymph node dissection. After SLN mapping and a detailed examination of the SLN, micrometastases may be found, and patients may receive adjuvant therapy. The National Comprehensive Cancer Network (NCCN) cervical cancer guideline presents SLN mapping as an alternative for the surgical management of early-stage cervical cancer less than 2 cm in diameter [11, 12]. Treatment guideline for cervical cancer version 2022 published by the Japan Society of Gynecologic Oncology (JSGO) indicated that a sentinel lymph node biopsy should be performed in institutions where pathologists cooperate with experienced surgical teams in clinical trials. The omission of pelvic lymph node dissection in patients with negative sentinel lymph node biopsy is approved in institutions in which accuracy and safety have been fully confirmed (level 2). As SLN biopsy and/or SLN mapping for the patients with cervical cancer has not been yet covered by public health insurance at the present time in Japan, the omission of pelvic lymph node dissection for patients with negative sentinel lymph node biopsy should be performed under the approval of the ethical review board at institutions where safety has been confirmed by clinical trials via a backup pelvic lymph node dissection. However, only 22% facilities have experience in SLN biopsy for gynecological cancers in Japan [12].

11.2 Principle and Indication

11.2.1 Detection Rate, Sensitivity of SLNs

In detecting SLNs in cervical cancer, the most commonly used tracers are indocyanine green (ICG), blue dyes, and 99TC [13–15]. Two types of tracers are commonly available for the detection of sentinel lymph nodes: radioactive isotopes injected into target organs 1 day preoperatively and where the sentinel lymph nodes can be imaged by scintigraphy in advance, or where the nodes are detected by a gamma probing during surgery. Among the vital dyes, three are commonly used, methylene blue, isosulfan blue, and patent blue violet, and they are injected at the start of the operation, thus allowing sentinel lymph node visualization during surgery. In a meta-analysis and systematic review of 2164 patients in 28 studies, the combined overall detection rate was 95% (95% CI; 93–97%), and the combined bilateral rate was 72% (95% CI: 67–78%) [16]. Moreover, in these studies, the sensitivity of the detection rate in SLN mapping was 94.99% (95% CI: 93.29–96.69%), with a sensitivity of 72.43% (95% CI; 67.36–77.50%) in bilateral sentinel node detection. The SLN overall detection rates using blue dye with Tc, Tc only, ICG were 96%, 95%, and 98%, respectively. The SLN bilateral detection rates using blue dye with Tc, Tc only, ICG were 76%, 63%, and 85%, respectively. The sensitivity of the SLN overall detection rate using blue dye with Tc, Tc only, and ICG was 95.52%, 94.99%, and 97.76%, while the bilateral detection rates were 75.82%, 63.45%, and 84.96%, respectively [16]. These results indicate that Tc combined with blue dye or ICG alone is a reliable SLN biopsy method with a high detection rate, sensitivity, and specificity, and that using blue dye alone as a tracer is not recommended for SLN biopsy in cervical cancer. Recently, several reports have shown that ICG has a feasible detection rate in patients with uterine cervical cancer, although SLN biopsy using ICG requires a fluorescence system [17–19]. SLN detection using ICG and near-infrared fluorescence was introduced in 2012 by Rossi et al. in cervical cancer [20]. ICG has several advantages, is easier to use, and does not require lymphoscintigraphy in terms of cost, ICG is cheaper than using Technetium-99 m [14]. Furthermore, a preoperative radiocolloid tracer injection may be painful, whereas ICG is injected after the induction of general anesthesia. Luhrs et al. reported bilateral SLN mapping rates of 98.5% using ICG and 60% using 99mTC ($p < 0.01$) in 65 cases of cervical cancer; however, the combination of ICG and TC did not increase the bilateral detection rate [21]. Recently, the randomized phase III FILM trial has demonstrated that an ICG tracer identified more SLNs (overall and bilateral) than did blue dye [22].

The injection of tracers to patients with a history of conization is difficult, and conization may hamper lymphatic flow. However, in line with the results of a previous study, we found that a history of conization was not associated with a lower detection rate [23]. The detection rates in patients who underwent laparoscopic surgery and open surgery were 93–96.1% and 87–90.2%, respectively. Moreover, the sensitivity in these patients was 89.8–93.2% and 86–91.7%, respectively [23–25]. These results suggest that laparoscopic procedures have excellent potential in the detection of SLNs in patients with early-stage cervical cancer. In our previous study, laparoscopy had a higher detection rate than laparotomy [26], and we believe that the wide and clear view attained by laparoscopy improves the detection rate. Therefore, in more patients with a higher detection rate under laparoscopy, a systematic pelvic lymphadenectomy could be omitted.

11.2.2 Lymphatic Drainage of the Cervical Cancer

The lymphatic system is an integral part of the body's anatomy and functionality. Pelvic uterine lymphatic drainage follows two major pathways: the upper paracervical pathway (UPP) and the lower paracervical pathway (LPP) [27] (Fig. 11.1). The UPP runs along the parauterine lymphovascular tissue parallel to the uterine artery and drains into lymph nodes usually located mediodorsal to the external iliac artery. The UPP thereafter continues laterally to the common iliac artery and consequently to the lower paraaortic and precaval area. Parallel lymphatic vessels are frequent, usually resulting in at least two SLNs, typically positioned medial of the bifurcation

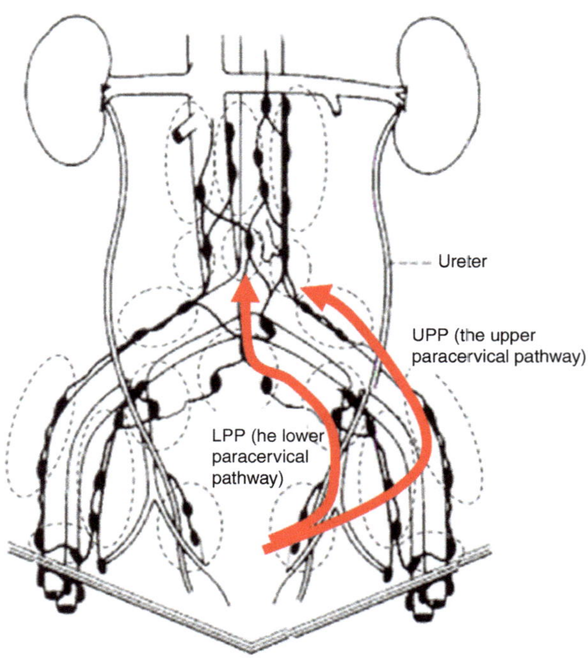

Fig. 11.1 Lymphatic drainage of the cervical cancer for SLN

of the external and internal iliac artery (interiliac position), and/or in the proximal obturator fossa ventral of the obturator nerve (proximal obturator position) [28]. The LPP runs medial of the internal iliac vessels, then continues presacrally medial to the common iliac artery and further to the lower precaval and paraaortic area. Contrary to the UPP, typical positions of SLNs cannot be defined due to a longitudinal variation of positions of the SLNs and latitudinal crossover of lymphatics. Mapping rates of the LPP are also lower than that of the UPP [17]. Moreover, Benedetti-Panici et al. [18] investigated the dissemination of cervical tumors through the parametrium with three main trunks: the lateral, the anterior, and the posterior. The lateral trunk runs through the lateral parametrium and is the main lymphatic drainage from the uterine cervix. As also described by Girardi et al. [19] and by Bonneau et al. [29], the lateral parametrium contains many lymph nodes and lymphatic vessels that can be a privileged pathway for tumor dissemination. In SLN mapping studies, the mapping rate of SLN was high, not only in the upper paracervical pathway, but also in the lower paracervical pathway in women with cervical cancer [30]. The prevalence of unusually located SLNs in cervical cancer has previously been reviewed in some studies. For example, Ouldamer et al. reported on 27 studies that included 1301 patients, and they concluded that 16.3% of SLNs were found at unusual locations, with 6.6% being found along the common iliac, 1.3% sacral, 4.3% parametrial, and 2.0% in the paraaortic area. All included studies utilized blue dye and/or technetium tracing techniques [31]. Balaya et al. analyzed the secondary data of the SENTICOL 1 and 2 studies and recently reported that the SLNs were mainly located in the interiliac or external iliac area in 83.2% of cervical cancer cases, and the other localizations were 9.2% in the common iliac area, 3.9% in the parametrium, 1.6% in the promontory area, 1.5% in the paraaortic area, and 0.5% in other areas [32].

11.2.3 Effect of Tumor Size

In the analysis of SENTICOL-1 and -2, a lower SLN mapping was also significantly associated with age > 70 years, tumor >2 cm, and a body-mass index >30 kg.m^2 [33]. In a systematic review and meta-analysis for cervical cancer, the pooled detection rate was 93.4% in tumors ≤2 cm and 73.9% in tumors >2 cm, whereas the pooled sensitivity was 94.7% in tumors ≤2 cm and 81.7% in tumors >2 cm [23]. Furthermore, in the retrospective SLN mapping study using ICG for 103 cases of cervical cancer cases, the false-negative rate was associated with a large tumor size (≥ 4 cm) [34]. In patients with a tumor size larger than 20 mm, usual lymphatic drainage may be altered. In some cases, the lymphatic tract may be destroyed, thus leading to a higher rate of lymph node metastasis. In such cases, non-involved lymph nodes may be detected as SLNs because the original SLN is completely replaced with cancer cells [35]. The reason for the failure of lymphatic mapping in large or locally advanced tumors, as compared to smaller tumors, is the higher possibility of lymph nodal involvement and lymphovascular invasion, which hampers lymphatic flow [23, 36]. Therefore, SLN mapping may not be well suited for large tumors (> 2 cm).

11.2.4 Preoperative Evaluation

11.2.4.1 Technique

All of the tracers were submucosally injected in four quadrants of the cervix at two to four sites of the cervix, as described in the NCCN guideline. The cervical injection was about 5 mm in all cases, as described previously [37, 38]. On the day before surgery, 2.0 mL of fluid containing 110 MBq 99 m-Technetium-labeled tin colloids (99mTc) was injected into the patient's cervix. The lymphoscintigraphy was performed within 6 h, and hot spots, indicating SLNs, were identified (Fig. 11.2). On the day of the operation, blue dye and/or indocyanine green (ICG) (50 μg/mL) was injected into the cervix at the start of surgery. SLNs were detected at 40 min after the injection of blue dye or ICG, and radioactive lymph nodes were located using a gamma-probe (Navigator GPS, RMD). The blue dye stained lymph nodes were detected by direct inspection. ICG fluorescence-positive lymph nodes were detected using a color fluorescence camera (Hyper Wye Medical System, MIZUHO Co., for laparotomy; Camera Control Unit JC300, MC Medical Co., for laparoscopy (Fig. 11.3) and robotic surgery (Fig. 11.4)). After the SLN biopsy, the area of pelvic lymph nodes was surveyed by direct observation and with a color fluorescence camera or a gamma-probe to confirm that no radioactive tissue remained.

An intraoperative pathological examination was then performed. The SLN was cut in half, parallel to the longest axis, to obtain a maximal section area. One half was used to create a frozen section. The specimen was cut with an interval of 2 mm and a 5 μm section, which was then stained with hematoxylin and eosin (H&E) and evaluated at the time that the frozen section was created. The other half and the non-SLN specimens were fixed in 10% formalin for a permanent section procedure; the

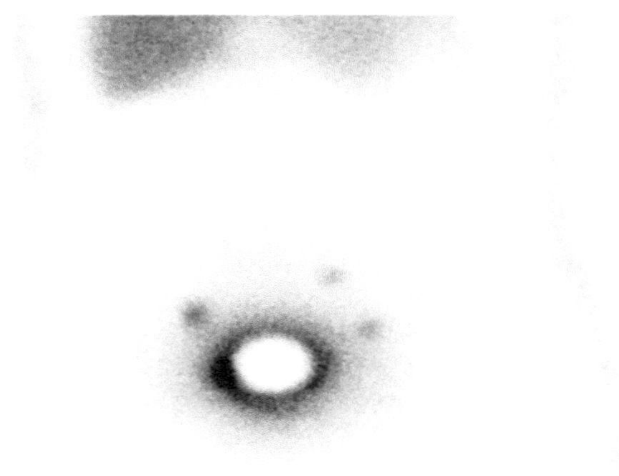

Fig. 11.2 Preoperative lymphoscintigram

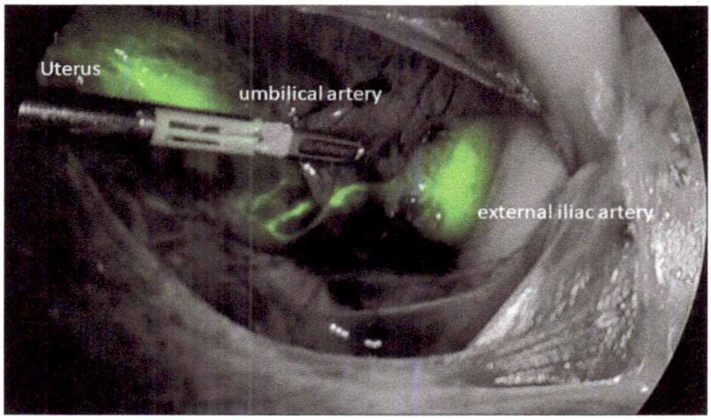

Fig. 11.3 SLN mapping for cervical cancer

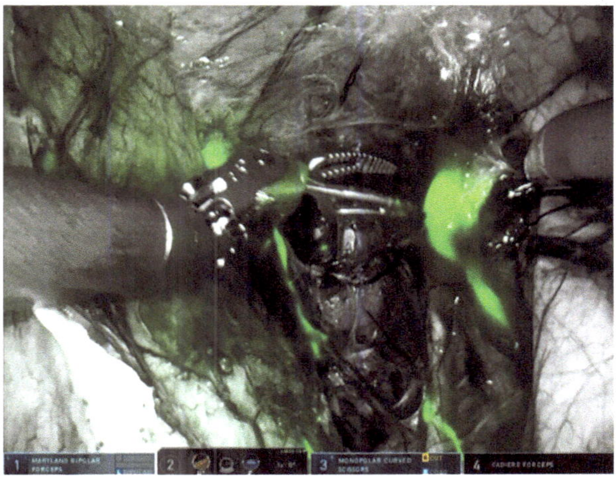

Fig. 11.4 SLN mapping for cervical cancer using robotic surgery

specimen was cut parallel to the longest axis with an interval of 2 mm. After fixation, the 5 μm-thick sections were stained with H&E and examined thereafter.

11.2.5 Morbidity

Recently, the results of the randomized multicenter trial in the treatment of early-stage cervical cancer patients in the SENTICOL II study were reported. The trial compared the effect of an SLN biopsy to that of an SLN biopsy with pelvic lymphadenectomy for patients at stage IA1-IIA1 (FIGO 2009) [39]. The disease-free survival (DFS) rate in the SLN biopsy and the SLN biopsy with pelvic lymphadenectomy groups was 89.5% and 93.1% ($p = 0.53$), respectively, with a mean follow-up duration of 50 months (3–89 months); the overall survival (OS) rates were 95.2% and 96.0% ($p = 0.97$), respectively [39]. Devaja et al. reported the prognosis of 103 stage IA1–IB1 cases (<2 cm) (FIGO 2009) with SLN biopsy without lymphadenectomy [40], and 7 of them (6.7%) had lymph node involvement. No pelvic or paraaortic lymph node recurrence was observed during a median follow-up of 53 months (8–120 months). In the report, the 3-year survival rate was 99.1%, and the 3-year recurrence-free survival (RFS) rate was 97.1%. Furthermore, Lennox et al. reported the survival data of 1188 node-negative stage IA-IB patients (FIGO 2009) with cervical cancer, including 110 cases of SLN biopsy and 1078 cases of lymphadenectomy. No significant difference was observed between SLN biopsy and lymphadenectomy in both the 2- and 5-year RFS rates (97% vs. 95% and 93% vs. 92%, respectively) [41]. In two Japanese single institution studies, Niikura et al. reported that no patients who underwent SLN biopsy without a systemic lymphadenectomy (the intraoperative frozen section identified negative for metastasis) had lymph node recurrence in the pelvic cavity [42]. Yhata et al. reported that patients who underwent SLN biopsy without a systemic lymphadenectomy (the intraoperative frozen section identified negative for metastasis) had only a 2.2% recurrence rate during a median follow-up period of 83.5 months (25–145 months) [43]. These findings suggest that SLN biopsy without a systemic lymphadenectomy seems feasible for patients with early-stage cervical cancer. However, the prospective survival data for SLN biopsy without a lymphadenectomy in those with cervical cancer remain lacking. To date, three prospective clinical trials, SENTIX [44], PHENIX [45], and SENTICOL III [46], which are aimed at evaluating the oncologic outcome of SLN biopsy in early-stage cervical cancer, are ongoing. The PHENIX trial (NCT02642471) is a multicenter, randomized, controlled trial comparing the oncologic outcomes of pelvic lymphadenectomy versus SLN biopsy in patients with (2-year DFS) and without (3-year DFS) SLN metastases. SENTICOL III is a prospective, multicenter, randomized trial designed to compare the 3-year DFS rates of SLN biopsy alone versus SLN biopsy and pelvic lymphadenectomy, and these results demonstrated the safety of omitting a systematic lymph node dissection in sentinel node-negative cases. These results are expected to establish the safety of omitting the procedure altogether.

11.3 Complications of SLN Biopsy

In the SENTICOL-2 study, a comparison of the frequency of complications up to 6 months postoperatively in the sentinel node biopsy-only group showed that it was significantly lower than in the group that underwent a systematic lymph node dissection [47]. As well, the frequency of lymphatic complications and neurological symptoms was significantly lower in the sentinel node biopsy-only group than in the group that underwent a systematic lymph node dissection; however, there was no difference between the two groups in the frequency of lymphedema. In other studies, the sentinel lymph node biopsy-only group had a significantly lower incidence of lymphedema and lymphocysts [42]. In a Japanese study, the sentinel node biopsy-only group had significantly shorter operative time and less intraoperative blood loss than the group that underwent a systematic lymph node dissection [48]. These results suggest that omitting a systematic lymph node dissection for patients with negative sentinel nodes may significantly reduce postoperative complications.

11.3.1 Ultrastaging

Another positive aspect of SLN mapping is the ultrastaging technique, which can increase the diagnosis of small-volume metastases in 19–22% of patients with cervical cancer, compared with routine histopathological processing [36, 49]. In the prospective SENTICOL study, 17 (60.7%) of 28 positive SLN cases presented only micrometastases (size >0.2 mm but ≤2 mm) or isolated tumor cells (ITC) [50]. Thus, ultrastaging can identify small metastatic lesions in a relatively large number of pN1 patients. In addition, an SLN biposy by histological ultrastaging enables the identification of metastases in unexpected anatomical locations that would have been otherwise undetected by a conventional histopathological assessment. Several studies reported that SLN biopsy was detected in areas not usually dissected (0.4–2.9% in the paraaortic and 0.4–1.9% in the presacral region) [34, 40, 51]. These studies demonstrate that SLN biopsy can lead to the excision of micrometastatic lymph nodes in unexpected regions, which may contribute to improved survival rates. A retrospective multicenter study demonstrated that overall survival rates were significantly reduced in patients with macro- and micro-metastasis. However, the presence of ITC was not associated with any significant risk for both RFS and OS [52, 53]. Patients with low-volume metastasis had a similar DFS (92.7%) to node-negative patients (93.6%) in SENTICOL1 and SENTICOL2 studies [53]. The FIGO 2018 classification considers only macro- and micrometastases, but not ITC, to be significant lymph node metastases.

Even if lymph node metastases are identified intraoperatively by a pathological examination of frozen sections, a scheduled radical hysterectomy and conventional lymphadenectomy are performed in Japanese institutions at present. It is debatable whether these procedures are necessary or not. In patients with lymph node metastasis detected intraoperatively, radiation therapy without a systematic lymphadenectomy is an option. Moreover, in cases with micrometastases (or ITCs) limited to the SLN, the efficacy of a hysterectomy and/or complete lymphadenectomy with adjuvant radiation therapy is not clear at present. Further studies are needed to clarify the necessity of a conventional lymphadenectomy and adjuvant therapy in such cases.

11.3.2 OSNA Assay

A one-step nucleic acid amplification (OSNA) assay, which is based on the RT loop- mediated isothermal amplification (RT-LAMP) technique, has been developed. The OSNA assay involves quantifying the number of cytokeratin-19 (CK19) mRNA copies [54, 55], without the requirement of RNA extraction, and allows for the simple and rapid (30–40 min) amplification of target genes. Since OSNA can screen the whole lymph node, it can also detect micrometastases localized within the nodes themselves. The effectiveness of the OSNA assay for many malignancies has been described [56–59]. In a multicenter study in Japan, the concordance rate between the OSNA assay and a histological examination, sensitivity, and specificity were 96.4% (95% CI: 92.7–98.5%), 90.3% (95% CI: 74.2–98.0%), and 97.6%

(95% CI: 93.8–99.4%) in cervical cancer, respectively [60]. However, previous studies have reported a 0–2.2% metastasis contamination rate caused by benign epithelial lesions, such as endosalpingiosis in the lymph nodes, and this may contribute to false-positive results in the OSNA assay. Hence, such cases should be treated with caution [61–63]. These findings suggest that the OSNA assay has an equivalent diagnostic ability for lymph node metastasis as a conventional histopathological examination of 2-mm interval slices of the lymph nodes in cervical cancer patients. As well, the OSNA assay might be a useful method for lymph node metastasis diagnosis in patients with cervical cancer.

11.4 Future and Prospect

Compared with systemic lymphadenectomy, SLN biopsy appears to be feasible for detecting lymph node metastasis in patients with early-stage cervical cancer. SLN without a systematic lymphadenectomy is a safe treatment modality for early-stage cervical cancer with a tumor size ≤2 cm. Compared with the open surgery, minimally invasive procedures have excellent potential in detecting SLNs in patients with early cervical cancer. The acceptance of SLN biopsy in gynecological cancer has become a recent trend worldwide. The LACC trial reported in 2018 has validated the problems with minimally invasive procedures for cervical cancer, reporting that laparoscopic total hysterectomy for cervical cancer has a higher recurrence rate than open surgery. At present, the standard technique is open surgery. However, in a recent meta-analysis, there are no differences in the rate or the pattern of relapse between the minimally invasive radical hysterectomy and open surgery in patients with stage IB1 cervical cancer and a tumor size under 2 cm [64]. SLN biopsy without a systematic lymphadenectomy is a safe treatment modality for early-stage cervical cancer and a tumor size ≤2 cm. We believe that the SLN biopsy using the laparoscopic or robotic radical hysterectomy, which can reduce surgical morbidities such as intraoperative blood loss and lower the risk of postoperative complications compared with open surgery, is well suited. Further prospective studies would be required for positive proof. Moreover, the three ongoing prospective studies previously mentioned will offer decisive data that will definitively validate SLN biopsy for lymph node staging in early-stage cervical cancer.

References

1. Sung H, et al. Global cancer statistics 2020: GLOBOCAN estimates of incidence and mortality worldwide for 36 cancers in 185 countries. CA Cancer J Clin. 2021;71(3):209–49.
2. Kim SM, Choi HS, Byun JS. Overall 5-year survival rate and prognostic factors in patients with stage IB and IIA cervical cancer treated by radical hysterectomy and pelvic lymph node dissection. Int J Gynecol Cancer. 2000;10(4):305–12.
3. Sakuragi N. Up-to-date management of lymph node metastasis and the role of tailored lymphadenectomy in cervical cancer. Int J Clin Oncol. 2007;12(3):165–75.

4. Kim SI, et al. Impact of lower limb lymphedema on quality of life in gynecologic cancer survivors after pelvic lymph node dissection. Eur J Obstet Gynecol Reprod Biol. 2015;192:31–6.
5. Carlson JW, et al. GOG 244-the lymphedema and gynecologic cancer (LEG) study: incidence and risk factors in newly diagnosed patients. Gynecol Oncol. 2020;156(2):467–74.
6. Cabanas RM. An approach for the treatment of penile carcinoma. Cancer. 1977;39(2):456–66.
7. Lyman GH, et al. American Society of Clinical Oncology guideline recommendations for sentinel lymph node biopsy in early-stage breast cancer. J Clin Oncol. 2005;23(30):7703–20.
8. Morton DL, et al. Sentinel-node biopsy or nodal observation in melanoma. N Engl J Med. 2006;355(13):1307–17.
9. Van der Zee AG, et al. Sentinel node dissection is safe in the treatment of early-stage vulvar cancer. J Clin Oncol. 2008;26(6):884–9.
10. Echt ML, et al. Detection of sentinel lymph nodes with lymphazurin in cervical, uterine, and vulvar malignancies. South Med J. 1999;92(2):204–8.
11. Koh WJ, et al. Cervical cancer, version 2.2015. J Natl Compr Cancer Netw. 2015;13(4): 395–404; quiz 404.
12. Togami S, et al. Survey of the clinical practice pattern of using sentinel lymph node biopsy in patients with gynecological cancers in Japan: the Japan Society of Gynecologic Oncology study. Int J Clin Oncol. 2021;26(5):971–9.
13. Beavis AL, et al. Sentinel lymph node detection rates using indocyanine green in women with early-stage cervical cancer. Gynecol Oncol. 2016;143(2):302–6.
14. Buda A, et al. Impact of indocyanine green for sentinel lymph node mapping in early stage endometrial and cervical cancer: comparison with conventional radiotracer (99m)Tc and/or blue dye. Ann Surg Oncol. 2016;23(7):2183–91.
15. Martínez-Palones JM, et al. Intraoperative sentinel node identification in early stage cervical cancer using a combination of radiolabeled albumin injection and isosulfan blue dye injection. Gynecol Oncol. 2004;92(3):845–50.
16. Wang L, et al. Sentinel lymph node mapping in early-stage cervical cancer: meta-analysis. Medicine (Baltimore). 2021;100(34):e27035.
17. Persson J, et al. Description of a reproducible anatomically based surgical algorithm for detection of pelvic sentinel lymph nodes in endometrial cancer. Gynecol Oncol. 2017;147(1):120–5.
18. Benedetti-Panici P, et al. Early cervical carcinoma: the natural history of lymph node involvement redefined on the basis of thorough parametrectomy and giant section study. Cancer. 2000;88(10):2267–74.
19. Girardi F, et al. The importance of parametrial lymph nodes in the treatment of cervical cancer. Gynecol Oncol. 1989;34(2):206–11.
20. Rossi EC, Ivanova A, Boggess JF. Robotically assisted fluorescence-guided lymph node mapping with ICG for gynecologic malignancies: a feasibility study. Gynecol Oncol. 2012;124(1):78–82.
21. Lührs O, et al. Combining indocyanine green and Tc(99)-nanocolloid does not increase the detection rate of sentinel lymph nodes in early stage cervical cancer compared to indocyanine green alone. Gynecol Oncol. 2020;156(2):335–40.
22. Frumovitz M, et al. Near-infrared fluorescence for detection of sentinel lymph nodes in women with cervical and uterine cancers (FILM): a randomised, phase 3, multicentre, non-inferiority trial. Lancet Oncol. 2018;19(10):1394–403.
23. Kadkhodayan S, et al. Sentinel node biopsy for lymph nodal staging of uterine cervix cancer: a systematic review and meta-analysis of the pertinent literature. Eur J Surg Oncol. 2015;41(1):1–20.
24. Wang XJ, Fang F, Li YF. Sentinel-lymph-node procedures in early stage cervical cancer: a systematic review and meta-analysis. Med Oncol. 2015;32(1):385.
25. Wu Y, et al. Sentinel lymph node biopsy in cervical cancer: a meta-analysis. Mol Clin Oncol. 2013;1(6):1025–30.
26. Tanaka T, et al. The detection of sentinel lymph nodes in laparoscopic surgery for uterine cervical cancer using 99m-technetium-tin colloid, indocyanine green, and blue dye. J Gynecol Oncol. 2017;28(2):e13.

27. Geppert B, et al. A study on uterine lymphatic anatomy for standardization of pelvic sentinel lymph node detection in endometrial cancer. Gynecol Oncol. 2017;145(2):256–61.
28. Bollino M, et al. Pelvic sentinel lymph node biopsy in endometrial cancer-a simplified algorithm based on histology and lymphatic anatomy. Int J Gynecol Cancer. 2020;30(3):339–45.
29. Bonneau C, et al. Lymphatic and nerve distribution throughout the parametrium. Gynecol Oncol. 2013;131(3):708–13.
30. Lührs O, et al. Similar distribution of pelvic sentinel lymph nodes and nodal metastases in cervical and endometrial cancer. A prospective study based on lymphatic anatomy. Gynecol Oncol. 2022;165(3):466–71.
31. Ouldamer L, et al. Unusual localizations of sentinel lymph nodes in early stage cervical cancer: a review. Surg Oncol. 2012;21(3):e153–7.
32. Balaya V, et al. Predictive factors of unexpected lymphatic drainage pathways in early-stage cervical cancer. Gynecol Oncol. 2019;154(1):102–9.
33. Balaya V, et al. Risk factors for failure of bilateral sentinel lymph node mapping in early-stage cervical cancer. Gynecol Oncol. 2020;156(1):93–9.
34. Kim JH, et al. The efficacy of sentinel lymph node mapping with indocyanine green in cervical cancer. World J Surg Oncol. 2018;16(1):52.
35. Leijte JA, et al. Visualization of tumor blockage and rerouting of lymphatic drainage in penile cancer patients by use of SPECT/CT. J Nucl Med. 2009;50(3):364–7.
36. Salvo G, et al. Sensitivity and negative predictive value for sentinel lymph node biopsy in women with early-stage cervical cancer. Gynecol Oncol. 2017;145(1):96–101.
37. Abu-Rustum NR, Khoury-Collado F, Gemignani ML. Techniques of sentinel lymph node identification for early-stage cervical and uterine cancer. Gynecol Oncol. 2008;111(2 Suppl):S44–50.
38. Eiriksson LR, Covens A. Sentinel lymph node mapping in cervical cancer: the future? BJOG. 2012;119(2):129–33.
39. Favre G, et al. Sentinel lymph-node biopsy in early-stage cervical cancer: the 4-year follow-up results of the senticol 2 trial. Front Oncol. 2020;10:621518.
40. Devaja O, et al. Sentinel lymph node biopsy alone in the management of early cervical carcinoma. Int J Gynecol Cancer. 2022;32(1):15–20.
41. Lennox GK, Covens A. Can sentinel lymph node biopsy replace pelvic lymphadenectomy for early cervical cancer? Gynecol Oncol. 2017;144(1):16–20.
42. Niikura H, et al. Prospective study of sentinel lymph node biopsy without further pelvic lymphadenectomy in patients with sentinel lymph node-negative cervical cancer. Int J Gynecol Cancer. 2012;22(7):1244–50.
43. Yahata H, et al. Long-term follow up after sentinel node biopsy alone for early-stage cervical cancer. Gynecol Oncol. 2022;165(1):149–54.
44. Cibula D, et al. A prospective multicenter trial on sentinel lymph node biopsy in patients with early-stage cervical cancer (SENTIX). Int J Gynecol Cancer. 2019;29(1):212–5.
45. Tu H, et al. Sentinel lymph node biopsy versus pelvic lymphadenectomy in early-stage cervical cancer: a multi-center randomized trial (PHENIX/CSEM 010). Int J Gynecol Cancer. 2020;30(11):1829–33.
46. Lecuru FR, et al. SENTICOL III: an international validation study of sentinel node biopsy in early cervical cancer. A GINECO, ENGOT, GCIG and multicenter study. Int J Gynecol Cancer. 2019;29(4):829–34.
47. Mathevet P, et al. Sentinel lymph node biopsy and morbidity outcomes in early cervical cancer: results of a multicentre randomised trial (SENTICOL-2). Eur J Cancer. 2021;148:307–15.
48. Yahata H, et al. Prognostic outcome and complications of sentinel lymph node navigation surgery for early-stage cervical cancer. Int J Clin Oncol. 2018;23(6):1167–72.
49. Devaja O, et al. A prospective single-center study of sentinel lymph node detection in cervical carcinoma: is there a place in clinical practice? Int J Gynecol Cancer. 2012;22(6):1044–9.
50. Bats AS, et al. The sentinel node technique detects unexpected drainage pathways and allows nodal ultrastaging in early cervical cancer: insights from the multicenter prospective SENTICOL study. Ann Surg Oncol. 2013;20(2):413–22.

51. Wuntakal R, et al. Location of sentinel lymph node in cervical carcinoma and factors associated with unilateral detection. Int J Gynecol Cancer. 2015;25(9):1663–8.
52. Nica A, et al. Does small volume metastatic lymph node disease affect long-term prognosis in early cervical cancer? Int J Gynecol Cancer. 2020;30(3):285–90.
53. Guani B, et al. The clinical impact of low-volume lymph nodal metastases in early-stage cervical cancer: the senticol 1 and senticol 2 trials. Cancers (Basel). 2020;12(5):1061.
54. Notomi T, et al. Loop-mediated isothermal amplification of DNA. Nucleic Acids Res. 2000;28(12):E63.
55. Tsujimoto M, et al. One-step nucleic acid amplification for intraoperative detection of lymph node metastasis in breast cancer patients. Clin Cancer Res. 2007;13(16):4807–16.
56. Creasman WT, et al. Surgical pathologic spread patterns of endometrial cancer. A gynecologic oncology group study. Cancer. 1987;60(8 Suppl):2035–41.
57. Kumagai K, et al. Multicenter study evaluating the clinical performance of the OSNA assay for the molecular detection of lymph node metastases in gastric cancer patients. Gastric Cancer. 2014;17(2):273–80.
58. Medas F, et al. Evaluation of accuracy of one-step nucleic acid amplification (OSNA) in diagnosis of lymph node metastases of papillary thyroid carcinoma. Diagnostic study. Ann Med Surg (Lond). 2019;46:17–22.
59. Shi F, et al. One-step nucleic acid amplification assay is an accurate technique for sentinel lymph node biopsy of breast cancer patients: a meta-analysis. Br J Cancer. 2017;117(8):1185–91.
60. Togami S, et al. Evaluation of the one-step nucleic acid amplification assay for detecting lymph node metastasis in patients with cervical and endometrial cancer: a multicenter prospective study. Gynecol Oncol. 2023;170:70–6.
61. Fanfani F, et al. One-step nucleic acid amplification (OSNA): a fast molecular test based on CK19 mRNA concentration for assessment of lymph-nodes metastases in early stage endometrial cancer. PLoS One. 2018;13(4):e0195877.
62. Kosťun J, et al. One-step nucleic acid amplification vs ultrastaging in the detection of sentinel lymph node metastasis in endometrial cancer patients. J Surg Oncol. 2019;119(3):361–9.
63. López-Ruiz ME, et al. One-step nucleic acid amplification (OSNA) for the detection of sentinel lymph node metastasis in endometrial cancer. Gynecol Oncol. 2016;143(1):54–9.
64. Manzour N, et al. Pattern of relapse in patients with stage IB1 cervical cancer after radical hysterectomy as primary treatment. Minimally invasive surgery vs. open approach. Systematic review and meta-analysis. Gynecol Oncol. 2022;164(2):455–60.

Part V

Multimodal Therapy for Cervical Cancer

Radiological Treatment of Cervical Cancer

12

Takashi Uno

Abstract

Radiation therapy is a definitive treatment for the uterine cervical cancer, and the treatment results are equivalent to those of surgery in stage IB1-II patients. Radiation therapy is also curative for patients with stage III or more advanced disease for whom surgery is not indicated. In addition, postoperative radiation therapy is performed when risk factors for recurrence are confirmed by histopathological examination after surgery. Concurrent chemoradiotherapy with cisplatin and other drugs is recommended for most patients except in the early stages. Standard radiation therapy is a combination of external beam radiation therapy and brachytherapy. External beam radiation therapy is followed by intracavitary brachytherapy, which is initiated when the primary tumor has shrunk to the extent within the high-dose area of brachytherapy. Postoperative radiation therapy is mainly performed with external beam radiation therapy alone, but intracavitary brachytherapy may be added when vaginal surgical margins are positive. External beam radiation therapy techniques such as intensity-modulated radiation therapy have been introduced, and image-guided brachytherapy has become the standard for brachytherapy. These techniques have made it possible to deliver higher doses that better conform the shape of the tumor and reduce the dose to risk organs and are further improving treatment outcomes.

Keywords

Radiation therapy · Brachytherapy · Chemoradiotherapy · Intensity-modulated radiation therapy · Image-guided brachytherapy

T. Uno (✉)
Diagnostic Radiology and Radiation Oncology, Graduate School of Medicine, Chiba University, Chiba, Japan
e-mail: unotakas@faculty.chiba-u.jp

D. Aoki (ed.), *Recent Topics on Prevention, Diagnosis, and Clinical Management of Cervical Cancer*, Comprehensive Gynecology and Obstetrics,
https://doi.org/10.1007/978-981-99-9396-3_12

12.1 Treatment Strategy

Definitive radiation therapy is indicated from stage IB1 to stage IVA (Table 12.1) [1]. Radiation therapy alone is recommended for stage I–II squamous cell carcinomas 4 cm or smaller. In a prospective, multicenter study conducted in Japan, the 2-year overall survival rate and 2-year recurrence-free survival rate for these patients treated with radiation therapy alone were very good (95% and 90%, respectively) [2]. Several randomized controlled trials (RCTs) have shown that concurrent chemoradiotherapy (CCRT) improves survival compared with radiation therapy alone in cases of locally advanced disease such as stages IIB to IVA, early stage with tumor size >4 cm (stages IB3 and IIA2), or positive pelvic lymph nodes [3]. In addition, concurrent chemoradiation therapy is recommended for stage I–II postoperative patients at high risk of recurrence [4].

The standard chemotherapy regimen for CCRT is 5–6 courses of weekly cisplatin (40 mg/m^2). The combination of high-dose cisplatin and 5FU (administered at 3- to 4-week intervals) is another regimen that has been shown to improve survival in randomized controlled trials. Other clinical trials of CCRT with various chemotherapy regimens have been conducted. A meta-analysis based on individual patient data showed that CCRT improved 5-year overall survival by 6% in all patients [3]. Recently, a large difference in survival has been demonstrated even in advanced cases such as IIIB [5]. CCRT has not been shown to increase late toxicity such as bladder or rectal bleeding compared with radiation therapy alone.

12.2 Radiation Therapy

Standard curative radiation therapy for cervical cancer is a combination of external beam radiation therapy and intracavitary brachytherapy. Usually, external beam radiation therapy is followed by intracavitary irradiation when the primary tumor has shrunk to the extent that it can be contained within the high-dose area of brachytherapy. Intracavitary irradiation is performed once or twice a week using a high-dose-rate remotely controlled after-loading intracavitary treatment device. When external beam radiation therapy is not sufficient to shrink the tumor, or when intracavitary irradiation cannot be performed due to difficulty in applicator insertion, additional irradiation may be performed using interstitial brachytherapy or external

Table 12.1 Radiological treatment by FIGO stage

FIGO stage[a]	Radiological treatment
• IB1–2, IIA1 (SqCC)	Radiation therapy alone
• IB3, IIA2 (SqCC) • I–II (adeno) • IIB, IIIA-C, IVA • I–II high-risk after surgery	Concurrent chemoradiation

[a]The International Federation of Gynaecology and Obstetrics (FIGO) staging of cancer of the cervix uteri (2018)

beam radiation therapy. However, the use of high-precision external irradiation as an alternative to brachytherapy is not recommended because it leads to poor outcomes [6]. Postoperative irradiation is mainly performed by external beam radiation therapy alone, but intracavitary irradiation may be added when vaginal surgical margins are positive.

12.2.1 External Beam Radiation Therapy

12.2.1.1 Target Volume

In radiation therapy, the gross tumor volume (GTV) is defined as the area of the primary tumor and enlarged pelvic lymph nodes that are visually, palpably, or radiographically evident. The clinical target volume (CTV) is defined as the area of microscopically suspected tumor invasion surrounding the GTV or pelvic lymph node area. The internal target volume (ITV) is defined in consideration of respiratory movement of the CTV, and the planning target volume (PTV) is defined as the target volume to which a setup margin is added to ensure that sufficient physical dose is delivered to the CTV. Around the GTV and CTV, organs at risk (OAR), such as rectum, sigmoid colon, small intestine, and bladder are defined as normal tissues that should be avoided irradiation as much as possible. In the past, whole pelvis irradiation was performed using the bone structure as a marker. A four-field "box" technique was used, where the anterior and posterior fields incorporate an upper border at the level of L4–5 interspace and an inferior border placed at the mid to lower obturator foramina or at least 3 cm below the lowest extent of clinically determined cervical or vaginal disease, and lateral borders are placed 1.5–2.0 cm beyond the bony margins of the true pelvis. The anterior border of lateral fields generally placed in front of symphysis pubis and the posterior border should carefully be determined to cover the presacral area without shielding tumors extending posteriorly along with the uterosacral ligaments. However, nowadays 3D treatment planning is performed by defining the GTV and CTV on the image, setting the PTV, creating a 3D dose distribution, and evaluating the dose-volume histogram (DVH) of the target and OARs. The PTV must be set with a certain margin around the CTV, but the size of this margin depends on the accuracy of each treatment due to breathing movements, differences in body position, the skill of the treating personnel, and the performance of each treatment device. In radiotherapy planning for cervical cancer, GTV is determined based on physical gynecological examination, CT, MRI T2-weighted images, FDG-PET findings, etc. CTV is the whole pelvic region including GTV, the whole uterine body, the proximal vagina and parametria, and the pelvic lymph node area (the external iliac, internal iliac, obturator, common iliac and presacral nodes). When there is clinically apparent para-aortic lymph node metastases or imaging findings strongly suspecting metastases are found on CT and/or PET-CT, an extended-field irradiation including the para-aortic lymph node area up to the renal vessels or even more cephalad is used.

Image-guided radiation therapy (IGRT), in which the position of irradiation is checked and corrected on the treatment couch just before each treatment session using a diagnostic imaging system installed in the treatment room, is now widely used. IGRT improves the reproducibility of each radiation treatment and reduces the setup margin. The reduction of the margin added to the CTV for PTV setting can reduce the dose to the OAR and even increase the dose to the CTV.

12.2.1.2 Dose Prescription

Generally, radiation therapy with high-energy X-rays of 6 MV or higher is performed using a linear accelerator. It is recommended to avoid OAR as much as possible by using customized multiple fields of irradiation. The treatment is delivered at 1.8–2 Gy once a day, 5 times a week for about 5 weeks. The total dose should be 45–50 Gy. In Japan, a central shield is generally inserted during external beam irradiation and an additional dose of 5–10 Gy may be added when there is a large lesion in the parametrium, such as primary tumor in stage IIIB cases. Recently, simultaneous integrated boost (SIB) irradiation using intensity-modulated radiotherapy, described below, has been used to irradiate the entire pelvic region with 45–50 Gy, and at the same time, a higher dose of 10–20 Gy is given to the enlarged lymph nodes.

12.2.1.3 Intensity-Modulated Radiation Therapy

Intensity-modulated radiation therapy (IMRT) is a highly complex treatment using advanced technology and is possible only in facilities that meet certain institutional standards for equipment and personnel. The target or OAR is carefully defined on the image, the dose to be administered to the target volume is prescribed, and DVH parameters meeting the dose constraint (the acceptable dose to a certain volume) of OARs are specified. The computer generates a plan to irradiate beams with spatially and temporally non-uniform radiation intensity from multiple directions to fulfill these conditions through inverse planning. This allows dose distribution that matches the geometry of the target volume and dose reduction to the OAR to be achieved. In conventional pelvic irradiation, OARs such as the rectum, bladder, and bone marrow receive almost same dose as the target. IMRT can reduce the dose to these OARs compared with conventional pelvic irradiation, such as four-field box irradiation, and thus reduces the incidence of acute and late adverse events. The use of IMRT has been standardized in the postoperative setting. IMRT allows greater sparing of normal tissues, especially the small bowel displaced into the pelvis after surgery and is reported to reduce the incidence of acute and late adverse events [7–9]. IMRT for intact cervical cancer requires careful attention to give wide margins to ensure full coverage of primary tumor. Inter- and intra-fractional target mobility, deformation, and tumor regression during a course of radiation therapy are of great concern in this setting. Recently, IMRT is increasingly used for external irradiation in definitive radiation therapy for cervical cancer. In the prospective EMBRACE II study for advanced cervical cancer, the most advanced radiation techniques currently available for cervix cancer treatment are applied including MRI guided adaptive IMRT for external beam radiotherapy with SIB to nodal disease [10]. The SIB method using IMRT can achieve a dose of 40–45 Gy to the entire pelvic region while at the same time delivering a higher dose of 10–20 Gy to the enlarged lymph nodes. In treatment planning, it is necessary to accurately delineate targets and risk

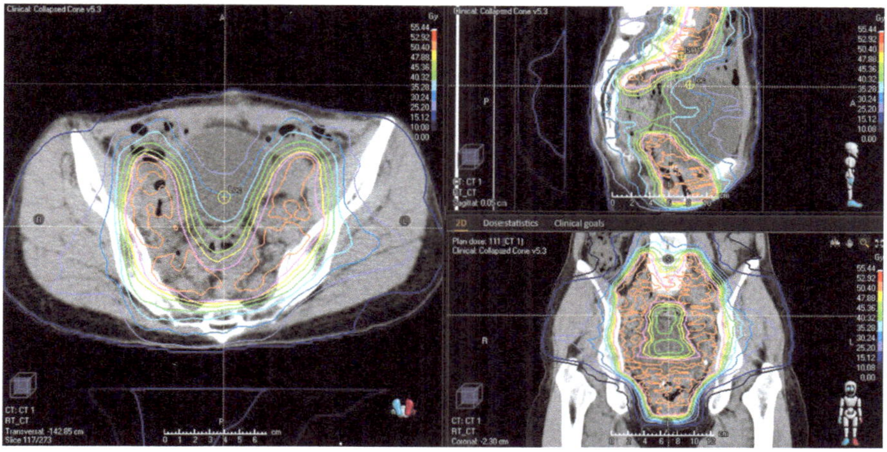

Fig. 12.1 Dose distribution in intensity-modulated radiation therapy (IMRT). Dose distribution of IMRT for postoperative pelvic irradiation of cervical cancer (bladder, obturator lymph node level). The dose to the clinical target volume (lymph node area) is sufficient, while the dose to risk organs such as the bladder and gastrointestinal tract is reduced

organs, and ideally, there should be no variation in these settings among treatment planners at different institutions or even within an institution. Guidelines for CTV setting for pelvic irradiation by IMRT for cervical cancer have been published and recently updated [11]. Figure 12.1 shows an example of dose distribution in a case of postoperative IMRT for cervical cancer.

12.2.2 Brachytherapy

Intracavitary irradiation is usually performed with a combination of a tandem applicator that is placed in the uterine cavity and an ovoid applicator positioned in vaginal fornix. Tandem and vaginal cylinders may be used in cases of severe vaginal invasion or in narrow vaginal cases. The remote after-loading system (RALS) is currently used for high-dose rate intracavitary irradiation in most centers worldwide. It is recommended that adequate preparation, such as the administration of analgesics and sedatives, be performed prior to the insertion of the applicator to reduce the patient's pain. It is also important to optimize the placement of the applicator to accomplish the dose to the tumor and to reduce the dose to the bladder, rectum, and other parts of the OAR by relieving the patient's pain and local tension. In the past, two-dimensional treatment planning was performed by taking anteroposterior and lateral radiographs after the applicator was inserted and then setting and evaluating the dose at the point A and the bladder/rectal evaluation points [12]. It was relatively simple and had clinical usefulness, as it showed some correlation between the point A dose and local control and between the rectal evaluation dose and the onset of late effects. However, it was considered extremely inadequate as today's medical technology because it did not depict actual tumors or organs, making it difficult to individualize treatment, and important treatment planning parameters such as DVH of tumors and risk organs were not available. Recently, a technique called image-guided brachytherapy (IGBT), in which MRI or CT is taken with the applicator inserted, the target volume and risk organs are defined, and three-dimensional treatment planning is performed in the same manner as external beam radiation therapy [13], is performed at many facilities. The applicator, tumor, and risk organs are visualized, and it is now possible to administer higher doses conforming the shape of the tumor and reduce the dose to OARs for each treatment.

When conventional tandem/ovoid applicators alone cannot adequately cover the extent of tumor extension, intracavitary irradiation with interstitial irradiation (IC/IS hybrid therapy) is also performed, in which separate needles are added (Fig. 12.2). Recently, applicators with a template function for inserting a needle for interstitial irradiation through the ovoids are commercially available. The direction and angle of the needle to be inserted are determined for each hole drilled in the half-moon shaped ovoids, making it possible to place interstitial needles in the desired location easily. A template-based interstitial brachytherapy is useful in specific clinical situations [14, 15]. Indications include patients with large residual disease after external beam radiation therapy, vaginal extension, anatomical distortion such as a narrow vagina or an obliterated endocervical canal, a prior supracervical hysterectomy, or recurrent tumor after radical hysterectomy. It is technically important to place a tandem with the interstitial implant, rather than just needles alone, in case other than post-hysterectomy.

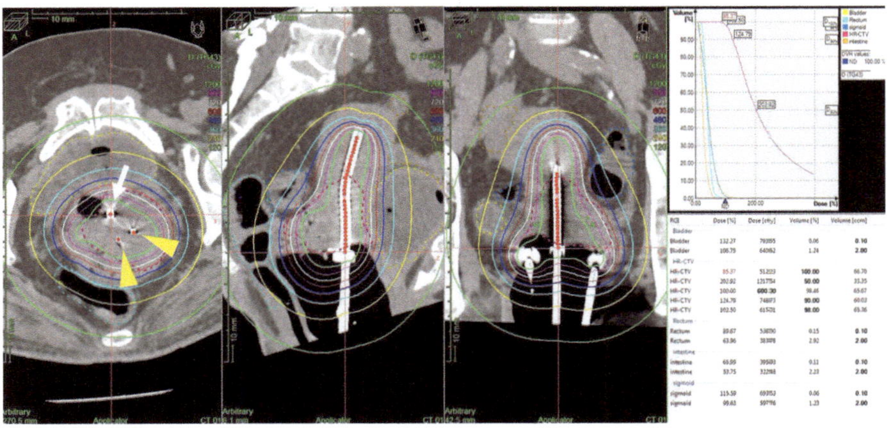

Fig. 12.2 Dose distribution in IC/IS hybrid therapy (intracavitary irradiation with interstitial irradiation). By adding two interstitial needles (yellow arrowheads) to intracavitary irradiation using tandem applicators (white arrows) and ovoid applicators, the area of tumor extension is covered while avoiding the rectum (light blue dotted line) and transverse colon (blue dotted line), and high-risk CTV (red dotted line) is included in the high-dose zone. HR-CTV D90 = 7.4 Gy, D98 = 6.1 Gy, and rectal D2cc = 2.9 Gy have been achieved by adding interstitial needles for large tumors

In patients with positive or close vaginal surgical margins after hysterectomy, vaginal brachytherapy using vaginal cylinder may be added as a boost to external beam radiation therapy. The dose prescription is usually to the vaginal surface or at 5 mm below the vaginal surface. Typical fractionation schedules include fractional dose of 5–6 Gy to the total of 10–12 Gy. In this treatment, CT or MRI based IGBT allows assessment of the placement of vaginal cylinder including the conformality of the vaginal surface to the applicator (especially at the vaginal apex) and the relationship to the OAR. It should be noted that an air gap between the applicator and the vaginal wall leads to a dose reduction to the target.

In IGBT, the dose to the tumor is evaluated using the dose (D90) to high-risk CTV (HR-CTV), which includes the entire cervix and the area suspected of having residual tumor in the primary tumor at the time of intracavitary irradiation as depicted by the MRI T2-weighted image. CT cannot accurately identify the upper margin of a cervical tumor. CT also provides inadequate contrast between the tumor and connective tissue in the pararectal tissue. Therefore, the contour of the tumor determined by CT tends to be larger than the contour determined by MR. The rectum, sigmoid colon, bladder, small intestine, and vagina are included as OARs, and the respective doses are evaluated using D2cc and others. Recently, favorable outcomes with IGBT [16] and indices of DVH parameters that correlate with prognosis and disorder development are also being demonstrated [17, 18]. For brachytherapy, a fractional dose of 7 Gy or more is recommended for D90 of the high-risk CTV. The linear-quadratic (LQ) model provides calculation estimates of biologically equivalent dose considering fractional dose of IGBT. The LQ model doses are normalized to an equivalent dose in 2 Gy (EQD2), where α/β ratio of 10 Gy is used for tumor and 3 Gy for normal tissues such as the rectum and bladder. The goals of total combined EQD2 for D90 of HR-CTV are 80–85 Gy and 87 Gy or higher for those with large tumors. EQD2 is recommended up to 65–70 Gy for D2cc in the rectum and 80–90 Gy for D2cc in the bladder. The total dose of external beam radiation therapy, the prescribed dose for high-risk CTV, and the dose parameters for the rectum and bladder recommended in 3D-IGBT in Japan are shown in Table 12.2.

Table 12.2 Recommended dose parameters for 3D-IGBT in Japan

	EBRT dose	Center block	HR-CTV D90	Rectum D2cc	Bladder D2cc
IB1–2	50 Gy	–	>7 Gy × 4	<6.5 Gy × 4	8 Gy × 4
<3- (4) cm	20 Gy	30 Gy			
IB3, IIA2	50 Gy	–	>7 Gy × 4	<6 Gy × 4	7 Gy × 4
IIB	30 Gy	20 Gy			
IIIB-IVA	45–50 Gy	–	>7 Gy × 4	<5 Gy × 4	6.3 Gy × 4
>5 cm[a]	40 Gy	10 Gy			

[a]Intracavitary irradiation with interstitial irradiation (hybrid therapy) is recommended

12.3 Prognosis

When standard definitive radiation therapy is performed, the 5-year survival rates by FIGO clinical stage are reported as follows: stage I: 80–90%, stage II: 70–80%, stage III: 50–70%, and stage IVA: 30–50%. A multicenter prospective clinical trial using the standard treatment schedule in Japan has confirmed the efficacy and safety of radiotherapy alone in the two-dimensional treatment for stage I–II (<4 cm) squamous cell carcinoma of the cervix. At 2 years, 96% pelvic control rate and 95% overall survival rate have been achieved [2]. Results of a multicenter prospective clinical trial of concurrent chemoradiotherapy for stage III–IVA using the standard treatment schedule in Japan are reported: at 2 years, progression-free survival rate was 66%, pelvic disease progression-free rate was 85% for tumors <5 cm, 72% for 5–7 cm, and 54% for >7 cm. The large tumor size limits the outcomes in the pre-IGBT era [19]. According to the recent RetroEMBRACE study, the 5-year local control was 98% for stage IB, 91% for stage IIB, and 75% for stage IIIB. The 5-year overall survival was 83% for stage IB, 70% for stage IIB, and 47% for stage IIIB [16]. The use of IC/IS increases D90 of HR-CTV and significantly improves the therapeutic ratio in locally advanced tumor with a HR-CTV volume equal to or more than 30 cm^3 [20]. In the 80 cases treated by Ohno et al. who incorporated 3D-IGBT earlier, local control exceeded 90% at 5 years, and the 5-year survival rate for stages III-IVA also exceeded 70%. In addition, there was only one case of grade 3 or higher late adverse event, urinary tract disorder [21]. Factors that influence prognosis include stage, tumor size, lymph node metastasis, parametrial invasion, stromal invasion, lymph-vascular space invasion, anemia, histologic types, and dose-volume parameters in radiation therapy. Recently, several artificial intelligence based prognostic analyses using MR images have been reported [22, 23].

12.4 Adverse Effects

Acute adverse events include nausea, decreased appetite, diarrhea, cystitis, dermatitis, and leukopenia. These are generally enhanced by concurrent chemotherapy but resolve mildly after treatment. During intracavitary irradiation, vaginal lacerations and perforation of the uterus caused by treatment procedures such as applicator insertion and packing are rarely encountered. Late adverse events include proctitis (bleeding), cystitis (bleeding, frequent urination), bladder atrophy, small bowel problems (abdominal pain, bowel obstruction), vaginitis (adhesions, bleeding, atrophy/stenosis), fistula formation, and bone fractures. Although no exacerbation of these symptoms with concurrent chemotherapy has been demonstrated, postoperative radiation therapy is associated with an increased risk of small bowel injury and lower extremity edema. Recently, IGBT has demonstrated DVH parameters associated with the development of failure, and the frequency of late adverse events is lower than in the past. The introduction of new techniques such as IMRT and IGBT in radiation therapy for cervical cancer is expected to further reduce adverse events.

References

1. NCCN guidelines version 1.2023 cervical cancer. National Comprehensive Cancer Network. https://www.nccn.org/professionals/physician_gls/pdf/cervical.pdf. Accessed 30 Jan 2023.
2. Toita T, Kato S, Niibe Y, et al. Prospective multi-institutional study of definitive radiotherapy with high-dose-rate intracavitary brachytherapy in patients with nonbulky (<4-cm) stage I and II uterine cervical cancer (JAROG0401/JROSG04-2). Int J Radiat Oncol Biol Phys. 2012;82:e49–56. https://doi.org/10.1016/j.ijrobp.2011.01.022.
3. Chemoradiotherapy for Cervical Cancer Meta-Analysis Collaboration. Reducing uncertainties about the effects of chemoradiotherapy for cervical cancer: a systematic review and meta-analysis of individual patient data from 18 randomized trials. J Clin Oncol. 2008;26:5802–12.
4. Peters WA III, Liu PY, Barrett RJ II, et al. Concurrent chemotherapy and pelvic radiation therapy compared with pelvic radiation therapy alone as adjuvant therapy after radical surgery in high-risk early-stage cancer of the cervix. J Clin Oncol. 2000;18:1606–0613. https://doi.org/10.1200/JCO.2000.18.8.1606.
5. Shirvastava S, Mahantshetty U, Engineer R, et al. Cisplatin chemoradiotherapy vs radiotherapy in FIGO stage IIIB squamous cell carcinoma of the uterine cervix: a randomized clinical trial. JAMA Oncol. 2018;4:506–13; https://jamanetwork.com/journals/jamaoncology/fullarticle/2671607.
6. Gill BS, Lin JF, Krivak TC, et al. National cancer data base analysis of radiation therapy consolidation modality for cervical cancer: the impact of new technological advancements. Int J Radiat Oncol Biol Phys. 2014;90:1083–90. https://doi.org/10.1016/j.ijrobp.2014.07.017.
7. Mundt AJ, Mell LK, Roeske JC. Preliminary analysis of chronic gastrointestinal toxicity in gynecology patients treated with intensity-modulated whole pelvic radiation therapy. Int J Radiat Oncol Biol Phys. 2003;56:1354–60. https://doi.org/10.1016/S0360-3016(03)00325-0.
8. Ahamad A, D'Souza W, Salehpour M, et al. Intensity-modulated radiation therapy after hysterectomy: comparison with conventional treatment and sensitivity of the normal-tissue-sparing effect to margin size. Int J Radiat Oncol Biol Phys. 2005;62:1117–24. https://doi.org/10.1016/j.ijrobp.2004.12.029.
9. Lin AJ, Kidd E, Dehdashti F, et al. Intensity modulated radiation therapy and image-guided adapted brachytherapy for cervix cancer. Int J Radiat Oncol Biol Phys. 2019;103:1088–97. https://doi.org/10.1016/j.ijrobp.2018.11.012.
10. Pötter R, Tanderup K, Kirisits C, et al. The EMBRACE II study: the outcome and prospect of two decades of evolution within the GEC-ESTRO GYN working group and the EMBRACE studies. Clin Transl Radiat Oncol. 2018;9:48–60. https://doi.org/10.1016/j.ctro.2018.01.001.
11. Small W Jr, Bosch WR, Harkenrider MM, et al. NRG oncology/RTOG consensus guidelines for delineation of clinical target volume for intensity modulated pelvic radiation therapy in postoperative treatment of endometrial and cervical cancer: an update. Int J Radiat Oncol Biol Phys. 2022;109:413–24. https://doi.org/10.1016/j.ijrobp.2020.08.061.
12. International Commission on Radiation Units and Measurement. Dose and volume specification for reporting intracavitary therapy in gynecology. Bethesda, MD: ICRU Report 38; 1985.
13. Haie-Meder C, Pötter R, Van Limbergen E, et al. Recommendations from Gynaecological (GYN) GEC-ESTRO working group (I): concepts and terms in 3D image based 3D treatment planning in cervix cancer brachytherapy with emphasis on MRI assessment of GTV and CTV. Radiother Oncol. 2005;74:235–45. https://doi.org/10.1016/j.radonc.2004.12.015.
14. Syed AM, Feder BH. Technique of after-loading interstitial implants. Radiol Clin. 1977;46:458–75.
15. Martinez A, Edmundson GK, Cox RS, et al. Combination of external beam irradiation and multiple-site perineal applicator (MUPIT) for treatment of locally advanced or recurrent prostatic, anorectal, and gynecological malignancies. Int J Radiat Oncol Biol Phys. 1985;11:391–8. https://doi.org/10.1016/0360-3016(85)90163-4.

16. Sturdza A, Pötter R, Fokdal LU, et al. Image guided brachytherapy in locally advanced cervical cancer: improved pelvic control and survival in RetroEMBRACE, a multicenter cohort study. Radiother Oncol. 2016;120:428–33. https://doi.org/10.1016/j.radonc.2016.03.011.
17. Mazeron R, Fokdal LU, Kirchheiner K, et al. Dose-volume effect relationships for late rectal morbidity in patients treated with chemoradiation and MRI-guided adaptive brachytherapy for locally advanced cervical cancer: results from the prospective multicenter EMBRACE study. Radiother Oncol. 2016;120:412–9. https://doi.org/10.1016/j.radonc.2016.06.006.
18. Okazaki S, Murata K, Noda S, et al. Dose-volume parameters and local tumor control in cervical cancer treated with central-shielding external-beam radiotherapy and CT-based image-guided brachytherapy. J Radiat Res. 2019;60:490–500. https://doi.org/10.1093/jrr/rrz023.
19. Toita T, Kitagawa R, Hamano T, et al. Phase II study of concurrent chemoradiotherapy with high-dose-rate intracavitary brachytherapy in patients with locally advanced uterine cervical cancer: efficacy and toxicity of a low cumulative radiation dose schedule. Gynecol Oncol. 2012;126:211–6. https://doi.org/10.1016/j.ygyno.2012.04.036.
20. Fokdal L, Sturdza A, Mazeron R, et al. Image guided adaptive brachytherapy with combined intracavitary and interstitial technique improves the therapeutic ratio in locally advanced cervical cancer: analysis from the retroEMBRACE study. Radiother Oncol. 2016;120:434–40. https://doi.org/10.1016/j.radonc.2016.03.020.
21. Ohno T, Noda SE, Okonogi N, et al. In-room computed tomography–based brachytherapy for uterine cervical cancer: results of a 5-year retrospective study. J Radiat Res. 2017;58:543–51. https://doi.org/10.1093/jrr/rrw121.
22. Takada A, Yokota H, Watanabe Nemoto M, et al. A multi-scanner study of MRI radiomics in uterine cervical cancer: prediction of in-field tumor control after definitive radiotherapy based on a machine learning method including peritumoral regions. Jpn J Radiol. 2020;38:265–73. https://doi.org/10.1007/s11604-019-00917-0.
23. Ikushima H, Haga A, Ando K, et al. Prediction of out-of-field recurrence after chemoradiotherapy for cervical cancer using a combination model of clinical parameters and magnetic resonance imaging radiomics: a multi-institutional study of the Japanese radiation oncology study group. J Radiat Res. 2022;63:98–106. https://doi.org/10.1093/jrr/rrab104.

13 Postoperative Adjuvant Therapy for Cervical Cancer

Munetaka Takekuma

Abstract

Treatment for most patients with early-stage cervical cancer involves radical hysterectomy and pelvic lymph node dissection. Indications for postoperative adjuvant therapy are determined by evaluating prognostic risk factors for recurrence in each individual case. Several clinicopathological factors, such as tumor size, lymphovascular space involvement, deep stromal invasion, parametrial involvement, and lymph node metastasis, have been identified as having prognostic significance in early-stage cervical cancer. However, these indicators remain controversial because there is substantial heterogeneity among patients after radical hysterectomy and lymphadenectomy and it is difficult to define clear risk groups. There is thus an unmet need to develop more accurate criteria to define risk groups and treat accordingly.

According to the currently available evidence, there remains the question of whether CCRT-P delivers a survival benefit superior to radiotherapy (RT) alone for patients with high-risk factors after radical surgery. In addition to this issue, patients with high-risk factors have a high incidence of distant metastasis, for whom systemic chemotherapy might be the key to improving overall survival.

Results from the pivotal study GOG092, that investigated the role of RT alone for patients with intermediate-risk factors after hysterectomy, also failed to resolve this issue. That trial did not show that postoperative RT significantly improved overall survival relative to no further treatment, even though a reduction in the risk of recurrence after RT was documented. However, the study did indicate that patients allocated to the RT group experienced an increase in severe toxicities compared with the NFT group. This could be why many physicians are

M. Takekuma (✉)
Shizuoka Cancer Center, Shizuoka, Japan
e-mail: m.takekuma@scchr.jp

D. Aoki (ed.), *Recent Topics on Prevention, Diagnosis, and Clinical Management of Cervical Cancer*, Comprehensive Gynecology and Obstetrics,
https://doi.org/10.1007/978-981-99-9396-3_13

reluctant to treat patients using this approach, although the guidelines recommend RT for patients with intermediate-risk factors.

Further improvement in adjuvant therapy will depend on more robust definition of prognostic risk factors, better patient selection, and refinements in both local and systemic therapies.

Keywords
Early-stage cervical cancer · Postoperative adjuvant therapy · Prognostic factors

13.1 Introduction

Worldwide, cervical cancer is the most common gynecologic malignancy, with nearly 570,000 new cases diagnosed in 2018 [1], causing a significant global burden of female cancers [2]. The disease disproportionately affects developing countries, essentially due to the absence of cervical cancer screening. In developed countries, the majority of cervical cancer patients is diagnosed at an early stage of the disease (stages I–II).

Early-stage cervical cancer has a relatively favorable prognosis, with a survival rate > 80% [3]. According to the Japanese guidelines [4], treatment options for stage IB1-IIB and some IIIC1r cervical cancers involve radical hysterectomy (RH) with pelvic lymph node dissection, or radiotherapy (RT) with concurrent chemoradiotherapy (CCRT). The indications for RH with pelvic lymph node dissection in Japan are broader than in many other countries. For that reason, the role of postoperative adjuvant therapy has been intensively discussed in Japan.

Postoperative adjuvant therapy with the aim of preventing recurrence is indicated after surgery depending on histopathological findings of the surgical specimen. Individual cases are classified into low-, intermediate-, and high-risk groups. The Japanese guidelines for cervical cancer [4] are that RT or CCRT is indicated for patients in the intermediate-group, and CCRT for the high-risk group.

The purpose of the current article is to raise and discuss the various issues that have not yet been resolved regarding prognostic risk factors and postoperative adjuvant therapy for this disease.

13.2 Prognostic Risk Factors for Recurrence

Risk factors for recurrence of early-stage cervical cancer after radical hysterectomy have been evaluated in many studies [5–10]. Risk groups, such as intermediate-risk and high-risk groups, have been defined according to the prognostic significance of each factor.

13.2.1 High-Risk Group

Peters et al. conducted a randomized trial that addressed the role of synchronous adjuvant RT and chemotherapy (CT) after radical hysterectomy and lymphadenectomy; patients with high-risk factors, which included positive pelvic lymph nodes, parametrial invasion, and a positive surgical margin, were enrolled in this trial [11].

Pelvic lymph node metastasis is a well-known high-risk factor [5–10]. Patients with lymph node metastasis have an increased recurrence rate of up to 40% for postoperative cervical cancer compared with those without this factor [12, 13], and node-positive patients have a greater rate of distant failure [14, 15]. The anatomic level of nodal involvement was also shown to be related to the risk of recurrence, with substantially higher recurrence rates being observed when common iliac or para-aortic nodal involvement was documented than when the involved nodes were confined to the pelvis. The number of nodes involved and their size could also be related to the risk of recurrence [14, 16].

Parametrial invasion has not been definitively recognized as a high-risk factor. Uno et al. showed that pelvic control of patients with parametrial invasion appeared identical to that of patients in other studies without parametrial invasion, and they suggested that pT2b without lymph node involvement should not be overestimated as a risk factor for recurrence outside the pelvis [17].

The prognostic significance of a positive surgical margin might have to be discussed separately from the other high-risk prognostic factors because these cases are outside the concept of adjuvant therapy after complete surgery. Hence, studies on high-risk patients that included a positive surgical margin as a prognostic factor should be interpreted cautiously.

13.2.2 Intermediate-Risk Group

The prognostic significance of intermediate-risk factors, such as lymphovascular space involvement (LVSI), deep stromal invasion (DSI), and large tumor size, remains controversial. No single one of these factors has been identified as causing a significant increase in the recurrence rate because sufficient power has not been obtained in statistical analyses, in part due to the interactions between them. However, when these factors are combined, the risk of recurrence increases by 15–20% [18–21].

Sedlis et al. defined the intermediate-risk group using various combinations of these three factors in a prospective study conducted by the Gynecologic Oncology Group (GOG) [18]. This approach resulted in the following GOG criteria: (a) positive capillary LVSI, deep and middle third penetration, and clinical tumor size ≥2 cm; (b) positive capillary LVSI, superficial third penetration and clinical tumor size ≥5 cm; and (c) negative capillary LVSI with middle or deep third penetration and clinical tumor size ≥4 cm. Despite their complexity, the use of these criteria in the GOG study by the participating institutions achieved a high acceptance rate, with only 7% of patients being found ineligible for the study. In addition, Putte et al.

also successfully validated these criteria and showed that they performed well [20]. In another study, Rogers et al. conducted a subgroup analysis of overall survival (OS) by prognostic category as defined by the GOG criteria and showed that post-operative adjuvant RT significantly reduced the mortality of patients with the combination of negative capillary LVSI, deep stromal invasion, and tumor size ≥4 cm [22]. However, Ryu et al. reported that the sensitivity of these criteria was only 50%, i.e. half of the recurrences occurred in patients not meeting the GOG criteria [23].

A model, referred to as Classic Criteria, proposed by Delagado et al., was established via a detailed GOG pathological study [19]. This prognostic model calculates the general relative risk (RR) by multiplying the RRs of three prognostic factors (LVSI, DSI, and tumor size). This makes it easy to classify patients into risk groups, so that appropriate therapeutic interventions can be planned accordingly. However, this model has low specificity and patients treated in accordance with it suffer a recurrence rate of 5–8%; in addition, many physicians avoid applying this model to their patients because of the possibility of overtreatment [23].

The two sets of criteria mentioned above leave an unresolved issue regarding the histological characteristics because they exclude patients with adenocarcinoma. A study has shown that the incidence of adenocarcinoma in cervical cancer has increased by 32.3% in the USA over a 35-year period [24], and the prognosis of patients with adenocarcinoma has been suggested to be poorer than that of those with squamous cell carcinoma [25, 26].

Ryu et al. conducted a retrospective study that aimed to define new criteria for the intermediate-risk group of patients with cervical cancer [21]; in that study, one-quarter of the patients had non-squamous cell carcinoma. The authors showed that four factors (adenocarcinoma, tumor size, DSI, and LVSI) were significantly associated with disease recurrence and identified a four-factor model, in which the presence of any two factors might be useful for predicting recurrence.

13.3 Treatment of Patients with High-Risk Factors After Radical Hysterectomy

Since the publication of five large, randomized trials that demonstrated a survival advantage in patients treated with CDDP-based CCRT in 1999 [11, 27–30], CCRT has become the standard therapy for cervical cancer. However, of these five studies, only one was a sufficiently powered, prospective, randomized trial that addressed the role of CCRT after radical hysterectomy and lymphadenectomy, namely the GOG0109/Southwest Oncology Group (SWOG) 8797/Radiation Therapy Oncology Group (RTOG) 91–12 trial [11]. This inter-group trial evaluated patients with positive pelvic lymph nodes and/or parametrial invasion and/or positive surgical margins, who were randomly allocated to receive either pelvic RT alone or CCRT-FP [RT in combination with CT (intravenous bolus of CDDP at 70 mg/m^2 and a 96-h infusion of fluorouracil (5-FU) at 1000 mg/m^2 every 3 weeks for four cycles)]. The results of this clinical trial demonstrated that progression-free survival (PFS) and OS were significantly improved by the addition of CT (hazard ratio (HR) 2.01,

$p = 0.003$, and 1.96, $p = 0.007$, respectively). However, CCRT-FP has not been applied in clinical practice because of its inconvenience and severe toxicities. Takekuma et al. reported their experience of this therapy and concluded that the toxicities remained problematic [31].

CCRT with CDDP administered weekly (CCRT-P), rather than CCRT-FP, is accepted as the standard therapy for patients with high-risk factors because the GOG0120 trial showed that CCRT-P is convenient and has equal effectiveness and favorable toxicities in comparison with CCRT-FP [27]. However, the rationale behind this might not be very robust because the GOG0120 trial investigated the usefulness of CCRT with radical irradiation for primary therapy in patients with stage IIB–IVA, not for postoperative adjuvant therapy, and the validity of CCRT-P in the postoperative setting could not be verified by this trial.

Patients with lymph node metastasis have been reported to exhibit a greater rate of distant failure [14, 15]. It is thus necessary for postoperative adjuvant therapy not only to control local recurrence, but also to prevent distant metastasis. In this context, systemic CT could play an important role in controlling distant metastasis and it has been hypothesized that the addition of further cycles of adjuvant CT following the completion of CCRT would decrease distant metastases and improve survival. To test this hypothesis directly, the GOG0724 trial evaluating patients with high-risk factors after surgery who were randomly allocated to receive either CCRT-P or CCRT-P followed by four cycles of paclitaxel and carboplatin has been ongoing since 2009 (NCT00980954).

It has been proposed that systemic CT alone could have a survival benefit even without RT. Postoperative RT would be expected to induce serious gastrointestinal toxicity, which could continue throughout the patient's life; this is because the region of the pelvis that would be targeted by RT has already been subjected to radical surgery [31, 32]. Takekuma et al. reported that the degree of invasiveness of the surgical procedure might be associated with toxicities of adjuvant CCRT and concluded that patients with ≥40 dissected lymph nodes would have significantly more non-hematological toxicities of adjuvant CCRT than those with <40. They suggested that, for patients undergoing CCRT, the use of this radical surgery to increase the possibility of a permanent cure has to be balanced against the possibility of developing a serious illness in association with the postoperative therapy. In this context, systemic CT alone could play an important role as postoperative adjuvant therapy for patients with high-risk cervical cancer [32].

Table 13.1 summarizes several studies of adjuvant therapy with systemic CT alone for patients with high-risk factors. Lahousen et al. conducted a randomized controlled trial to evaluate the efficacy of CT alone compared with external pelvic radiotherapy or no further treatment (NFT) for patients with risk factors after hysterectomy [12]. However, this trial was stopped because the number of recruited patients was far below expectations, and the validity of the results was unclear because of low statistical power.

In Japan, there has been a tendency to apply postoperative adjuvant CT alone because Okabayashi's radical hysterectomy, which is a superior method in terms of radicality compared to the other methods, is common and disease control in the pelvic area seems often to have already been achieved. Several retrospective studies have reported non-inferiority of CT alone compared to RT or CCRT [32–34]. Two phase II studies were reported in 2018. Matoda et al. conducted a prospective study (JGOG1067) for high-risk patients to test efficacy of a combination of irinotecan plus nedaplatin in a postoperative adjuvant setting. They reported that 2-year and 5-year recurrence-free survival (RFS) rates were 87.1% and 77.2%, respectively [35]. Takekuma et al. also conducted a phase II study to test the efficacy of a combination of paclitaxel plus nedaplatin in the same setting as the JGOG1067 study and showed that the 2-year RFS and 2-year OS were 79.0% and 93.5%, respectively [36]. Both trials met the statistical requirement of their primary endpoint. Enthusiasm for postoperative adjuvant CT alone has also spread to the USA. Mastuo et al. showed the results of analyses using the SEER database, in which the utilization of systemic CT without RT significantly increased over time by a multivariable analysis (adjusted odds ratio per one-year increment 1.06, 95% confidence interval 1.02–1.09) in the USA. Systemic CT alone was associated with more all-cause mortality than CCRT [37]. The authors concluded that the impact of systemic CT alone on survival may vary according to patient and tumor factors, and that its use without RT should be considered with caution [37]. Currently, a randomized phase III trial, JGOG1082, evaluating patients with high-risk factors after surgery who were

Table 13.1 Summary of studies on adjuvant therapy with systemic chemotherapy for patients with high-risk factors

Authors	Year	Study design	Treatment	Regimen of CT	Recurrence rate	Survival	
Lahousen et al. [12]	1999	phase III	CT alone	BLM/CDDP	28.6%	5y OS 86%	
			RT		16.7%	80%	
			NFT		25%	81%	n.s.
Takeshima et al. [33]	2006	Retrospective	CT alone	BOMP	14.3%	5y DFS 85.7%	
Hosaka et al. [34]	2012	Retrospective	CT alone	PTX/CDDP	21.9%	3y OS 93.8%	
			RT		32.7%	69.4%	$p = 0.02$
Takekuma et al. [32]	2016	Retrospective	CT alone	Platinum combination[a]	27%	4y OS 76.0%	
			CCRT-FP		31.1%	82.7%	$p = 0.782$
Matod et al. [35]	2018	Phase II	CT alone	CPT11/NDP	N/A	2y RFS 87.1%	
						5y RFS 77.2%	
						5y OS 86.5%	
Takekua et al. [36]	2018	Phase II	CT alone	PTX/NDP	N/A	2y RFS 79.0%	
						2y OS 93.5%	

NFT no further treatment, *n. s* not significant, *N/A* not applicable, *OS* overall survival, *DFS* disease free survival, *RFS* relapse free survival, *BLM* bleomycin, *CDDP* cisplatin, *BOMP* bleomycin, vincristine, mitomycin, and CDDP, *PTX* paclitaxel, *CPT11* irinotecan, *NDP* nedaplatin

[a]PTX + platinum, etoposide+platinum and irinotecan hydrochloride+platinum

randomly allocated to receive either CCRT-P or CT alone, has been ongoing since 2019 (jRCTs041190042) [38].

13.4 Treatment for Patients with Intermediate-Risk Factors after Radical Hysterectomy

A pivotal study, the GOG092 trial, investigated the role of RT alone for patients with intermediate-risk factors after radical hysterectomy [18]. Of 277 patients, 137 were randomly allocated to receive pelvic RT and 140 to receive NFT. Twenty-one patients (15%) in the RT group and 39 (28%) in the NFT group had cancer recurrence, of which 18 and 27, respectively, recurred in the vagina and pelvis. This difference translated into a 47% reduction in the risk of recurrence (RR = 0.53, $p = 0.008$) after RT, with two-year recurrence-free rates of 88% vs. 79%. Rotman et al. reported the final results of the survival analysis for this trial and updated the results on recurrence-free interval, based on an extended follow-up period [39]. They showed that the use of adjuvant RT was associated with an HR of 0.54 for recurrence ($p = 0.007$) and of 0.58 for progression or death ($p = 0.009$). However, the improvement in OS with RT did not reach statistical significance (HR: 0.70, $p = 0.074$), but patients allocated to the RT group did experience an increase in severe toxicities compared with the NFT group. There are several potential reasons why this study did not achieve statistically significant results regarding survival despite the significant benefit regarding local recurrence. First, the sample size might have been too small. This trial was planned to have 80% power to detect risk reductions of 46% or greater in OS; however, patients with RT had only a 30% reduction in the risk of mortality, so significance was not reached. Second, compliance with adjuvant RT in the RT group was insufficient. The proportion of patients who received no RT in the RT arm was 6.7%, and the proportion of those who received less than the planned protocol RT dose was 19.7% [39]. Third, there were some deficiencies in the technique of RT used in this study. For example, Zunino et al. showed that the posterior border of the lateral field in the four-field technique used in this GOG trial was inadequate in 50% of FIGO IB patients [40]. In fact, the recurrence rate in the GOG092 trial was still significant (15%, 21 of 137 cases) in the RT group, even though it was reduced with the use of adjuvant RT.

The results of the GOG092 trial mean that the role of adjuvant RT in improving survival is still controversial although it significantly reduced recurrence. Many physicians might be reluctant to treat patients in this group using this approach because of concerns about overtreatment. A retrospective study including 127 patients with intermediate risk, conducted by Cibula et al., showed that the recurrence rate, local control, or overall survival of patients with no further treatment after surgery did not differ from patients with postoperative CCRT [41]. They concluded that for patients with intermediate risk, radical surgery alone could achieve survival benefit equal to that achieved by combining the surgery with adjuvant therapy. Cao et al. also compared the prognosis of patients who underwent no adjuvant treatment, pelvic RT alone, or CCRT after radical hysterectomy for intermediate-risk, early-stage cervical cancer [42]. They reported that radical hysterectomy alone without adjuvant treatment may achieve favorable survival for patients with intermediate-risk cervical cancer as defined by the Sedlis criteria and suggested that the criteria for adjuvant treatment in patients without high-risk factors need to be further evaluated. Based on these results, a phase III randomized study, the CERVANTES study, has been ongoing nation-wide since 2022 (NCT04989647) [43].

Conversely, it has been hypothesized that, as in the high-risk group, CCRT could be more effective than RT alone as an adjuvant therapy in the intermediate-risk group. From their multivariate analysis, Ho et al. reported that in patients with LVSI and deep stromal invasion, the three-year recurrence-free survival of the CCRT group was significantly greater than that of the RT alone group [44]. A Cochrane review suggested that the addition of platinum-based CT to adjuvant RT may improve survival in patients with early-stage (IA2-IIA) cervical cancer with risk factors [45].

Table 13.2 shows the results of the GOG92 trial and two retrospective studies on adjuvant CCRT for patients with intermediate-risk factors. Ryu et al. retrospectively investigated whether weekly CCRT-P increases three-year recurrence-free interval in patients with two or more intermediate-risk factors [23]. Patients were categorized into the following groups: NFT ($n = 34$), RT ($n = 49$), and CCRT ($n = 89$). The three-year recurrence-free interval increased to 90.5% (RT) from 67.5% (NFT) and further increased to 97.5% (CCRT), making the disease almost completely curable by adding chemotherapy. Kim et al. also showed in their retrospective study that CCRT was significantly more effective regarding five-year recurrence-free survival and had similar toxicities to RT alone [46]. Given these results, a trial that is now ongoing, the GOG0263 trial, was established to evaluate patients with intermediate-risk factors after surgery who were randomly allocated to receive RT alone or CCRT-P (NCT01101451).

13.5 Toxicities of Adjuvant Radiotherapy or Concurrent Chemoradiotherapy

RT is a key modality in the treatment strategy of cervical cancer and it could be considered necessary as an adjuvant postoperative therapy for patients with intermediate- or high-risk factors. However, this would be problematic because adjuvant RT or CCRT would be expected to induce serious toxicities. The organs in the pelvis have already been subjected to radical surgery and RT would start at a stage when complete recovery from the damage associated with this would not yet have occurred. Several studies have reported the incidence of morbidity associated with adjuvant RT or CCRT [11, 18, 23, 31, 39, 47–51]. With regard to acute toxicities, the rates of gastrointestinal toxicities, urinary toxicities, and hematologic toxicities of grades 2/3+ were 2.3–94%/0–56%, 0–26%/0–3.1%, and 14.3–84%/2.3–54.8%, respectively. With regard to late toxicities, the rates of gastrointestinal toxicities and

Table 13.2 Summary of studies on adjuvant CCRT for patients with intermediate-risk factors

Authors	Year	Study design	Treatment	Regimen of CT	Recurrence rate		Survival	
GOG092	1999 and 2006	phase III	RT alone	–	17.5%		80.3%	
Sedlis [18] and Rotman [39]			NFT		30.7%	$p = 0.007$	71.4%	$p = 0.074$
Ryu et al. [23]	2011	Retrospective	CCRT	Weekly CDDP or tri-weekly CP[a]	2.2%		3y RFS 97.5%	
			RT alone	–	8.1%		97.6%	
			NFT		17.6%	$p = 0.009$	94.1%	$p < 0.05$
Kim et al. [46]	2009	Retrospective	CCRT	5FU or PTX/CDDP	7.3%		5y RFS 89%	
			RT alone	–	33.3%	NA	67%	$p = 0.01$

NFT no further treatment, *NA* no analysis

[a] Tri-weekly CP, cyclophosphamide at 500 mg/m^2 + CDDP at 50 mg/m^2, every 3 weeks

urinary toxicities of grades 2/3+ were 4.0–28%/2.2–19% and 3.0–6%/1.0–8.6%, respectively.

Late toxicities would be more problematic than acute toxicities because some of the former could continue for the rest of the patient's life. For example, Barter et al. reported that 30% of patients treated with RT had serious complications, with small bowel obstruction being one of the severe problems [52]. In addition, Ohba et al. [53] and Oda et al. [54] investigated risk factors for lower-limb lymphedema and persistent lower bladder compliance after radical hysterectomy, respectively; they showed that adjuvant RT was an independent risk factor for both. Furthermore, Takekuma et al. reported that the level of invasiveness of the surgical procedure might be associated with the toxicities of adjuvant CCRT. In their report, as mentioned above, patients who had ≥40 dissected lymph nodes had significantly more non-hematological toxicities compared with those who had <40 [31].

The use of intensity-modulated radiotherapy (IMRT) has been considered with the aim of reducing RT toxicities [47, 55]. A phase II trial of postoperative IMRT (RTOG0418) was conducted in the USA in patients with uterine body cancer and cervical cancer, and its feasibility and association with the onset of early adverse events were reported [56, 57]. The JCOG1402 study, which investigated the utility and safety of postoperative CCRT with IMRT, has been conducted in Japan (jRCTs031180194). We will report the results of this trial and we expect that adjuvant IMRT or concurrent chemotherapy with IMRT will become the standard treatment for patients with some risk factors also in Japan.

13.6 Conclusions

As the several topics discussed in this article, there have been some issue which should be resolved. Currently, a number of randomized phase III studies is ongoing to clarify some of these issues. Further improvements in adjuvant therapy should emerge from an improved definition of prognostic risk factors, better patient selection, and refinements in both local and systemic therapies.

References

1. Arbyn M, Weiderpass E, Bruni L, et al. Estimates of incidence and mortality of cervical cancer in 2018: a worldwide analysis. Lancet Glob Health. 2020;8:e191-e 203.
2. Ginsburg O, Bray M, Coleman MP, et al. The global burden of women' cancers: a grand challenge in global health. Lancet. 2017;389:847–60.
3. Benedet JL, Odicino F, Maisonneuve P, et al. Carcinoma of the cervix uteri. J Epidemiol Biostat. 2001;6:7–43.
4. Ebina Y, Mikami M, Nagase S, et al. Japan Society of Gynecologic Oncology guidelines 2017 for the treatment of uterine cervical cancer. Int J Clin Oncol. 2019;24:1–19.
5. Fuller AF Jr, Elliott N, Kosloff C, et al. Determinants of increased risk for recurrence in patients undergoing radical hysterectomy for stage IB and IIA carcinoma of the cervix. Gynecol Oncol. 1989;33:34–9.
6. Piver MS, Chung WS. Prognostic significance of cervical lesion size and pelvic node metastases in cervical carcinoma. Obstet Gynecol. 1975;46:507–10.
7. Sevin BU, Lu Y, Bloch DA, et al. Surgically defined prognostic parameters in patients with early cervical carcinoma. A multivariate survival tree analysis. Cancer. 1996;78:1438–46.
8. Snijders-Keilholz A, Hellebrekers BW, Zwinderman AH, et al. Adjuvant radiotherapy following radical hysterectomy for patients with early-stage cervical carcinoma (1984–1996). Radiother Oncol. 1999;51:161–7.
9. Soisson AP, Soper JT, Clarke-Pearson DL, et al. Adjuvant radiotherapy following radical hysterectomy for patients with stage IB and IIA cervical cancer. Gynecol Oncol. 1990;37:390–5.
10. Stock RG, Chen AS, Flickinger JC, et al. Node-positive cervical cancer: impact of pelvic irradiation and patterns of failure. Int J Radiat Oncol Biol Phys. 1995;31:31–6.
11. Peters WA III, Liu PY, Barrett RJ II, et al. Concurrent chemotherapy and pelvic radiation therapy compared with pelvic radiation therapy alone as adjuvant therapy after radical surgery in high-risk early-stage cancer of cervix. J Clin Oncol. 2000;18:1606–13.
12. Lahousen M, Haas J, Pickel H, et al. Chemotherapy versus radiotherapy versus observation for high-risk cervical carcinoma after radical hysterectomy: a randomized, prospective, multicenter trial. Gynecol Oncol. 1999;73:196–201.
13. Rose PG. Advances in the management of cervical cancer. J Reprod Med. 2000;45:971–8.
14. Thomas GT, Dembo AJ. Is there a role for adjuvant pelvic radiotherapy after radical hysterectomy in early stage cervical cancer? Int J Gynecol Cancer. 1991;1:1–8.
15. Uno T, Isobe K, Yamamoto S, et al. Postoperative radiation therapy for carcinoma of the uterine cervix. Radiat Med. 2006;24:91–7.
16. Monk BJ, Wang J, Im S, et al. Rethinking the use of radiation and chemotherapy after radical hysterectomy: a clinical-pathologic analysis of a gynecologic oncology group/southwest oncology group/radiation therapy oncology group trial. Gynecol Oncol. 2005;96:721–8.
17. Uno T, Ito H, Isobe K, et al. Postoperative pelvic radiotherapy for cervical cancer patients with positive parametrial invasion. Gynecol Oncol. 2005;96:335–40.
18. Sedlis A, Bundy BN, Rotman MZ, et al. A randomized trial of pelvic radiation therapy versus no further therapy in selected patients with stage IB carcinoma of the cervix after radical

hysterectomy and pelvic lymphadenectomy: a gynecologic oncology group study. Gynecol Oncol. 1999;73:177–83.
19. Delgado G, Bundy B, Zaino R, et al. Prospective surgical-pathological study of disease-free interval in patients with stage IB squamous cell carcinoma of the cervix: a gynecologic oncology group study. Gynecol Oncol. 1990;38:352–7.
20. Putte G, Lie AK, Vach W, et al. Risk grouping in stage IB squamous cell cervical carcinoma. Gynecol Oncol. 2005;99:106–12.
21. Ryu SY, Kim MH, Nam BH, et al. Intermediate-risk grouping of cervical cancer patients treated with radical hysterectomy: a Korean gynecologic oncology group study. Br J Cancer. 2014;110:278–85.
22. Rogers L, Ss S, Luesley D, et al. Radiotherapy and chemoradiation after surgery for early cervical cancer. Cochrane Database Syst Rev. 2012;5:CD007583. https://doi.org/10.1002/14651858. http://www.ncbi.nlm.nih.gov/pubmed/22592722.
23. Ryu SY, Park SI, Nam BH, et al. Is adjuvant chemoradiotherapy overtreatment in cervical cancer patients with intermediate risk factors? Int J Radiat Oncol Biol Phys. 2011;79:794–9.
24. Adegoke O, Kulasingam A, Virnig B. Cervical cancer trends in the United States: a 35-year population-based analysis. J Women's Health. 2012;21:1031–7.
25. Eifel PJ, Burke TW, Morris M, et al. Adenocarcinoma as an independent risk factor for disease recurrence in patients with stage IB cervical carcinoma. Gynecol Oncol. 1995;59:38–44.
26. Lai C, Hsueh S, Hog JH, et al. Are adenocarcinomas and adenosquamous carcinomas different from squamous carcinomas in stage IB and II cervical cancer patients undergoing primary radical surgery? Int J Gynecol Cancer. 1999;9:28–36.
27. Rose PG, Bundy BN, Watkins EB, et al. Concurrent cisplatin-based radiotherapy and chemotherapy for locally advanced cervical cancer. New Engl J Med. 1999;340:1144–53.
28. Morris M, Eifel PJ, Lu J, et al. Pelvic radiation with concurrent chemotherapy compared with pelvic and para-aortic radiation for high-risk cervical cancer. New Engl J Med. 1999;340:1137–43.
29. Keys HM, Bundy BN, Stehman FB, et al. Cisplatin, radiation and adjuvant hysterectomy compared with radiation and adjuvant hysterectomy for bulky stage IB cervical carcinoma. New Engl J Med. 1999;340:1154–61.
30. Whitney CW, Sause W, Bundy BN, et al. Randomized comparison of fluorouracil plus cisplatin versus hydroxyurea as an adjunct to radiation therapy in stage IIB-IVA carcinoma of the cervix with negative para-aortic lymph nodes: a gynecologic oncology group and southwest oncology group study. J Clin Oncol. 1999;17:1339–148.
31. Takekuma M, Kasamatsu Y, Kado N, et al. Reconsideration of postoperative concurrent chemoradiotherapy with fluorouracil and cisplatin for uterine cervical cancer. J Obstet Gynaecol Res. 2015;41:1638–43.
32. Takekuma M, Kasamatsu Y, Kado N, et al. Adjuvant chemotherapy versus concurrent chemoradiotherapy for high-risk cervical cancer after radical hysterectomy and systematic lymphadenectomy. Int J Clin Oncol. 2016;21:741–7.
33. Takeshima N, Umayahara K, Fujiwara K, et al. Treatment results of adjuvant chemotherapy after radical hysterectomy for intermediate- and high-risk stage IB-IIA cervical cancer. Gynecol Oncol. 2006;103:618–22.
34. Hosaka M, WatariH KT, et al. Clinical efficacy of paclitaxel/cisplatin as an adjuvant chemotherapy for patients with cervical cancer who underwent radical hysterectomy and systematic lymphadenectomy. J Surg Oncol. 2012;105:612–6.
35. Matoda MM, Takeshima N, Michimae H, et al. Postoperative chemotherapy for node-positive cervical cancer: results of a multicenter phase II trial (JGOG1067). Gynecol Oncol. 2018;149:513–9.
36. Takekuma M, Shimokawa M, Nishio S, et al. Phase II study of adjuvant chemotherapy with paclitaxel and nedaplatin for uterine cervical cancer with lymph node metastasis. Cancer Sci. 2018;109:1602–8.

37. Matsuo K, Nusbaum DJ, Matsuzaki S, et al. Utilization and outcomes of adjuvant systemic chemotherapy alone in high risk, early stage cervical cancer in the United States. Int J Gynecol Cancer. 2021;31:991–1000.
38. Furusawa A, Takekuma M, Mori K, et al. A randomized phase III trial of adjuvant chemotherapy versus concurrent chemoradiotherapy for postoperative cervical cancer: Japanese gynecologic oncology group study (JGOG1082). Int J Gynecol Cancer. 2021;31:623–6.
39. Rotman M, Sedlis A, Piedmonte MR, et al. A phase III randomized trial of postoperative pelvic irradiation in stage IB cervical carcinoma with poor prognostic factors: follow-up of a gynecologic oncology group study. Int J Radiat Oncol Biol Phys. 2006;65:169–76.
40. Zunino S, Rosto O, Lucino S, et al. Anatomic study of the pelvis in carcinoma of the uterine cervix as related to the box technique. Int J Radiat Oncol Biol Phys. 1999;44:53–9.
41. Cibula D, Abu-Rustum NR, Fischerova D, et al. Surgical treatment of "intermediate risk" lymph node negative cervical cancer patients without adjuvant radiotherapy- a retrospective cohort study and review of the literature. Gynecol Oncol. 2018;151:438–43.
42. Cao L, Wen H, Feng Z, et al. Role of adjuvant therapy after radical hysterectomy in intermediate-risk, early-stage cervical cancer. Int J Gynecol Cancer. 2021;31:52–8.
43. Cibula D, Borcinova M, Kocian R, et al. CERVANTES: an international randomized trial of radical surgery followed by adjuvant (chemo)radiation versus no further treatment in patients with early-stage, intermediate-risk cervical cancer (CEEGOG-CX-05; ENGOT-CX16). Int J Gynecol Cancer. 2022;32:1327. https://doi.org/10.1136/ijgc-2022-003918.
44. Ho CM, Chien TY, Huang SH, et al. Multivariate analysis of the prognostic factors and outcomes in early cervical cancer patients undergoing radical hysterectomy. Gynecol Oncol. 2004;93:458–64.
45. Rosa DD, Medeiros LR, Edelweiss ML, et al. Adjuvant platinum-based chemotherapy for early stage cervical cancer. Cochrane Database Syst Rev. 2012;5:CD007583.
46. Kim K, Kang SB, Chung HH, et al. Comparison of chemoradiation with radiation as postoperative adjuvant therapy in cervical cancer patients with intermediate-risk factors. Eur J Surg Oncol. 2009;35:192–6.
47. Chen MF, Tseng CJ, Tseng CC, et al. Clinical outcome in posthysterectomy cervical cancer patients treated with concurrent cisplatin and intensity modulated pelvic radiotherapy: comparison with conventional radiotherapy. Int J Radiat Oncol Biol Phys. 2007;67:1438–44.
48. Mitsuhashi A, Uno T, Usui H, et al. Postoperative concurrent daily low-dose cisplatin-based chemoradiation improves the prognosis of patients with pathologic T2b or N1 cervical cancer. Anticancer Res. 2010;30:2341–6.
49. Heinzelmann F, Henke G, von Grafensten M, et al. Adjuvant radiochemotherapy in patients with locally advanced high-risk cervical cancer. Strahlenther Onkol. 2012;18:568–75.
50. Pu J, Qin SS, Ding JX, et al. A randomized controlled study of single-agent cisplatin and radiotherapy versus docetaxel/cisplatin and radiotherapy in high-risk early-stage cervical cancer after radical surgery. J Cancer Res Clin Oncol. 2013;139:703–8.
51. Isohashi F, Yoshioka Y, Mabuchi S, et al. Intensity-modulated radiation therapy versus three-dimensional conformal radiation therapy with concurrent nedaplatin-based chemotherapy after radical hysterectomy for uterine cervical cancer: comparison of outcome, complications, and dose-volume histogram parameters. Radiat Oncol. 2015;10:180. https://doi.org/10.1186/s13014-015-0486-5.
52. Barter JF, Soong SJ, Shingleton HM, et al. Complications of combined radical hysterectomy-postoperative radiation therapy in women with early stage cervical cancer. Gynecol Oncol. 1989;32:292–6.
53. Ohba Y, Todo Y, Kobayashi N, et al. Risk factors for lower-limb lymphedema after surgery for cervical cancer. Int J Clin Oncol. 2011;16:238–43.
54. Oda Y, Todo Y, Hanley S, et al. Risk factors for persistent low bladder compliance after radical hysterectomy. Int J Clin Oncol. 2011;21:167–72.
55. Folkert MR, Shin KK, Abu-Rustum NR, et al. Postoperative pelvic intensity-modulated radiotherapy and concurrent chemotherapy in intermediate- and high-risk cervical cancer. Gynecol Oncol. 2013;128:288–93.

56. Jhingran A, Winter K, Portelance L, et al. A phase II study of intensity modulated radiation therapy to the pelvis for postoperative patients with endometrial carcinoma: radiation therapy oncology group trial 0418. Int J Radiat Oncol Biol Phys. 2012;84:e23–8.
57. Klopp AH, Moughan J, Portelance L, et al. Hematologic toxicity in RTOG0418: a phase 2 study of postoperative IMRT for gynecologic cancer. Int J Radiat Oncol Biol Phys. 2013;86:83–90.

Chemotherapy for Advanced and Recurrent Cervical Cancer

14

Shin Nishio

Abstract

For patients with advanced and recurrent cervical cancer, chemotherapy remains the standard treatment, although it is neither curative nor associated with long-term disease control. In this chapter, we summarized the history of treatment of advanced and recurrent cervical cancer and the current recommendation for chemotherapy and anti-angiogenic therapy. Since cisplatin every 21 days was considered as the historical standard treatment for recurrent cervical cancer, subsequent trials have evaluated and demonstrated activity for other agents including paclitaxel, gemcitabine, topotecan, and vinorelbine, among others. Accordingly, promising agents were incorporated into phase III trials. To examine the best agent to combine with cisplatin, several landmark phase III clinical trials were conducted by Gynecologic Oncology Group (GOG) and Japan Clinical Oncology Group (JCOG). Through GOG204 and JCOG0505, paclitaxel/cisplatin (TP) and paclitaxel/carboplatin (TC) are now considered to be the recommended therapies for recurrent cervical cancer patients. However, the prognosis of patients who are already resistant to chemotherapy is very poor. Therefore new therapeutic strategies are urgently required. Molecular-targeted therapy will be the most hopeful candidate of these strategies. From the results of GOG240, bevacizumab combined with TP reached its primary endpoint of improving overall survival (OS). Although the prognosis for recurrent cervical cancer patients is still poor, the results of GOG240 shed light on the usefulness of molecular target agents to chemotherapy in cancer patients. Recurrent cervical cancer is generally considered incurable and current chemotherapy regiments offer only modest gains in OS, particularly for patients with multiple poor

S. Nishio (✉)
Department of Obstetrics and Gynecology, Kurume University School of Medicine, Kurume, Japan
e-mail: shinshin@med.kurume-u.ac.jp

D. Aoki (ed.), *Recent Topics on Prevention, Diagnosis, and Clinical Management of Cervical Cancer*, Comprehensive Gynecology and Obstetrics,
https://doi.org/10.1007/978-981-99-9396-3_14

prognostic factors. Therefore, it is crucial to consider not only the survival benefit but also the minimization of treatment toxicity and maximization of quality of life (QOL).

Keywords
Advanced and recurrent cervical cancer · Chemotherapy · Anti-angiogenic therapy

14.1 Introduction

Despite effective screening programs in most countries, women who lack access to health care and/or those failing to participate in screening are at an increased risk of developing cervical cancer [1]. The prognosis for advanced or recurrent cervical cancer is poor, with a one-year survival rate between 10 and 15% [2]. Chemotherapy remains the standard treatment for patients with advanced and recurrent cervical cancer. However, it is neither curative nor associated with long-term disease control [3]. Therefore, there is an urgent need for effective therapy against cervical cancer, as the optimal treatment is yet to be defined.

In this chapter, we summarized the history of medical treatment for recurrent cervical cancer and the current recommendations for chemotherapy and anti-angiogenic therapy.

14.2 Single-Agent Chemotherapy

14.2.1 Cisplatin

Cisplatin is the primary chemotherapy used for patients with advanced cervical cancer. The Gynecologic Oncology Group (GOG) study revealed that the overall response rate (ORR) among 34 patients with advanced or recurrent cervical squamous cell carcinoma treated with cisplatin (50 mg/m^2) every 3 weeks [4] was 38%; however, three complete responses (CR) and eight partial responses (PR) were observed in 22 previously untreated patients, with an ORR of 50%. Only two PR were observed in 12 patients who had received prior chemotherapy.

Based on its antitumor effect, toxicity, and feasibility, a dose of 50 mg/m^2 every 21 days became the standard administration method for cisplatin.

14.2.2 Topotecan

Topotecan inhibits topoisomerase-I, an intranuclear enzyme that relieves torsional stress in DNA [5]. The binding of topotecan to topoisomerase-I creates a stabilized cleavable complex, leading to single-strand DNA breaks, which are converted to lethal double-strand breaks during DNA replication. In addition to these direct effects, topotecan can potentiate cisplatin activity by inhibiting DNA repair [6].

The GOG evaluated the activity and toxicity of topotecan in a multicenter phase II study of patients with previously treated squamous cell carcinoma of the uterine cervix [7]. Topotecan was administered at 1.5 mg/m^2 daily for five consecutive days on a 21-day cycle. Among the 40 patients evaluated, the ORR was 12.5%, with stable disease (SD) in an additional 37.5%. The median progression-free survival (PFS) was 2.1 months. As a single agent, topotecan exhibited modest antitumor activity in patients with previously treated squamous cell carcinoma of the cervix. These results led the GOG to include a combination of topotecan and cisplatin in phase III trials.

14.2.3 Irinotecan

A phase II study was performed to evaluate the antitumor activity and toxicity of irinotecan, a water-soluble derivative of camptothecin, in patients with prior chemotherapy-treated squamous cell cancer of the cervix [8]. The initial dose of CPT-11 was 125 mg/m2, administered as a weekly 90-min intravenous infusion for 4 weeks, every 6 weeks. Monitoring the responses of 42 patients revealed that the ORR was 21%, and the median time to response and response duration were 6 and 12 weeks, respectively. The median overall survival was 6.4 months. A statistically significant survival advantage (median of 12.6 vs. 5.1 months) was observed in patients whose disease responded to irinotecan.

14.2.4 Paclitaxel

A phase II trial of paclitaxel was initiated in advanced non-squamous carcinoma of the cervix to determine its efficacy in patients who had failed standard chemotherapy [9]. The starting dose of paclitaxel was 170 mg/m^2 (135 mg/m^2 for patients with prior pelvic radiation), administered as a 24-h continuous intravenous infusion with courses repeated every 3 weeks. Among the 42 assessable patients enrolled, 13 responses were observed: four patients had a CR, whereas nine patients had a PR. The ORR was 31%. The primary and dose-limiting toxicity was neutropenia. Thus, paclitaxel was deemed to be effective for non-squamous carcinoma of the cervix.

14.2.5 Nab-Paclitaxel

Nab-paclitaxel is a nanoparticle formulation of albumin-bound paclitaxel [10]. No premedication was required for the risk of hypersensitivity [11].

The GOG conducted a phase II trial of nab-paclitaxel in the treatment of recurrent or persistent advanced cervical cancer [12]. Nab-paclitaxel was administered at 125 mg/m^2 over 30 min on days 1, 8, and 15 of each 28-day cycle to 37 women with metastatic or recurrent cervical cancer that had progressed or relapsed following first-line cytotoxic drug treatment. Thirty-five eligible patients were evaluated for response and tolerability. All eligible patients had one prior chemotherapy regimen, among whom 27 had prior radiation therapy with concomitant cisplatin. The median number of nab-paclitaxel cycles was four (range, 1–15). Ten (28.6%; 95% confidence interval [CI], 14.6–46.3%] of the 35 patients had PR, and another 15 patients (42.9%) had SD. The median PFS and overall survival (OS) were 5.0 and 9.4 months, respectively. Notably, the 28.6% ORR in the 35 eligible patients is the most effective record in the GOG for a single agent against drug-refractory, platinum-resistant disease [13–28]. Thus, nab-paclitaxel may be considered a leading candidate for future studies on combinations of agents in adjuvant and advanced disease settings, especially when evaluating weekly dosing schedules.

Table 14.1 presents the ORR of single-agent chemotherapy [29, 30].

14.3 Combination Chemotherapy: Phase II Clinical Trials

In combination chemotherapy trials, other active agents were selected for combination with cisplatin. Therefore, several agents that exhibited modest-to-good responses were used in combination with cisplatin, and their activities were evaluated in a phase II trial. Furthermore, cisplatin analogs (such as carboplatin) were evaluated to identify those that could reduce the adverse effects of cisplatin.

14.3.1 Topotecan + Cisplatin

Fiorica et al. conducted a phase II trial to evaluate the efficacy of cisplatin + topotecan in patients with persistent or recurrent cervical cancer [31]. Cisplatin (50 mg/m^2) and topotecan (0.75 mg/m^2) were administered on day 1 and days 1, 2, and 3, respectively, of a 21-day cycle for six cycles or until disease progression. The toxicity and tumor response were monitored in 32 of the 35 enrolled patients, among

Table 14.1 Overall response rate (ORR) to cervical cancer (single-agent chemotherapy)

Agent (reference number)	ORR (%)
Cisplatin [4]	38
Carboplatin [30]	15
Paclitaxel [9, 14]	17–31
Nab-paclitaxel [11]	28
Docetaxel [24]	8
Topotecan [7, 20]	12–18
Irinotecan [8, 21]	13–21
Etoposide [16, 17]	11–12
5-fluorouracil [22, 23]	4–9
Ifosfamide [13]	15
Gemcitabine [18, 19]	4–8
Liposomal doxorubicin [26]	11
Vinorelbine [27–29]	7–17

whom all but two evaluable patients had previously received radiotherapy. None of the patients had previously received chemotherapy. The most common toxicities were hematologic, with grade 3 and 4 neutropenia and thrombocytopenia reported in 30% and 10% of the cycles, respectively. The ORR was 28% (9/32), with three CR and six PR. Nine patients (28%) experienced SD. The antitumor response in the non-irradiated fields (30%) was similar to that observed in the previously irradiated fields (33%), suggesting optimal drug penetration. The median response duration was 5 months (range, 2–15 months). An additional nine (28%) patients achieved SD. The median OS was 10 months. Thus, the cisplatin/topotecan combination was considered safe, well-tolerated, and active in patients with cervical cancer.

14.3.2 Paclitaxel + Cisplatin

Based on the activity of paclitaxel as a single agent in chemotherapy for naive squamous cell carcinoma of the cervix in a prior GOG trial, a phase II study of paclitaxel and cisplatin as first-line therapy was conducted by the GOG [32].

The patients received paclitaxel 135 mg/m^2 over 24 h, followed by cisplatin 75 mg/m^2 every 21 days. Overall, the responses in 41 patients were monitored. Forty patients (90.9%) had previously received radiation therapy. Of the 41 assessable patients, 5 (12.2%) achieved CR, and 14 (34.1%) achieved PR for an ORR of 46.3%. The median PFS and OS were 5.4 and 10.0 months, respectively (range, 0.9–22.2 months). The response was relatively frequent in patients with disease at non-irradiated sites (70% vs. 23%, $P = 0.008$). Collectively, this regimen appeared to be highly active, and these results led to the development of GOG 169 in phase III randomized study to compare the combinations of paclitaxel/cisplatin with cisplatin alone.

14.3.3 Paclitaxel + Carboplatin

Patients with advanced or recurrent cervical carcinoma were treated with carboplatin/paclitaxel every 28 days [33]. The initial doses of carboplatin/paclitaxel were: AUC 5–6 and 155–175 mg/m^2. Among the 25 women treated with this combination, 23 (92%) had prior treatment with pelvic radiotherapy, and 14 (56%) had concurrent radiosensitizing cisplatin. There was a 20% PR and 20% CR (10/25). The median PFS and OS for the entire study group were 3 and 21 months, respectively. Thus, carboplatin/paclitaxel is considered an active combination for advanced and recurrent cervical cancer.

14.4 Combination Chemotherapy: Phase III Clinical Trials

A cisplatin dose of 50 mg/m^2 every 21 days is considered the historical standard treatment for recurrent cervical cancer [4]. Subsequent trials have evaluated and demonstrated the activity of other agents, including mitolactol, ifosfamide, paclitaxel, gemcitabine, topotecan, and vinorelbine [7, 9, 13, 14, 18–20, 27, 28, 34]. Accordingly, promising agents have been incorporated into phase III trials. In this section, we summarize the landmark phase III clinical trials conducted by the GOG and Japan Clinical Oncology Group (JCOG). Table 14.2 presents the results of representative phase III clinical trials [35–37].

14.4.1 GOG 169

Previous GOG phase II trials demonstrated that the paclitaxel/cisplatin combination was highly active in cervical cancer. Therefore, a phase III trial was conducted to compare the efficacy of paclitaxel/cisplatin with cisplatin alone [38].

Among the 264 eligible patients, 134 received cisplatin and 130 received cisplatin/paclitaxel. Most patients had prior radiation therapy (cisplatin, 92%; cisplatin/paclitaxel, 91%). The ORR in patients receiving cisplatin and those receiving cisplatin/paclitaxel was 19% (6% CR plus 13% PR) and 36% (15% CR plus 21% PR), respectively ($P = 0.002$). The median PFS for cisplatin vs. cisplatin/paclitaxel was 2.8 and 4.8 months, respectively ($P < 0.001$). Conversely, the median OS did not significantly differ (8.8 vs. 9.7 months). Notably, this trial prospectively collected quality of life (QOL) assessment data before each treatment cycle. Despite similar QOL scores in both groups, the dropout rate, as determined by the completion of the survey, was higher in the cisplatin group, suggesting stable rather than worsening QOL for patients receiving combination therapy. Collectively, cisplatin/paclitaxel is considered superior to cisplatin alone in terms of response rate and PFS with sustained QOL.

14.4.2 GOG 179

Following the GOG 169 closure, a replacement trial was conducted to compare single-agent cisplatin with other active regimens from previous phase II trials. Patients were randomized into one of three treatment arms: (I) cisplatin; (II) cisplatin/topotecan; and (III) methotrexate, vinblastine, doxorubicin, and cisplatin (MVAC) [39]. The MVAC arm was closed by the Data Safety Monitoring Board after four treatment-related deaths occurred among 63 patients and were excluded from the analysis. Improvements in ORR (27% vs. 13%; P=0.004) and PFS (4.6 vs. 2.9 months; P=0.014) favored cisplatin/topotecan regimens over cisplatin alone. OS was higher for the combination regimen compared with that for cisplatin alone (9.4 vs. 6.5 months; P=0.017). This was the first randomized phase III trial to demonstrate a survival advantage of combination chemotherapy over cisplatin alone in

Table 14.2 Phase III clinical trials for stage IVB and recurrent cervical cancers

Author	Regimen	OS (months)	PFS (months)	ORR (%)
GOG43 Bobomi [35]	CDDP 50 mg/m^2 vs. CDDP 100 mg/m^2 Vs. CDDP 20 mg/m^2 × 5 days	7.1 vs. 7.0 Vs. 6.1 (NS)	3.7 vs. 4.6 Vs. 3.9 (NS)	21.0 vs. 31.0 vs. 25.0 ($P < 0.05$)
GOG110, Omura [36]	CDDP 50 mg/m^2 vs. CDDP 50 mg/m^2 + IFM 5 g/m^2	8.0 vs. 8.3 (NS)	3.2 vs. 4.6 ($P < 0.01$)	18.0 vs. 31.0 ($P < 0.01$)
GOG149, Bloss [37]	CDDP 50 mg/m^2 + IFM 5 g/m^2 vs. CDDP 50 mg/m^2 + IFM 5 g/m^2 + BLM 30 U	8.5 vs. 8.4 (NS)	4.6 vs. 5.1 (NS)	32.0 vs. 31.0 (NS)
GOG169 Moore [38]	CDDP 50 mg/m^2 vs. CDDP 50 mg/m^2 + PTX 135 mg/m^2	8.8 vs. 9.7 (NS)	2.8 vs. 4.8 ($P < 0.01$)	19.0 vs. 36.0 ($P < 0.01$)
GOG179, Long [39]	CDDP 50 mg/m^2 vs. CDDP 50 mg/m^2 + TPO 0.75 mg/m^2	7.0 vs. 9.2 ($P < 0.05$)	2.9 vs. 4.6 ($P < 0.01$)	13.0 vs. 26.0 ($P < 0.01$)
GOG204, Monk [40]	CDDP 50 mg/m^2 + PTX 135 mg/m^2 vs. CDDP 50 mg/m^2 + TPO 0.75 mg/m^2 vs. CDDP 50 mg/m^2 + GEM 1000 mg/m^2 vs. CDDP 50 mg/m^2 + VNR 30 mg/m^2	12.9 vs. 10.3 vs. 10.3 vs. 10.0 (NS)	5.8 vs. 4.6 Vs. 4.7 vs. 4.0 (NS)	29.1 vs. 23.4 Vs. 22.3 vs. 25.9 (NS)
GOG240, Tewari [54]	CDDP 50 mg/m^2 + PTX 135 mg/m^2 with or without BEV 15 mg/kg vs. CDDP 50 mg/m^2 + TOP 0.75 mg/m^2 with or without BEV 15 mg/kg	BEV+: 17.5 or BEV−: 14.3 ($P < 0.05$) vs. BEV+: 16.2 or BEV−: 12.7 (NS)		50.0 or 45.0 (NS) vs. 47.0 or 27.0 (P < 0.05)
JCOG0505, Kitagawa [41]	CDDP 50 mg/m^2 + PTX 135 mg/m^2 Vs. CBDCA AUC5 + PTX 175 mg/m^2	18.3 vs. 17.5 (NS)	6.9 vs. 6.2 (NS)	58.8 vs. 62.6 (NS)

OS overall survival, *PFS* progression-free survival, *CDDP* cisplatin, *IFM* ifosfamide, *BLM* bleomycin, *PTX* paclitaxel, *TPO* topotecan, *GEM* gemcitabine, *VNR* vinorelbine, *Bev* bevacizumab, *CBDCA* carboplatin, *GOG* Gynecologic Oncology Group, *JCOG* Japan Clinical Oncology Group, *NS* not significant

advanced cervical cancer. The ORR of single-agent cisplatin was only 13%. Compared with GOG 169, where 30% of patients received chemoradiation in the cisplatin-alone control arm, 56% of patients in the control arm in GOG 179 had been treated with prior chemoradiation therapy, potentially explaining the benefit observed in the experimental arm. Owing to these promising improvements in OS, the topotecan and cisplatin combination was added to GOG 204.

14.4.3 GOG 204

GOG 204 assessed the winning cisplatin doublets from two preceding trials, cisplatin/paclitaxel (GOG 169) and cisplatin/topotecan (GOG 179). The combination regimens, gemcitabine/cisplatin and vinorelbine/cisplatin, were also evaluated in this crucial phase III trial [40]. Among the 513 patients enrolled before a planned interim analysis, 70% had been treated with prior cisplatin chemoradiation. The trial was prematurely closed after the analysis revealed that the three control arms were not superior to cisplatin/paclitaxel. The ORR was statistically similar for each of the four arms, ranging from 22.3% for gemcitabine/cisplatin to 29.1% for paclitaxel/cisplatin. PFS (4–5.8 months) and OS (10–12.9 months) were similar between the arms; however, paclitaxel was noted to have the highest response rate at 29.1% and OS of 12.9 months.

Vinorelbine/cisplatin, gemcitabine/cisplatin, and topotecan/cisplatin regimens were not superior to paclitaxel/cisplatin in terms of OS. However, the trends in ORR, PFS, and OS favor paclitaxel/cisplatin as the standard care. GOG 204 represented a significant step forward in defining optional therapy; however, low ORR (29.1%) and relatively short OS (12.9 months) were unsatisfactory. The OS was significantly worse in patients who had undergone previous concurrent chemoradiotherapy (CCRT) than in those who had undergone radiotherapy alone (hazard ratio [HR) =1.148; 95% CI, 0.90–1.47]. These results suggest that CCRT contributes to improving the prognosis of advanced cervical cancer; however, treating recurrent disease after CCRT remains challenging because both chemotherapy and radiation therapy have already been administered.

14.4.4 JCOG0505

Patients with recurrent or advanced cervical cancer often have urinary tract problems, which can induce renal dysfunction. For such patients, cisplatin administration is counterproductive owing to its nephrotoxic effects. Despite being a derivative of cisplatin, carboplatin has gained attention owing to its low renal toxicity and reduced hydration requirement.

The JCOG conducted a randomized phase III study to evaluate the clinical benefits of carboplatin/paclitaxel compared with that of cisplatin/paclitaxel in patients with advanced or recurrent disease.

Of the 253 enrolled patients, 246 were evaluable, including 201 with disease assessable for response [41]. The ORRs were 60% and 62% for cisplatin/paclitaxel and carboplatin/paclitaxel, respectively. The median OS and PFS were 18.3 and 6.9 months, respectively, for GOG 169, and 17.5 and 6.2 months, respectively, for carboplatin/paclitaxel. Thus, the antitumor activity of carboplatin/paclitaxel was similar to that of cisplatin/paclitaxel. Carboplatin/paclitaxel was less toxic than cisplatin/paclitaxel in inducing febrile neutropenia, creatinine elevation, and nausea/vomiting. Notably, the interim analysis demonstrated that substituting carboplatin with cisplatin did not result in an inferior outcome. The observed toxicities were similar in severity and frequency based on previous experience with these compounds.

Notably, in the secondary analysis of 117 patients who had not received prior platinum, cisplatin/paclitaxel doublet appeared to be superior to carboplatin/paclitaxel, with a median OS of 23.2 vs. 13.0 months (HR =1.57; 95% CI, 1.06–2.32).

Without evidence of inferiority, carboplatin/ paclitaxel may become the new standard for patients with the recurrent disease unless they have not received prior chemoradiation therapy, where they may benefit from cisplatin/paclitaxel.

14.5 Anti-Angiogenic Therapy

The prognosis of patients who experience recurrence after prior chemotherapy is relatively poor; therefore, new therapeutic strategies are urgently required. Molecular-targeted therapy is the most promising candidate for these strategies. Compared with other cancers, few clinical trials of molecularly targeted agents have been conducted. However, the results of bevacizumab therapeutic trials for cervical cancer have suggested that targeting the vascular endothelial growth factor (VEGF) pathway is a viable therapeutic strategy.

14.5.1 VEGF Pathway

Angiogenesis, the process leading to the formation of new blood vessels from the pre-existing vascular network, is necessary for tumor growth, invasion, metastasis, and survival. It has been generally considered a highly attractive target for cancer therapy. VEGF plays a pivotal role in regulating angiogenesis, tumor growth, and metastasis [42–44]. The binding of VEGF to its receptors activates a signaling cascade that ultimately increases endothelial cell survival, proliferation, vascular permeability, migration, and invasion [45]. Cervical cancer heavily depends on angiogenesis, perhaps even more than most solid tumors, because human papillomavirus infection and ongoing hypoxia (associated with increased expression of hypoxia-inducible factor-1 alpha) are associated with increased levels of VEGF, a common target for anti-angiogenesis therapy. VEGF overexpression has been associated with tumor progression and poor prognosis in several tumors, including cervical cancer [46]. The cytosolic VEGF levels are reportedly increased in cervical cancer compared with that in normal cervical tissue [47–50]. Monoclonal antibodies, such as bevacizumab, and small-molecule tyrosine kinase inhibitors (TKIs), such as pazopanib, are promising candidates for specific treatments against VEGF.

14.5.2 Bevacizumab

Bevacizumab is a humanized antibody that recognizes and neutralizes all major VEGF isoforms, prevents receptor binding, and inhibits endothelial cell proliferation and vessel formation [51]. Bevacizumab was the first FDA-approved drug designed to inhibit angiogenesis in patients with advanced colorectal, non-small lung, and renal cancers [52]. Bevacizumab targets VEGF-A, which is increased in malignant cervical cancer cells and is correlated with advanced stages of cervical cancer. The findings of the phase II multicenter trial revealed a relatively better PFS (24% probability to survive over 6 months; 90% CI, 14–37%), median OS (7.29 months; 95% CI, 6.11–10.41 months), and ORR (10.9%; 90% CI, 4.4–21.5%) [53].

14.5.3 GOG 240

In GOG 240, a phase III, randomized trial performed in the USA and Spain through GOG and the Spanish Research Group for Ovarian Cancer, the administration of bevacizumab and the use of non-platinum combination chemotherapy in the treatment of advanced cervical cancer were investigated [54]. In this trial, 452 patients were randomly assigned to receive chemotherapy with or without bevacizumab at a dose of 15 mg/kg. Chemotherapy consisted of cisplatin plus paclitaxel at doses of 50 mg/m^2 and 135 or 175 mg/m^2, respectively, or topotecan at a dose of 0.75 mg/m^2 on days 1–3, plus paclitaxel at a dose of 175 mg/m^2 on day 1. The cycles were repeated every 21 days until the disease progressed. Most patients (72%) had recurrent disease, whereas 11% had persistent disease. Over 70% of the patients in each group had previously received platinum-based chemoradiotherapy.

Topotecan/paclitaxel was not superior to cisplatin/ paclitaxel (HR for death =1.20). The data for the two chemotherapy regimens combined suggested that the addition of bevacizumab to chemotherapy was associated with increased OS (17.0 vs. 13.3 months; HR for death =0.71; 98% CI, 0.54–0.95; $P = 0.004$ in a one-sided test) and higher ORR (48% vs. 36%, $P = 0.008$). Among the patients who received bevacizumab, 28 had CR, and among those who received chemotherapy alone, 14 had CR ($P = 0.03$). Compared with chemotherapy alone, bevacizumab was associated with an increased incidence of grade 2 hypertension or higher (25% vs. 2%; $P < 0.001$), grade 3 or higher thromboembolic events (8% vs. 1%; $P = 0.001$), and grade 3 or higher gastrointestinal fistulas (6% vs. 0%; $P = 0.002$). Bevacizumab-containing regimens were associated with a reduced hazard of disease progression and an increased probability of response. Bevacizumab-containing therapy was effective even in the presence of target lesions in the previously irradiated pelvis. The addition of bevacizumab to combination chemotherapy in patients with recurrent, persistent, or metastatic cervical cancer was associated with an improvement of 3.7 months in median OS. GOG 240 is a landmark trial because it is the first time a targeted agent has reached its primary endpoint of improving OS in gynecological cancer.

14.5.4 JCOG1311

To evaluate the efficacy and safety of dose-dense weekly paclitaxel plus carboplatin (ddTC), with or without bevacizumab, compared with conventional tri-weekly paclitaxel plus carboplatin (cTC), with or without bevacizumab, in metastatic or recurrent cervical cancer that is refractory to curative local therapy [55]. Patients were randomly assigned to either the cTC or ddTC arm. The cTC regimen consisted of paclitaxel 175 mg/m^2 and carboplatin at an area under the curve (AUC) of 5 on day 1. The ddTC regimen was paclitaxel 80 mg/m^2 on days 1, 8, and 15 and carboplatin at an AUC of 5 on day 1. Both cTC and ddTC treatments were repeated every 3 weeks for up to nine cycles. After bevacizumab was approved in Japan, patients in both arms received 15 mg/kg of bevacizumab if not contraindicated. The primary endpoint of phase II was response rate (RR). An RR of ddTC+bevacizumab at least 5% higher than that of cTC + bevacizumab was considered the criterion for proceeding to phase III, which had OS as its primary endpoint. Among the 122 patients who were randomly assigned to either the cTC arm (cTC + bevacizumab, 32; cTC, 29) or the ddTC arm (ddTC+bevacizumab: 30; ddTC: 31), the RR for patients on cTC + bevacizumab, ddTC+bevacizumab, cTC, and ddTC was 67.9%, 60.7%, 55.2%, and 50.0%, respectively. However, the study did not meet the primary endpoint of phase II. Therefore, dose-dense weekly paclitaxel plus carboplatin is not promising for metastatic or recurrent cervical cancer.

14.6 Other Anti-Angiogenic Therapy

Following the results of the GOG 240 trial, additional studies were conducted to explore the efficacy of bevacizumab in combination with other therapies in patients with cervical cancer. The CECILIA study is currently underway to investigate the efficacy of adding bevacizumab to another commonly used platinum doublet, carboplatin and paclitaxel. Trial enrollment has been completed, and the interim results suggest that this combination is well tolerated, with adverse events comparable with those documented in GOG 240. The outcomes of this trial are expected in the near future [56].

Bevacizumab has been incorporated into the standard of care for the management of metastatic and recurrent cervical cancer; however, other pro-angiogenic factors have been studied as potential targets for additional therapy. EGFR and HER2/neu have been associated with poor outcomes in patients with cervical cancer [57, 58]. Pazopanib is an oral multi-targeted anti-vascular agent that targets VEGFR, and lapatinib is a dual anti-EGFR and anti-Her2/neu tyrosine kinase inhibitor [59]. The efficacy of these two agents has been investigated in a phase II trial for metastatic cervical cancer. Initially, patients were randomized to receive pazopanib versus lapatinib versus the combination of the two; however, at the time of interim analysis, the combination arm was closed owing to futility. Nonetheless, both agents were deemed tolerable as monotherapy, with an equal number of grade 3/4 toxicities experienced in each arm. Median PFS was 18.1 vs. 17.1 weeks in pazopanib and lapatinib, respectively. OS was increased by 11.6 weeks in pazopanib compared with that in lapatinib (50.7 weeks vs. 39.1 weeks). These results suggested that pazopanib and lapatinib are well-tolerated as monotherapies, with modest activity in patients with advanced and recurrent cervical cancer [59].

Neratinib, another tyrosine kinase inhibitor, has recently been demonstrated to have activity against cervical cancer. The SUMMIT Trial is an open-label phase II study conducted to evaluate the safety and efficacy of neratinib in patients with solid tumors with various mutations, including those in *Her2* (NCT01953926). The interim results of the cervical cancer arm were presented at the 2019 SGO Annual Meeting. Of the nine eligible patients (eight with adenocarcinoma) who had undergone prior chemotherapy for cervical cancer, four achieved an objective response rate (ORR 44%), including one complete response. The most common adverse event was diarrhea; however, the drug was well tolerated, and no patient discontinued the therapy owing to side effects [60].

The CIRCCa trial was conducted to investigate the combination of cediranib, a potent inhibitor of VEGFR 1, 2, and 3, with carboplatin and paclitaxel. This small, double-blind, placebo-controlled, phase II trial included 69 patients. The addition of cediranib to carboplatin/paclitaxel increased PFS from 6.7 months to 8.1 months compared with that of placebo (HR 0.58, 80% CI 0.40–0.85, $p = 0.032$). Concordantly, the addition of cediranib to cytotoxic therapy resulted in a significant increase in grade 3/4 adverse events, including diarrhea, fatigue, leukopenia, neutropenia, and febrile neutropenia.

The findings of this study confirmed that cediranib provided partial benefit when combined with carboplatin/paclitaxel in patients with advanced and metastatic cervical cancer; however, this was accompanied by increased toxicity [61].

Cetuximab, an antibody that targets EGFR, has been evaluated in combination with cisplatin in women with advanced, persistent, or recurrent cervical cancer. Combination therapy was well tolerated. PFS with cetuximab and cisplatin was comparable with that of historical controls in patients treated with cisplatin alone in GOG 169 and GOG 179. The response to cisplatin plus cetuximab was similar to that of cisplatin alone, as demonstrated in previous studies [62].

The efficacy of sunitinib, another multi-target VEGF tyrosine kinase inhibitor, for treating locally advanced or metastatic cervical cancer was evaluated in a phase II trial. Nineteen patients were evaluated, with a median time to progression of 3.5 months (range 2.7–7.0 months). No objective responses were observed in these 19 patients, although 16 had stable disease with a median duration of 4.4 months (range 2.3–17.0 months). Five of 19 patients (26.3%) developed a fistula; thus, sunitinib was considered to exhibit minimal benefit with a higher rate of fistulalization and did not warrant additional study [63]. Other non-bevacizumab anti-angiogenic therapies currently being evaluated include nimotuzumab in combination with concurrent chemoradiation therapy [64, 65], nintedanib with carboplatin and paclitaxel [66], and apatinib with a platinum doublet [67].

References

1. Safaeian M, Solomon D, Castle PE. Cervical cancer prevention-cervical screening: science in evolution. Obstet Gynecol Clin N Am. 2007;34:739–60.
2. Greer BE, Koh WJ, Abu-Rustum NR, Apte SM, Campos SM, Chan J, Cho KR, Copeland L, Crispens MA, Dupont N, Eifel PJ, Gaffney DK, Huh WK, Kapp DS, Lurain JR 3rd, Martin L, Morgan MA, Morgan RJ Jr, Mutch D, Remmenga SW, Reynolds RK, Small W Jr, Teng N, Valea FA, National Comprehensive Cancer Networks. Cervical cancer. J Natl Compr Cancer Netw. 2010;8:1388–416.
3. DiSaia PJ, Creasman WT. Clinical gynecologic oncology. 6th ed. St. Louis: Mosby; 2002.
4. Thigpen T, Shingleton H, Homesley H, Lagasse L, Blessing J. Cis- platinum in treatment of advanced or recurrent squamous cell carcinoma of the cervix: a phase II study of the gynecologic oncology group. Cancer. 1981;48:899–903.
5. Hsiang YH, Liu LF. Identification of mammalian DNA topoisomerase I as intracellular targets of the anticancer drug camptothecin. Cancer Res. 1988;48:1722–6.
6. Chou TC, Motzer RJ, Tong Y, Bosl GJ. Computerized quantitation of synergism and antagonism of taxol, topotecan, and cisplatin against human teratocarcinoma cell growth: a rational approach to clinical protocol design. J Natl Cancer Inst. 1994;86:1517–24.
7. Bookman MA, Blessing JA, Hanjani P, Herzog TJ, Andersen WA. Topotecan in squamous cell carcinoma of the cervix: a phase II study of the gynecologic oncology group. Gynecol Oncol. 2000;77:446–9.
8. Verschraegen CF, Levy T, Kudelka AP, Llerena E, Ende K, Freedman RS, Edwards CL, Hord M, Steger M, Kaplan AL, Kieback D, Fishman A, Kavanagh JJ. Phase II study of irinotecan in prior chemotherapy-treated squamous cell carcinoma of the cervix. J Clin Oncol. 1997;15:625–31.
9. Curtin JP, Blessing JA, Webster KD, Rose PG, Mayer AR, Fowler WC Jr, Malfetano JH, Alvarez RD. Paclitaxel, an active agent in nonsquamous carcinomas of the uterine cervix: a gynecologic oncology group study. J Clin Oncol. 2001;19:1275–8.
10. Gradishar WJ. Albumin-bound paclitaxel: a next-generation taxane. Expert Opin Pharmacother. 2006;7:1041–53.
11. Micha JP, Goldstein BH, Birk CL, Rettenmaier MA, Brown JV 3rd. Abraxane in the treatment of ovarian cancer: the absence of hypersensitivity reactions. Gynecol Oncol. 2006;100:437–8.
12. Alberts DS, Blessing JA, Landrum LM, Warshal DP, Martin LP, Rose SL, Bonebrake AJ, Ramondetta LM. Phase II trial of nab-paclitaxel in the treatment of recurrent or persistent advanced cervix cancer: a gynecologic oncology group study. Gynecol Oncol. 2012;127:451–5.
13. Sutton GP, Blessing JA, DiSaia PJ, McGuire WP, Adcock L. Phase II study of ifosfamide and mesna in nonsquamous carcinoma of the cervix: a gynecologic oncology group study. Gynecol Oncol. 1993;49:48–50.
14. McGuire WP, Blessing JA, Moore D, Lentz SS, Photopulos G. Paclitaxel has moderate activity in squamous cervix cancer. A gynecologic oncology group study. J Clin Oncol. 1996;14:792–5.
15. Rose PG, Blessing JA, Arseneau J. Phase II evaluation of altretamine for advanced and recurrent squamous cell carcinoma of the cervix: a gynecologic oncology group study. Gynecol Oncol. 1996;62:100–2.
16. Rose PG, Blessing JA, Van Le L, Waggoner S. Prolonged oral etoposide in recurrent or advanced squamous cell carcinoma of the cervix: a gynecologic oncology group study. Gynecol Oncol. 1998;70:263–6.
17. Rose PG, Blessing JA, Buller RE, Mannel RS, Webster KD. Prolonged oral etoposide in recurrent or advanced non-squamous cell carcinoma of the cervix: a gynecologic oncology group study. Gynecol Oncol. 2003;89:267–70.
18. Schilder RJ, Blessing JA, Morgan M, Mangan CE, Rader JS. Evaluation of gemcitabine in patients with squamous cell carcinoma of the cervix: a phase II study of the gynecologic oncology group. Gynecol Oncol. 2000;76:204–7.

19. Schilder RJ, Blessing J, Cohn DE. Evaluation of gemcitabine in previously treated patients with non-squamous cell carcinoma of the cervix: a phase II study of the gynecologic oncology group. Gynecol Oncol. 2005;96:103–7.
20. Muderspach LI, Blessing JA, Levenback C, Moore JL Jr. V a phase II study of topotecan in patients with squamous cell carcinoma of the cervix: a gynecologic oncology group study. Gynecol Oncol. 2001;8:213–5.
21. Look KY, Blessing JA, Levenback C, Kohler M, Chafe W, Roman LD. A phase II trial of CPT-11 in recurrent squamous carcinoma of the cervix: a gynecologic oncology group study. Gynecol Oncol. 1998;70:334–8.
22. Look KY, Blessing JA, Valea FA, McGehee R, Manetta A, Webster KD, Andersen WA. Phase II trial of 5-fluorouracil and high-dose leucovorin in recurrent adenocarcinoma of the cervix: a gynecologic oncology group study. Gynecol Oncol. 1997;67:255–8.
23. Look KY, Blessing JA, Gallup DG, Lentz SS. A phase II trial of 5-fluorouracil and high-dose leucovorin in patients with recurrent squamous cell carcinoma of the cervix: a gynecologic oncology group study. Am J Clin Oncol. 1996;19:439–41.
24. Garcia AA, Blessing JA, Vaccarello L, Roman LD, Gynecologic Oncology Group Study. Phase II clinical trial of docetaxel in refractory squamous cell carcinoma of the cervix: a gynecologic oncology group study. Am J Clin Oncol. 2007;30:428–31.
25. Garcia AA, Blessing JA, Darcy KM, Lenz HJ, Zhang W, Hannigan E, Moore DH. Phase II clinical trial of capecitabine in the treatment of advanced, persistent or recurrent squamous cell carcinoma of the cervix with translational research: a gynecologic oncology group study. Gynecol Oncol. 2007;104:572–9.
26. Rose PG, Blessing JA, Lele S, Abulafia O. Evaluation of pegylated liposomal doxorubicin (Doxil) as second-line chemotherapy of squamous cell carcinoma of the cervix: a phase II study of the gynecologic oncology group. Gynecol Oncol. 2006;102:210–3.
27. Muggia FM, Blessing JA, Method M, Miller DS, Johnson GA, Lee RB, Menzin A. Gynecologic oncology group study. Evaluation of vinorelbine in persistent or recurrent squamous cell carcinoma of the cervix: a gynecologic oncology group study. Gynecol Oncol. 2004;92:639–43.
28. Muggia FM, Blessing JA, Waggoner S, Berek JS, Monk BJ, Sorosky J, Pearl ML. Evaluation of vinorelbine in persistent or recurrent nonsquamous carcinoma of the cervix: a gynecologic oncology group study. Gynecol Oncol. 2005;96:108–11.
29. Lhommé C, Vermorken JB, Mickiewicz E, Chevalier B, Alvarez A, Mendiola C, Pawinski A, Lentz MA, Pecorelli S. Phase II trial of vinorelbine in patients with advanced and/or recurrent cervical carcinoma: an EORTC Gynaecological cancer cooperative group study. Eur J Cancer. 2000;36:194–9.
30. Weiss GR, Green S, Hannigan EV, Boutselis JG, Surwit EA, Wallace DL, Alberts DS. A phase II trial of carboplatin for recurrent or metastatic squamous carcinoma of the uterine cervix: a southwest oncology group study. Gynecol Oncol. 1990;39:332–6.
31. Fiorica J, Holloway R, Ndubisi B, Orr J, Grendys E, Boothby R, DeCesare S, LaPolla J, Hoffman M, Patel J. Phase II trial of topotecan and cisplatin in persistent or recurrent squamous and nonsquamous carcinomas of the cervix. Gynecol Oncol. 2002;85:89–94.
32. Rose PG, Blessing JA, Gershenson DM, McGehee R. Paclitaxel and cisplatin as first-line therapy in recurrent or advanced squamous cell carcinoma of the cervix: a gynecologic oncology group study. J Clin Oncol. 1999;17:2676–80.
33. Tinker AV, Bhagat K, Swenerton KD, Hoskins PJ. Carboplatin and paclitaxel for advanced and recurrent cervical carcinoma: the British Columbia Cancer Agency experience. Gynecol Oncol. 2005;98:54–8.
34. Stehman FB, Blessing JA, McGehee R, Barrett RJ. A phase II evaluation of mitolactol in patients with advanced squamous cell carcinoma of the cervix: a gynecologic oncology group study. J Clin Oncol. 1989;7:1892–5.
35. Bonomi P, Blessing JA, Stehman FB, DiSaia PJ, Walton L, Major FJ. Randomized trial of three cisplatin dose schedules in squamous-cell carcinoma of the cervix: a gynecologic oncology group study. J Clin Oncol. 1985;3:1079–85.

36. Omura GA, Blessing JA, Vaccarello L, Berman ML, Clarke-Pearson DL, Mutch DG, Anderson B. Randomized trial of cisplatin versus cisplatin plus mitolactol versus cisplatin plus ifosfamide in advanced squamous carcinoma of the cervix: a gynecologic oncology group study. J Clin Oncol. 1997;15:165–71.
37. Bloss JD, Blessing JA, Behrens BC, Mannel RS, Rader JS, Sood AK, Markman M, Benda J. Randomized trial of cisplatin and ifosfamide with or without bleomycin in squamous carcinoma of the cervix: a gynecologic oncology group study. J Clin Oncol. 2002;20:1832–7.
38. Moore DH, Blessing JA, McQuellon RP, Thaler HT, Cella D, Benda J, Miller DS, Olt G, King S, Boggess JF, Rocereto TF. Phase III study of cisplatin with or without paclitaxel in stage IVB, recurrent, or persistent squamous cell carcinoma of the cervix: a gynecologic oncology group study. J Clin Oncol. 2004;22:3113–9.
39. Long HJ III, Bundy BN, Grendys EC Jr, Benda JA, McMeekin DS, Sorosky J, Miller DS, Eaton LA, Fiorica JV. Gynecologic oncology group study. Randomized phase III trial of cisplatin with or without topotecan in carcinoma of the uterine cervix: a gynecologic oncology group study. J Clin Oncol. 2005;23:4626–33.
40. Monk BJ, Sill MW, McMeekin DS, Cohn DE, Ramondetta LM, Boardman CH, Benda J, Cella D. Phase III trial of four cisplatin-containing doublet combinations in stage IVB, recurrent, or persistent cervical carcinoma: a gynecologic oncology group study. J Clin Oncol. 2009;27:4649–55.
41. Kitagawa R, Katsumata N, Shibata T, Kamura T, Kasamatsu T, Nakanishi T, Nishimura S, Ushijima K, Takano M, Satoh T, Yoshikawa H. Paclitaxel plus carboplatin versus paclitaxel plus cisplatin in metastatic or recurrent cervical cancer: the open-label randomized phase III trial (JCOG0505). J Clin Oncol. 2015;33:2129–35.
42. Rahimi N. The ubiquitin-proteasome system meets angiogenesis. Mol Cancer Ther. 2012;11:538–48.
43. Wahl O, Oswald M, Tretzel L, Herres E, Arend J, Efferth T. Inhibition of tumor angiogenesis by antibodies, synthetic small molecules and natural products. Curr Med Chem. 2011;18:3136–55.
44. Folkman J. Tumor angiogenesis: therapeutic implications. N Engl J Med. 1971;285:1182–6.
45. Gasparini G. Prognostic value of vascular endothelial growth factor in breast cancer. Oncologist. 2000;5(Suppl 1):37–44.
46. Ferrara N. Vascular endothelial growth factor: basic science and clinical progress. Endocr Rev. 2004;25:581–611.
47. Cheng WF, Chen CA, Lee CN, Wei LH, Hsieh FJ, Hsieh CY. Vascular endothelial growth factor and prognosis of cervical carcinoma. Obstet Gynecol. 2000;96:721–6.
48. Lee CM, Shrieve DC, Zempolich KA, Lee RJ, Hammond E, Handrahan DL, Gaffney DK. Correlation between human epidermal growth factor receptor family (EGFR, HER2, HER3, HER4), phosphorylated Akt (P-Akt), and clinical outcomes after radiation therapy in carcinoma of the cervix. Gynecol Oncol. 2005;99:415–21.
49. Loncaster JA, Cooper RA, Logue JP, Davidson SE, Hunter RD, West CM. Vascular endothelial growth factor (VEGF) expression is a prognostic factor for radiotherapy outcome in advanced carcinoma of the cervix. Br J Cancer. 2000;83:620–5.
50. Guidi AJ, Abu-Jawdeh G, Berse B, Jackman RW, Tognazzi K, Dvorak HF, Brown LF. Vascular permeability factor (vascular endothelial growth factor) expression and angiogenesis in cervical neoplasia. J Natl Cancer Inst. 1995;87:1237–45.
51. Ferrara N, Hillan KJ, Gerber HP, Novotny W. Discovery and development of bevacizumab, an anti-VEGF antibody for treating cancer. Nat Rev Drug Discov. 2004;3:391–400.
52. Presta LG, Chen H, O'Connor SJ, Chisholm V, Meng YG, Krummen L, Winkler M, Ferrara N. Humanization of an anti-vascular endothelial growth factor monoclonal antibody for the therapy of solid tumors and other disorders. Cancer Res. 1997;57:4593–9.
53. Monk BJ, Sill MW, Burger RA, Gray HJ, Buekers TE, Roman LD. Phase II trial of bevacizumab in the treatment of persistent or recurrent squamous cell carcinoma of the cervix: a gynecologic oncology group study. J Clin Oncol. 2009;27:1069–74.

54. Tewari KS, Sill MW, Long HJ 3rd, Penson RT, Huang H, Ramondetta LM, Landrum LM, Oaknin A, Reid TJ, Leitao MM, Michael HE, Monk BJ. Improved survival with bevacizumab in advanced cervical cancer. N Engl J Med. 2014;370:734–43.
55. Ishikawa M, Shibata T, Iwata T, Nishio S, Takada T, Suzuki S, Horie K, Kudaka W, Kagabu M, Tanikawa M, Kitagawa R, Takekuma M, Kobayashi H, Yaegashi N, Japan Clinical Oncology Group. A randomized phase II/III trial of conventional paclitaxel and carboplatin with or without bevacizumab versus dose-dense paclitaxel and carboplatin with or without bevacizumab, in stage IVB, recurrent, or persistent cervical carcinoma (JCOG1311): primary analysis. Gynecol Oncol. 2021;162:292–8.
56. Redondo A, Colombo N, McCormack M, Dreosti L, Nogueira-Rodrigues A, Scambia G, Lorusso D, Joly F, Schenker M, Ruff P, Estevez-Diz M, Irahara N, Donica M, Gonzalez-Martín A. Primary results from CECILIA, a global single-arm phase II study evaluating bevacizumab, carboplatin and paclitaxel for advanced cervical cancer. Gynecol Oncol. 2020;159:142–9.
57. Yamashita H, Murakami N, Asari T, Okuma K, Ohtomo K, Nakagawa K. Correlation among six biologic factors (p53, p21WAF1, MIB-1, EGFR, HER2, and Bcl-2) and clinical outcomes after curative chemoradiation therapy in squamous cell cervical cancer. Int J Radiat Oncol Biol Phys. 2009;74:1165–72.
58. Pérez-Regadera J, Sánchez-Muñoz A, De-la-Cruz J, Ballestín C, Lora D, García-Martín R, Mendiola C, Alonso L, Alba E, Lanzós E. Negative prognostic impact of the coexpression of epidermal growth factor receptor and c-erbB-2 in locally advanced cervical cancer. Oncology. 2009;76:133–41.
59. Monk BJ, Lopez LM, Zarba JJ, Oaknin A, Tarpin C, Termrungruanglert W, Alber JA, Ding J, Stutts MW, Pandite LN. Phase II, open-label study of pazopanib or lapatinib monotherapy compared with pazopanib plus lapatinib combination therapy in patients with advanced and recurrent cervical cancer. J Clin Oncol. 2010;28:3562–9.
60. Oaknin A, Friedman CF, Roman LD, D'Souza A, Brana I, Bidard FC, Goldman J, Alvarez EA, Boni V, ElNaggar AC, Passalacqua R, Do KTM, Santin AD, Keyvanjah K, Xu F, Eli LD, Lalani AS, Bryce RP, Hyman DM, Meric-Bernstam F, Solit DB, Monk BJ. Neratinib in patients with HER2-mutant, metastatic cervical cancer: findings from the phase 2 SUMMIT basket trial. Gynecol Oncol. 2020;159:150–6.
61. Symonds RP, Gourley C, Davidson S, Carty K, McCartney E, Rai D, Banerjee S, Jackson D, Lord R, McCormack M, Hudson E, Reed N, Flubacher M, Jankowska P, Powell M, Dive C, West CML, Paul J. Cediranib combined with carboplatin and paclitaxel in patients with metastatic or recurrent cervical cancer (CIRCCa): a randomised, double-blind, placebo-controlled phase 2 trial. Lancet Oncol. 2015;16:1515–24.
62. Farley J, Sill MW, Birrer M, Walker J, Schilder RJ, Thigpen JT, Coleman RL, Miller BE, Rose PG, Lankes HA. Phase II study of cisplatin plus cetuximab in advanced, recurrent, and previously treated cancers of the cervix and evaluation of epidermal growth factor receptor immunohistochemical expression: a gynecologic oncology group study. Gynecol Oncol. 2011;121:303–8.
63. Mackay HJ, Tinker A, Winquist E, Thomas G, Swenerton K, Oza A, Sederias J, Ivy P, Eisenhauer EA. A phase II study of sunitinib in patients with locally advanced or metastatic cervical carcinoma: NCIC CTG trial IND.184. Gynecol Oncol. 2010;116:163–7.
64. Evaluate efficacy of the association nimotuzumab(HR3)/cisplatin vinorelbine on patients with cervical carcinoma (CIMAHOPE). https://ClinicalTrials.gov/show/NCT03413579.
65. Study of nimotuzumab combined with concurrent chemoradiotherapy for locally advanced cervical cancer. https://ClinicalTrials.gov/show/NCT03469531.
66. ENGOT-cx1/BGOG-cx1: 3 weekly carboplatin/paclitaxel with or without nintedanib in cervix cancer. https://ClinicalTrials.gov/show/NCT02009579.
67. Apatinib and chemotherapy sequential treatment with cervical cancer. https://ClinicalTrials.gov/show/NCT03029013.

New Therapeutic Strategies for Cervical Cancer with Special Reference to Immunotherapy

15

Takashi Iwata

Abstract

Immunotherapy has emerged as a promising treatment option for advanced cervical cancer, which has limited surgical and radiation therapy indications. The immunosuppressive environment in tumor tissues, caused by cancer cells, has a crucial role in immune evasion. Mechanisms such as the downregulation of antigen-presenting molecules, recruitment of immune suppressor cells, and T cell exhaustion contribute to immune resistance. Immune checkpoint inhibitors (ICIs) block inhibitory signals and enhance anti-tumor immune responses. Among ICIs, anti-programmed cell death 1 (anti-PD-1) has shown particularly good clinical outcomes compared with conventional chemotherapy. Adoptive T cell therapy (ACT) utilizing tumor-infiltrating lymphocytes has shown durable complete responses in advanced cervical cancer patients. Therapeutic vaccines targeting human papillomavirus antigens, such as *Listeria monocytogenes*-based vaccines and DNA vaccines, have demonstrated encouraging results in preclinical and clinical studies. Ongoing trials are evaluating the efficacy of ICIs, ACT, and therapeutic vaccines in various settings, including first-line treatment and combination approaches. The use of immunotherapy strategies is revolutionizing the treatment of cervical cancer and offers new hope for patients with advanced disease.

Keywords

Immunotherapy · Immune checkpoint inhibitor · Anti-PDL-1 · Anti-CTLA4 · Adaptive T cell therapy · Therapeutic vaccine

T. Iwata (✉)
Department of Obstetrics and Gynecology, Keio University School of Medicine, Tokyo, Japan
e-mail: iwata@a8.keio.jp

D. Aoki (ed.), *Recent Topics on Prevention, Diagnosis, and Clinical Management of Cervical Cancer*, Comprehensive Gynecology and Obstetrics,
https://doi.org/10.1007/978-981-99-9396-3_15

15.1 Introduction

The indications for surgery and radiation therapy for advanced cervical cancer patients are limited, and until recently, chemotherapy has been the mainstay of treatment. Currently, the most effective regimen for advanced cervical cancer is a combination of cisplatin, paclitaxel, and bevacizumab, with an overall response rate (RR) of 48% and a median survival of 17 months [1]. Furthermore, if this treatment is ineffective, there is no alternative effective therapy, and no consensus has yet been reached on second-line chemotherapy. Immunotherapy as a treatment consists of using the patient's own immune cells to recognize and kill tumor cells. For several decades, there have been attempts to induce anti-tumor immune responses to kill cancer cells, but these have been extremely ineffective. However, since the recent discovery of immune checkpoint molecules, drugs targeting programmed cell death 1 (PD-1) [2, 3], its ligand programmed death ligand 1 (PD-L1) [4], and cytotoxic T cell lymphocyte-associated antigen 4 (CTLA-4) [5] have been investigated clinically for various tumor types and have achieved better clinical outcomes than conventional chemotherapy. These agents, called immune checkpoint inhibitors (ICIs), promote endogenous anti-tumor immunity and, because of their broad spectrum of activity, are considered key cancer therapies, even in patients with inoperable advanced cancer [6]. Thus, recently developed cancer immunotherapy strategies are revolutionizing cancer therapy.

Most cervical cancers are caused by infection with human papillomavirus (HPV) [7]. HPV infects the basal cells of the cervical epidermis, but in most cases the infection is transient and HPV is cleared by the host immune response. However, in cases of high-risk HPV, the infection often persists, HPV genes integrate into the host genome, and oncoproteins E6 and E7 are overexpressed. These oncoproteins interfere with natural immune responses by downregulating critical pathways involved in interferon production, the STING pathway, and the expression of HPV antigens by class I major histocompatibility complex (MHC) molecules [8]. The suppression of the immune system is an important step in the development of cervical cancer. However, the expression of viral antigens in cervical cancer may be recognized as foreign antigens by the host immune system leading to tumor elimination. Thus, immunotherapy appears to be an attractive treatment option for patients with advanced cervical cancer.

The rationale for the efficacy of immunotherapy in cervical cancer is strongly supported by several molecular features including high tumor mutation burden (TMB), microsatellite instability (MSI), high expression of programmed cell death ligand 1(PD-L1), and high tumor inflammatory state. Currently, cervical cancer is considered a tumor with TMB high. The number of somatic mutations per DNA megabase is used as a proxy for the neoantigen burden, which is a newly established independent predictor of immune checkpoint inhibitor (ICI) treatment outcomes [9]. Furthermore, it is estimated that 8% of cervical cancer cases have high MSI [10], and as with other cancers, immunotherapy may be effective in such cases [11]. As mentioned above, HPV-positive cells escape the immune system if inflammatory responses are acute and by inhibiting immune recognition. Recent studies showed that the carcinogenic environment caused by a virus and inflammation may be involved in the expression of PD-L1 [12], which has an important role in suppressing T cell activity and allowing cancer cells to escape from the immune system [13]. A high expression of PD-L1 was reported in 35–96% of cervical cancer cases [13, 14], making it a good target for ICIs.

Recently developed cancer immunotherapy strategies have revolutionized the treatment of cancer. In this chapter, the current status of cancer immunotherapy for cervical cancer is discussed.

Mechanisms related to the immunosuppressive environment in tumor tissues.

Cancer cells can evade the immune system by various mechanisms that suppress or evade the immune response.

1. Cancer cells downregulate immune responses by decreasing the expression of antigen-presenting molecules or co-stimulatory molecules that are required for T cell activation [15]. Additionally, cancer cells produce immunosuppressive cytokines, such as IL-10 and TGF-β, that inhibit immune responses [16].
2. Tumors recruit various types of immune cells, such as regulatory T cells (Tregs), myeloid-derived suppressor cells, and tumor-associated macrophages, that suppress immune responses. These cells inhibit the function of effector T cells and promote angiogenesis, tumor growth, and metastasis [17].
3. Chronic exposure to antigens can cause T cells to become exhausted and lose their effector function. In cancer, this can be caused by a high level of antigen exposure and the immunosuppressive environment of a tumor [18].

Under these circumstances, immunosuppressive mechanisms induce changes in tumor immunogenicity and the acquisition of immune resistance. This is the major reason why immunotherapies that only stimulate the autoimmune system have shown low clinical efficacy in previous studies, and strategies to release immunosuppression have been attempted to overcome these obstacles. One such approach is the blocking of inhibitory molecules such as PD-1, PD-L1, and CTLA-4.

This chapter describes ICIs, such as anti-PD-1 and anti-CTLA-4 antibodies, adoptive T cell therapy (ACT) utilizing chimeric antigen receptor T cells and tumor-infiltrating T cells, as well as therapeutic vaccines targeting HPV.

15.2 ICIs

Among the many immune checkpoint molecules, PD-1/PD-L1, PD-L2, and CTLA-4 have already been used clinically in cancer therapy. PD-1 and CTLA-4 are immune checkpoint proteins that have a key role in regulating immune responses. They are part of the mechanism involved in preventing excessive immune responses, which can lead to autoimmune disease or tissue damage [19]. The location of the two molecules differs: PD-1 is present on T cells, B cells, and myeloid cells, whereas CTLA-4 is limited to T lymphocytes. Ligands of PD-1 are also widely expressed, with PD-L1 and PD-L2 expressed on non-hematopoietic cells and non-lymphoid tissues as it is induced by proinflammatory and tumorigenic signals [20]. Cancer cells can hijack these pathways to evade the immune system and promote their survival.

PD-1 and its ligands, PD-L1 and PD-L2, are often upregulated in tumor cells and in the tumor microenvironment. When PD-1 on the surface of CD4 and CD8 T cells binds to its ligand, PD-L1 and PD-L2 send an inhibitory signal to the T cell, leading to a reduction in T cell activation and function [21]. This mechanism is an important pathway that allows cancer cells to evade the immune system.

Similarly, CTLA-4 is an inhibitory protein expressed on the surface of T cells. T cells are activated by a series of signals, among which the binding of CD28 to B7 on antigen-presenting cells (APCs) is important. CTLA-4 is a homolog of CD28 but has a higher affinity than CD28 for B7. When CTLA-4-B7 binding is relatively stronger than CD28-B7 binding, interleukin-2 (IL-2) production is reduced and inhibitory signals opposing TCR-MHC binding are elicited, which prevents T cell activation [22]. CTLA-4 regulates effector T cells through other pathways, including its constitutional expression on Tregs, which downregulates B7 expression on APCs. In cancer cells, the expression of CTLA-4 can be upregulated, leading to the increased inhibition of T cell activation and function, which promotes their growth and survival and allows them to evade immune surveillance.

Therapies that target PD-1 and CTLA-4 have been developed to reverse this immunosuppression and enhance the anti-tumor immune response. These therapies, called ICIs, have shown significant promise in the treatment of a variety of cancers by blocking the interaction between these proteins and their ligands, releasing the brakes on the immune system and allowing T cells to attack cancer cells more effectively. Because of the dramatic clinical effects of ICIs, several clinical trials have been launched to assess their effects against various cancers.

15.3 Anti-PD-1/Anti-PD-L1 Therapy

The use of ICIs in cervical cancer has received a lot of attention in the past few years, with many trials for advanced or recurrent cervical cancer. ICIs currently approved by the Food and Drug Administration (FDA) include pembrolizumab and cemiplimab, which were approved as a single agent for patients with progressing or persistent PD-L1-positive cervical cancer during or after chemotherapy. The approval of pembrolizumab was based on the phase II Keynote-158 basket study [23], which enrolled 98 patients with cervical cancer who had unresectable or metastatic solid tumors that were not responding to standard therapy. At a median follow-up of 10.2 months, the objective response rate (ORR) was 12.2% (95% CI, 6.5%–20.4%), with 3 patients achieving a complete response (CR) and 9 patients achieving a partial response (PR). All 12 responses were in patients with PD-L1-positive tumors.

Following the Keynote-158 study, the Keynote-826 double-blind, phase III trial of pembrolizumab plus the standard regimen of platinum plus paclitaxel ± bevacizumab for patients with first relapse or advanced stage was conducted [24]. In the

Keynote-826 study, 617 patients with persistent, recurrent, or metastatic cervical cancer were randomly assigned at a 1:1 ratio to receive pembrolizumab (200 mg) or placebo. The primary endpoints were progression-free survival (PFS) and overall survival (OS). The median PFS was 10.4 months in the pembrolizumab group and 8.2 months in the placebo group (hazard ratio 0.65, $P < 0.001$), and the median OS was 24.4 months in the pembrolizumab group and 16.5 months in the placebo group (hazard ratio 0.67, $P < 0.001$). In a subgroup analysis based on the combined positive score (CPS), there was no significant difference in the PFS and OS for patients with CPS < 1 (hazard ratio PFS: 0.94, OS: 1.00). Of note, there were no significant differences in the PFS and OS between stage IVB patients and patients older than 65 years. The main grade 3–5 adverse events (AEs) were myelosuppression, including anemia and neutropenia, and these AEs were chemotherapy-induced. Potential immune-mediated adverse events occurred in 33.9% of patients in the pembrolizumab group and in 15.2% of those in the placebo group, including 11.4% and 2.9%, respectively, who had grade 3–5 AEs. One patient in the pembrolizumab group died from an immune-mediated adverse event (encephalitis). Infusion reactions occurred in 13.4% of patients in the pembrolizumab group and in 12.6% of those in the placebo group; events of grade 3–5 severity occurred in 2.3% of patients in each group. The results of the Keynote-826 trial have led to the approval for use in combination with chemotherapy for persistent, recurrent, or metastatic cervical cancer in the USA in 2021 and in Europe and Japan in 2022.

Cemiplimab is an anti-PD-1 antibody approved for single-agent use in persistent, recurrent, or metastatic cervical cancer. The Empower-Cervical 1 phase 3 trial included patients with disease progression after primary platinum-containing chemotherapy [25]. Patients were randomly assigned (1:1) to receive cemiplimab (350 mg every 3 weeks) or the investigator's choice of single-agent chemotherapy. The primary endpoint was OS, and PFS and safety were also assessed. Overall, 608 women were enrolled (304 in each group). In the overall trial population, the median OS was longer in the cemiplimab group than in the chemotherapy group (12.0 months vs 8.5 months; hazard ratio for death, 0.69, $P < 0.001$). The OS benefit was consistent in both histologic subgroups (squamous-cell carcinoma and adenocarcinoma). The PFS was also longer in the cemiplimab group than in the chemotherapy group in the overall population (hazard ratio for disease progression or death, 0.75, $P < 0.001$). In this trial, there was no significant difference between cemiplimab and chemotherapy in the group with low PD-L1 expression (<1%), indicating that PL-L1 expression in tumor cells is a predictive biomarker for ICI response.

The CALLA trial (NCT03830866) and Keynote A18 trial (NCT04221945) are being conducted as first-line treatment for cervical cancer. The CALLA trial studied the anti-PD-L1 antibody durvalumab, and the Keynote A18 trial investigated the anti-PD-1 antibody pembrolizumab in combination with concurrent chemoradiotherapy (CCRT). Results of the CALLA trial showed no significant difference in the PFS, OS, or ORR between the durvalumab and placebo groups. The Keynote A18 trial is ongoing as of March 2023. The use of ICIs in combination with CCRT for locally advanced cervical cancer needs further investigation.

15.4 Anti-CTLA4 Therapy

CTLA-4 is expressed on activated T cells and regulatory T cells (Treg) and inhibits T cell activation by binding to B7 (CD80/CD86) on APCs. Anti-CTLA-4 antibodies reactivate T cells by inhibiting the binding of CTLA-4 to B7 (CD80/CD86), allowing the binding of CD28 and B7 (CD80/CD86), which are co-stimulatory molecules on T cells. Anti-CTLA-4 antibodies not only bind to CTLA-4 on Tregs to reduce their immunosuppressive functions but also decrease the number of Tregs in tumor tissues by antibody-dependent cellular cytotoxicity, thereby maturing APCs and promoting cytotoxic T cell activation.

CTLA-4 blockade was shown to overcome local tumor immune escape in HPV-related cancers [26]. A phase I trial (NCT01711515) in patients with stage IB2-IIB or IIIB-IVA cervical cancer receiving ipilimumab after chemoradiotherapy and a phase II trial (NCT01693783) in patients with metastatic or recurrent HPV-related cervical cancer are ongoing. Both of these trials have completed patient recruitment and results are pending publication.

15.5 Combination of Anti-PD-1 and Anti-CTLA4 Therapy

Nivolumab, an anti-PD-1 antibody, in combination with ipilimumab, an anti-CTLA-4 antibody, is approved for the treatment of several solid tumors. In the Checkmate-358 trial, nivolumab alone and in combination with other anticancer agents was tested as a treatment for virus-associated tumors in 91 cervical cancer patients who were untreated or had failed up to two systemic therapies. At European Society for Medical Oncology (ESMO) 2019, the interim results of two regimens of nivolumab + ipilimumab (Combo A: nivolumab 3 mg/kg Q2W + ipilimumab 1 mg/kg Q6W; Combo B: nivolumab 1 mg/kg + ipilimumab 3 mg/kg Q3W [nivolumab 240 mg Q2W after 4 doses]) were presented [27]. Previously untreated patients had a numerically higher ORR for both regimens (Combo A and B untreated: 32% and 46%; previously treated: 23% and 36%). This trend was also evident for the median PFS and OS (PFS for untreated Combo A and Combo B: 13.8 and 8.5 months; previously treated: 3.6 and 5.8 months; OS untreated: both not reached; previously treated: 10.3 and 25.4 months, respectively). Primary endpoint completion was expected in September 2021, but the results have not been published to date.

Cadonilimab (AK104) is a first-in-class anti-PD-1/CTLA-4 bispecific monoclonal antibody being used as monotherapy for patients with recurrent or metastatic cervical cancer after failed platinum-based chemotherapy. It has FDA fast-track and orphan drug designation, as well as breakthrough therapy designation from the National Medical Products Administration of China [28]. A phase II single-arm study of cadonilimab monotherapy in platinum-resistant cervical cancer patients reported an ORR of 33.0% (12.0% CR) in 100 patients treated with cadonilimab [29]. The ORR for patients considered PD-L1 positive ($n = 64$) was 43.8%. In addition, a phase 3 trial (NCT04982237) of platinum-based chemotherapy ±

cadonilimab vs placebo combined with bevacizumab for first-line persistent or advanced cervical cancer has been initiated.

15.6 Adoptive T Cell Therapy

Adoptive T cell therapy (ACT) is an immunotherapy that involves removing T cells from a patient, modifying or expanding them to target tumor antigens more effectively, and then reinfusing them into the patient. The goal is to promote tumor regression by enhancing the immune system's ability to recognize and attack cancer cells. There are three main categories of ACT: tumor-infiltrating lymphocytes (TILs), engineered T cell receptor (TCR) T cells, and chimeric antigen receptor (CAR) T cells [30]. Cervical cancer is an HPV-associated tumor and theoretically a good candidate for ACT therapy. ACT requires tumor-specific antigens that are targeted by T cells, and cervical cancer expresses HPV proteins. Because these HPV proteins are not present in normal tissues, the targeting of HPV proteins by ACT allows only cancer cells to be attacked without triggering an autoimmune response, a common side effect of ACTs [31]. Engineered TCR and CAR-T therapies targeting HPV E6 and E7 have been investigated in patients with cervical cancer [32, 33]. Although these two therapies are highly effective in hematologic cancers, they have yet to be commercialized for use on solid tumors [33]. Even in cervical cancer, high-quality clinically applicable engineered TCR and CAR-T have not yet been developed.

Currently, the most promising ACT is TIL therapy. Using an established protocol, TILs are isolated and extracted from surgically excised lesions, followed by initial outgrowth and rapid expansion steps, which generate over 1000-fold TILs from the initial phase, which are finally reinfused into the patient (Fig. 15.1). An initial preliminary clinical report on TILs was published in 1988 by Rosenberg et al. at the National Cancer Institute (NCI). In that study, 20 melanoma patients were treated by TILs and IL-2 after receiving one dose of cyclophosphamide intravenously, and an objective response was noted in 11 patients, with 1 CR [34]. Since then, several more clinical trials have been performed at the NCI, with a total of 194 melanoma patients treated by TILs extracted from individual tumor fragments, and of these, over 55% of patients reported an OR [35]. Recently, an investigational, autologous cell therapy derived from TILs, ITIL-168, was granted approval by the FDA in April 2021 as an orphan drug for advanced-stage melanoma treatment, which was the first TIL therapy approved by the FDA [36]. A phase I trial by Stevanovic et al. between 2012 and 2014 with 9 patients using TILs cultured from cervical cancer tumor tissues reported durable CR in 2 patients [37]. A follow-up phase II study showed that, including the above 9 patients, of 18 patients with cervical cancer who received TIL treatment, 2 achieved CR, 3 achieved PR, and 1 achieved SD. The two CR patients maintained complete remission with no recurrence for more than 4 years (median: 58.5 months) after treatment [38]. Recently, a multicenter phase II clinical trial of 27 advanced cervical cancer patients using the same protocol reported that the ORR was 44%, the disease control rate was 89%,

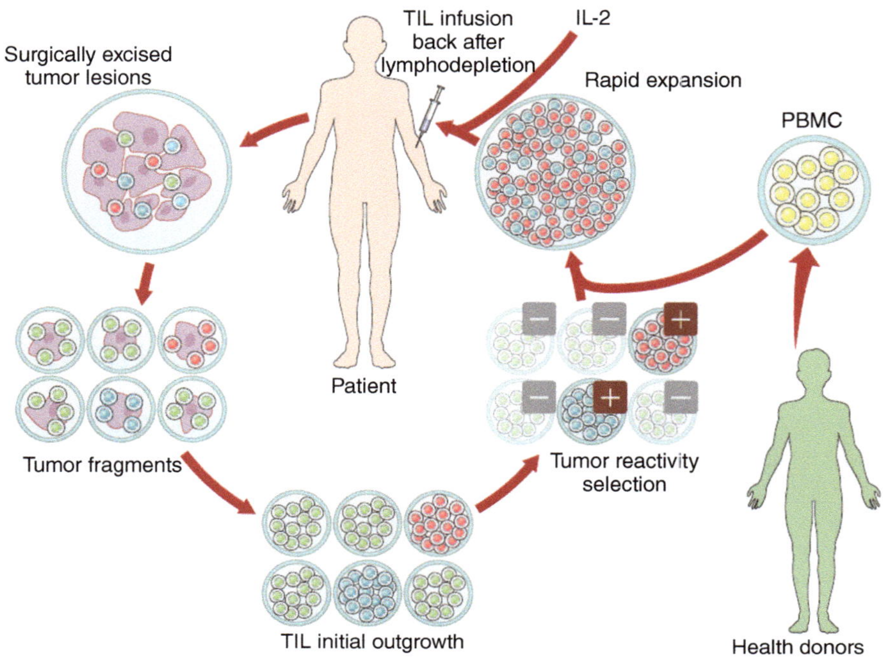

Fig. 15.1 Schematic of standard TIL therapy. Tumor tissue isolated from a surgically excised lesion is sliced into 2–3 mm^2 fragments, plated individually in culture medium, and cultured in a good manufacturing practice production facility. After several weeks of initial outgrowth, TILs from each fragment are co-cultured with tumor cells or an HLA-matched tumor cell line to confirm tumor reactivity, then collected for rapid expansion with allogeneic PBMC feeder cells from healthy donors for 14 days. Prior to TIL infusion, a non-myeloablative chemotherapy regimen for lymphodepletion is performed. After TIL infusion, the patient promptly receives a high-dose IL-2 intravenous infusion. *IL-2* interleukin-2, *PBMC* peripheral blood mononuclear cell, *TIL* tumor-infiltrating lymphocytes

with a median of 3.5 months in duration of response [39]. These data promoted the further investigation of TIL therapy for cervical cancer. Currently, a phase II trial (NCT03108495) with 138 participants is opening at multiple locations worldwide to evaluate the efficacy and safety of TILs for recurrent, metastatic, or persistent cervical carcinoma. In addition, the combination immunotherapy of TILs and ICI (anti-PD-1) improved the prognosis of metastatic cervical cancer patients with low levels of microsatellite instability who were PD-L1 negative, which might be an effective treatment for patients with poor responses to anti-PD-1 alone [40].

15.7 Therapeutic Vaccines

Human papillomavirus (HPV) infection is a major cause of cervical cancer and is present in 95% of cases. This provides a clear target antigen for immunotherapeutic approaches, because HPV antigens are consistently expressed in infected cells but absent in healthy tissues. This simplifies the development of antigen-specific immunotherapies for cervical cancer compared with other cancers without well-defined and consistently expressed antigens. Therapeutic vaccination aims to stimulate cell-mediated immunity against the HPV E6 and E7 oncoproteins in cervical cancer. *Listeria monocytogenes* (*Lm*) has gained attention as a live bacterial vector vaccine. *Lm* can infect APCs, replicate in their cytosol, and generate potent CD8 and CD4 T cell-mediated immune responses. Axalimogene filolisbac (ADXS11–001) is an engineered *Lm* vaccine fused to the HPV-16 E7 oncoprotein. Preclinical studies have shown promising results, and a phase II trial demonstrated a 12-month OS rate of 38% and a median OS of 6.1 months in advanced cervical cancer patients [41]. Another phase II study evaluated the safety and efficacy of ADXS11–001 with or without cisplatin in recurrent or refractory cervical cancer patients, showing comparable OS and PFS between the groups. Among 69 women, the group that received AXAL11–001 alone had a median OS (8.28 months; 95% CI, 5.85–10.5 months) that was comparable with the combination therapy group (8.78 months; 95% CI, 7.4–13.3 months). The median PFS (6.10 versus 6.08 months) and overall RR (17.1% versus 14.7%) were similar for both groups [42].

Therapeutic genetic vaccines, also known as naked-DNA vaccines, can be engineered to incorporate targeting and co-stimulatory genes. GX-188E is an intramuscular DNA vaccine targeting HPV E6/E7, which is administered via electroporation. In a phase II study of patients with cervical intraepithelial neoplasia (CIN) III positive for HPV type 16/18, GX-188E demonstrated 52% and 67% of patients had regression to ≤ CIN I at 20 weeks and 36 weeks after injection, respectively. Among patients who experienced regression, the HPV clearance rates were 73% at 20 weeks and 77% at 36 weeks [43]. A phase I/II trial (NCT03444376) is evaluating GX-188E in combination with pembrolizumab for advanced, inoperable, or metastatic HPV type 16/18 positive cervical cancer patients. The estimated study completion date is December 2023.

15.8 Future Directions

Various immunotherapies, including ICIs, ACT, and therapeutic vaccines, have been extensively investigated for the treatment of cervical cancer. Although pembrolizumab and cemiplimab are currently the only immunotherapies approved for clinical use in advanced cervical cancer patients, ongoing clinical trials and preclinical investigations are exploring the potential of immunotherapy for cervical cancer. The approval of pembrolizumab and cemiplimab by the FDA represents a significant milestone and opens doors for the development of other immunotherapeutic approaches targeting different aspects of the immune environment. These treatments focus on two main strategies: generating cancer-specific T cells and modulating the tumor microenvironment. By stimulating the immune system to generate cancer antigen-specific T cells, the immune response against cervical cancer cells can be enhanced. Additionally, targeting the tumor microenvironment aims to modify its immunosuppressive nature, allowing for a more effective immune response against cancer cells. These novel therapies have the potential to improve overall disease control and patient outcomes while minimizing adverse effects.

Combination therapies are also being explored to maximize the effectiveness of immunotherapy in cervical cancer. The integration of immunotherapy with other standard-of-care treatments, such as chemotherapy or radiation, has shown promise in improving treatment responses and patient outcomes. These combination approaches have the potential to enhance the immune response while simultaneously targeting cancer cells through different mechanisms, providing a more comprehensive and synergistic treatment strategy.

In conclusion, the future of cervical cancer immunotherapy holds significant potential. With the development of novel treatments that focus on generating cancer-specific T cells and modulating the tumor microenvironment, there is hope for improved disease control and patient outcomes. Ongoing research, clinical trials, and the exploration of combination therapies will have a crucial role in advancing the field of cervical cancer immunotherapy and addressing the remaining challenges.

Acknowledgments We thank J. Ludovic Croxford, PhD, from Edanz (https://jp.edanz.com/ac) for editing a draft of this manuscript.

References

1. Tewari KS, et al. Improved survival with bevacizumab in advanced cervical cancer. N Engl J Med. 2014;370:734–43. https://doi.org/10.1056/NEJMoa1309748.
2. Topalian SL, et al. Safety, activity, and immune correlates of anti-PD-1 antibody in cancer. N Engl J Med. 2012;366:2443–54. https://doi.org/10.1056/NEJMoa1200690.
3. Topalian SL, et al. Five-year survival and correlates among patients with advanced melanoma, renal cell carcinoma, or non-small cell lung cancer treated with Nivolumab. JAMA Oncol. 2019;5:1411–20. https://doi.org/10.1001/jamaoncol.2019.2187.
4. Brahmer JR, et al. Safety and activity of anti-PD-L1 antibody in patients with advanced cancer. N Engl J Med. 2012;366:2455–65. https://doi.org/10.1056/NEJMoa1200694.
5. Hodi FS, et al. Improved survival with ipilimumab in patients with metastatic melanoma. N Engl J Med. 2010;363:711–23. https://doi.org/10.1056/NEJMoa1003466.
6. Topalian SL, Drake CG, Pardoll DM. Immune checkpoint blockade: a common denominator approach to cancer therapy. Cancer Cell. 2015;27:450–61. https://doi.org/10.1016/j.ccell.2015.03.001.
7. Walboomers JM, et al. Human papillomavirus is a necessary cause of invasive cervical cancer worldwide. J Pathol. 1999;189:12–9. https://doi.org/10.1002/(SICI)1096-9896(199909)189:1<12::AID-PATH431>3.0.CO;2-F.
8. Zhou C, Tuong ZK, Frazer IH. Papillomavirus immune evasion strategies target the infected cell and the local immune system. Front Oncol. 2019;9:682. https://doi.org/10.3389/fonc.2019.00682.

9. Klempner SJ, et al. Tumor mutational burden as a predictive biomarker for response to immune checkpoint inhibitors: a review of current evidence. Oncologist. 2020;25:e147–59. https://doi.org/10.1634/theoncologist.2019-0244.
10. Lazo PA. The molecular genetics of cervical carcinoma. Br J Cancer. 1999;80:2008–18. https://doi.org/10.1038/sj.bjc.6690635.
11. Le DT, et al. PD-1 blockade in tumors with mismatch-repair deficiency. N Engl J Med. 2015;372:2509–20. https://doi.org/10.1056/NEJMoa1500596.
12. Wang J, et al. HPV-positive status associated with inflamed immune microenvironment and improved response to anti-PD-1 therapy in head and neck squamous cell carcinoma. Sci Rep. 2019;9:13404. https://doi.org/10.1038/s41598-019-49771-0.
13. Mezache L, Paniccia B, Nyinawabera A, Nuovo GJ. Enhanced expression of PD L1 in cervical intraepithelial neoplasia and cervical cancers. Mod Pathol. 2015;28:1594–602. https://doi.org/10.1038/modpathol.2015.108.
14. Enwere EK, et al. Expression of PD-L1 and presence of CD8-positive T cells in pre-treatment specimens of locally advanced cervical cancer. Mod Pathol. 2017;30:577–86. https://doi.org/10.1038/modpathol.2016.221.
15. Taylor BC, Balko JM. Mechanisms of MHC-I downregulation and role in immunotherapy response. Front Immunol. 2022;13:844866. https://doi.org/10.3389/fimmu.2022.844866.
16. Landskron G, De la Fuente M, Thuwajit P, Thuwajit C, Hermoso MA. Chronic inflammation and cytokines in the tumor microenvironment. J Immunol Res. 2014;2014:149185. https://doi.org/10.1155/2014/149185.
17. Marvel D, Gabrilovich DI. Myeloid-derived suppressor cells in the tumor microenvironment: expect the unexpected. J Clin Invest. 2015;125:3356–64. https://doi.org/10.1172/JCI80005.
18. Kamphorst AO, et al. Rescue of exhausted CD8 T cells by PD-1-targeted therapies is CD28-dependent. Science. 2017;355:1423–7. https://doi.org/10.1126/science.aaf0683.
19. Ishida Y, Agata Y, Shibahara K, Honjo T. Induced expression of PD-1, a novel member of the immunoglobulin gene superfamily, upon programmed cell death. EMBO J. 1992;11:3887–95. https://doi.org/10.1002/j.1460-2075.1992.tb05481.x.
20. Jenkins RW, Barbie DA, Flaherty KT. Mechanisms of resistance to immune checkpoint inhibitors. Br J Cancer. 2018;118:9–16. https://doi.org/10.1038/bjc.2017.434.
21. Chamoto K, Hatae R, Honjo T. Current issues and perspectives in PD-1 blockade cancer immunotherapy. Int J Clin Oncol. 2020;25:790–800. https://doi.org/10.1007/s10147-019-01588-7.
22. Buchbinder EI, Desai A. CTLA-4 and PD-1 pathways: similarities, differences, and implications of their inhibition. Am J Clin Oncol. 2016;39:98–106. https://doi.org/10.1097/COC.0000000000000239.
23. Chung HC, et al. Efficacy and safety of Pembrolizumab in previously treated advanced cervical cancer: results from the phase II KEYNOTE-158 study. J Clin Oncol. 2019;37:1470–8. https://doi.org/10.1200/JCO.18.01265.
24. Colombo N, et al. Pembrolizumab for persistent, recurrent, or metastatic cervical cancer. N Engl J Med. 2021;385:1856–67. https://doi.org/10 1056/NEJMoa2112435.
25. Tewari KS, et al. Survival with Cemiplimab in recurrent cervical cancer. N Engl J Med. 2022;386:544–55. https://doi.org/10.1056/NEJMoa2112187.
26. Callahan MK, Wolchok JD. At the bedside: CTLA-4- and PD-1-blocking antibodies in cancer immunotherapy. J Leukoc Biol. 2013;94:41–53. https://doi.org/10.1189/jlb.1212631.
27. Naumann RW, Oaknin A, Meyer T, Lopez-Picazo JM, Lao C, Bang Y-J. Efficacy and safety of nivolumab (Nivo) + ipilimumab (Ipi) in patients (pts) with recurrent/metastatic (R/M) cervical cancer: results from CheckMate 358. Ann Oncol. 2019;30:v898–9.
28. Keam SJ. Cadonilimab: first approval. Drugs. 2022;82:1333–9. https://doi.org/10.1007/s40265-022-01761-9.
29. X, W. in Society of Gynecologic Oncology Annual Meeting on Womens' cancer. Phoenix, AZ. 2022.
30. Draper LM, et al. Targeting of HPV-16+ epithelial cancer cells by TCR gene engineered T cells directed against E6. Clin Cancer Res. 2015;21:4431–9. https://doi.org/10.1158/1078-0432.CCR-14-3341.

31. Rohaan MW, Wilgenhof S, Haanen J. Adoptive cellular therapies: the current landscape. Virchows Arch. 2019;474:449–61. https://doi.org/10.1007/s00428-018-2484-0.
32. Dai H, Wang Y, Lu X, Han W. Chimeric antigen receptors modified T-cells for cancer therapy. J Natl Cancer Inst. 2016;108:djv439. https://doi.org/10.1093/jnci/djv439.
33. Norberg SM, Hinrichs CS. Engineered T cell therapy for viral and non-viral epithelial cancers. Cancer Cell. 2023;41:58–69. https://doi.org/10.1016/j.ccell.2022.10.016.
34. Rosenberg SA, et al. Use of tumor-infiltrating lymphocytes and interleukin-2 in the immunotherapy of patients with metastatic melanoma. A preliminary report. N Engl J Med. 1988;319:1676–80. https://doi.org/10.1056/NEJM198812223192527.
35. Rosenberg SA, Restifo NP. Adoptive cell transfer as personalized immunotherapy for human cancer. Science. 2015;348:62–8. https://doi.org/10.1126/science.aaa4967.
36. FDA Grants Orphan Drug Designation to Novel TIL Therapy for Advanced-Stage Melanoma. 2021.
37. Stevanovic S, et al. Complete regression of metastatic cervical cancer after treatment with human papillomavirus-targeted tumor-infiltrating T cells. J Clin Oncol. 2015;33:1543–50. https://doi.org/10.1200/JCO.2014.58.9093.
38. Stevanovic S, et al. Landscape of immunogenic tumor antigens in successful immunotherapy of virally induced epithelial cancer. Science. 2017;356:200–5. https://doi.org/10.1126/science.aak9510.
39. Stevanovic S, et al. A phase II study of tumor-infiltrating lymphocyte therapy for human papillomavirus-associated epithelial cancers. Clin Cancer Res. 2019;25:1486–93. https://doi.org/10.1158/1078-0432.CCR-18-2722.
40. Yin H, et al. TILs and anti-PD1 therapy: an alternative combination therapy for PDL1 negative metastatic cervical cancer. J Immunol Res. 2020;2020:8345235. https://doi.org/10.1155/2020/8345235.
41. Huh WK, et al. Phase II study of axalimogene filolisbac (ADXS-HPV) for platinum-refractory cervical carcinoma: an NRG oncology/gynecologic oncology group study. Gynecol Oncol. 2020;158:562–9. https://doi.org/10.1016/j.ygyno.2020.06.493.
42. Basu P, et al. A randomized phase 2 study of ADXS11-001 listeria monocytogenes-Listeriolysin O immunotherapy with or without cisplatin in treatment of advanced cervical cancer. Int J Gynecol Cancer. 2018;28:764–72. https://doi.org/10.1097/IGC.0000000000001235.
43. Choi YJ, et al. A phase II, prospective, randomized, multicenter, open-label study of GX-188E, an HPV DNA vaccine, in patients with cervical intraepithelial neoplasia 3. Clin Cancer Res. 2020;26:1616–23. https://doi.org/10.1158/1078-0432.CCR-19-1513.

Molecular Target Drug for Cervical Cancer

16

Kazunori Nagasaka

Abstract

Cervical cancer is the fourth most common malignant tumor in women worldwide in terms of incidence and mortality. Although cervical cancer is a disease whose morbidity and mortality rates have decreased over the past few decades in some developed countries due to the widespread use of cervical cancer screening and HPV vaccination with the introduction of HPV testing, no significant progress has been made in terms of treatment options. Chemotherapy, represented by platinum-based drugs such as cisplatin, is still the mainstay of treatment, but its efficiency is low, and new drugs, such as molecularly targeted therapies, are urgently needed. With the development of molecular biology and genomic medicine, molecular-targeted therapeutics have made groundbreaking progress in many cancer tumors. Effective therapies such as angiogenesis inhibitors and immune checkpoint inhibitors have been developed for cervical cancer. This review summarizes new targeted therapeutics in clinical trials to treat cervical cancer. Furthermore, it aims to summarize novel agents with a focus on their therapeutic efficacy in preclinical studies.

Keyword

Cervical cancer · Angiogenesis inhibitors · Immune checkpoint inhibitors · PARP inhibitors · Tisotumab vedotin

K. Nagasaka (✉)
Department of Obstetrics and Gynecology, Teikyo University School of Medicine, Tokyo, Japan
e-mail: nagasakak@med.teikyo-u.ac.jp

D. Aoki (ed.), *Recent Topics on Prevention, Diagnosis, and Clinical Management of Cervical Cancer*, Comprehensive Gynecology and Obstetrics,
https://doi.org/10.1007/978-981-99-9396-3_16

16.1 Introduction

Advanced, recurrent cervical cancer cervical cancer is one of the few cancers for which survival has not improved significantly since 1970s, reflecting the fact that few advances have been made in the treatment of this cancer. The concept of chemotherapy was first proposed by Paul Ehrlich in the early 1900s [1]. Since then, many anti-cancer drugs have been developed, and now, 100 years later, the use of humanized monoclonal antibodies and small molecule compounds targeting signaling pathways has become a reality. For advanced, recurrent cervical cancer, chemotherapy with the angiogenesis inhibitor bevacizumab and the single use of anti-PD-1 antibody pembrolizumab for some patients with high-frequency microsatellite instability (MSI-H) is now available for use as insurance coverage. However, advanced, recurrent cervical cancer is very frequently refractory to treatment. The worldwide clinical trials have also shown the efficacy of treatment with immune checkpoint inhibitors such as the anti-PD-1 antibody cemiplimab, PARP inhibitors, the tissue factor-directed antibody-microtubule inhibitor complex tisotumab vedotin, and even therapeutic vaccines targeting HPV in combination. In recent years, cancer genome medicine has also led to the search for targeted therapeutic agents. A number of drugs are being developed to address unmet clinical needs, and we would like to introduce a few in this report.

16.2 Development of Angiogenesis Inhibitors

Angiogenesis is essential for tumor growth and metastasis development. Vascular endothelial growth factor (VEGF), which promotes angiogenesis, is thought to be a mediator of disease progression in cervical cancer, and pathology has shown that microvessel density within tumor tissue correlates with survival [2]. The VEGF family comprises signaling proteins (VEGF-A, B, C, D, E) and its cell surface receptors (VEGFR-1, 2, 3), which in turn reduce signaling required for receptor activation, endothelial cell proliferation, and migration, and thus angiogenesis [3]. In cervical cancer, both VEGF expression and microvessel density are associated with poor prognosis, making angiogenesis inhibitors a promising option [4, 5].

Molecular biology shows that aberrant expression of the human papillomavirus (HPV)-derived E6 and E7 genes inhibits human tumor suppressor genes: the E6 gene promotes ubiquitination of p53, and the E7 gene activates HIF1-α, which inactivates retinoblastoma proteins and induces hypoxia. The E7 gene activates HIF1-α, which inactivates retinoblastoma proteins and induces hypoxia. These actions increase VEGF expression and promote angiogenesis [6]. The efficacy of treatment with bevacizumab, a human monoclonal antibody targeting VEGF, in combination with chemotherapy was demonstrated in a phase III study, GOG240. Compared to chemotherapy alone, both median PFS (2.2 months longer) and median OS (3.5 months longer) were shown to be improved, and it is currently the first-line treatment for advanced, recurrent cervical cancer [7]. As expected, the bevacizumab arm had a higher incidence of hypertension, thromboembolism, and fistulae in this study, but the toxicity profile was similar to the previous study, manageable, and this treatment approach was accepted worldwide as the standard molecular-targeted chemotherapy.

Furthermore, for locally advanced cervical cancer, a phase II trial (NCT00369122) showed an objective response rate (ORR) of 68.7% when bevacizumab was administered concurrently with cisplatin-based chemoradiation [8]. It should be noted, however, that although bevacizumab improved the median overall survival of patients with advanced, recurrent cervical cancer, it only lasted 17 months [8]. Other angiogenesis inhibitors than bevacizumab, such as cediranib, apatinib, pazopanib, and lapatinib, have not demonstrated improved survival [9]. Therefore, there are high expectations for developing molecular agents that target other growth factor pathways and personalized therapy by supplementing circulating tumor cells (CTCs) in patient's blood samples to identify molecular biomarkers for predicting the therapeutic efficacy of angiogenesis inhibitors [10]. Given the frequency of PIK3CA mutations in cervical cancer and the importance of the PI3K/Akt/mTOR pathway, clinical trials investigating the efficacy of PI3K inhibitors [11], mTOR inhibitors [12], and mTOR/PI3K dual inhibitors [13], which also inhibit angiogenesis, may become promising molecular targets.

16.3 Development of Immune Checkpoint Inhibitors

Immune checkpoint inhibitors can target cancer cells that have acquired immune escape mechanisms by activating cytotoxic T-cells. In cervical cancer, PD-L1 expression is observed in 34.4–96% of tissues, while expression is rarely observed in normal tissues [14]. It has also been shown that HPV positivity is positively correlated with increased PD-L1 expression [15], which is attributed to somatic mutations caused by HPV infection and the induction of immune checkpoint-related genes such as CTLA-4, PD-1, and PD-L1 by many neoantigens that play an inhibitory role in the tumor microenvironment [16]. It has also been shown that increased PD-L1 expression is positively associated with tumor metastasis, progression, and poor prognosis [17]. Therefore, based on the results of KEYNOTE-158 (NCT02628067), the US FDA has determined that a patient is PD-L1 positive by immunohistochemistry (CPS: Combined Positive Score (PD-L1-expressing tumour cells, lymphocytes and macrophages)/total tumour cells x 100) of 1 or greater for advanced, recurrent or metastatic cervical cancer that has been previously treated with chemotherapy [18]. Furthermore, the KEYNOTE-826 (NCT0335567) trial evaluated the effect of adding pembrolizumab to paclitaxel and platinum combination therapy with or without bevacizumab for recurrent, residual, or metastatic cervical cancer that had not previously been treated with chemotherapy, except in cases of concurrent radiation therapy. The study showed improvement in overall survival (OS; HR = 0.64; $p = 0.0001$) and progression-free survival (PFS; HR = 0.62; $p < 0.0001$), respectively. Therefore, in October 2021, the U.S. FDA approved chemotherapy ± bevacizumab plus pembrolizumab as a combination therapy [19]. Next, in the EMPOWER-Cervical 1/GOG-3016/ENGOT-cx9 trial [20], although the comparator was single-agentchemotherapy of the physician's choice (pemetrexed, vinorelbine, gemcitabine, irinotecan, topotecan), the anti-PD-1 antibody cemiplimab recurrent or metastatic cervical cancer, cemiplimab in recurrent or metastatic cervical cancer (all histological types) that worsened after paclitaxel and cisplatin combination chemotherapy" reduced the risk of death by 31% regardless of PD-L1 positivity (median OS 12.0 months with cemiplimab versus 8.5 months with single-agent chemotherapy; HR=0.69; p<0.001) [20]. Notably, it was effective "regardless of PD-L1 positivity". Perhaps future theoretical investigations into the efficacy of cemiplimab will lead to the search for clinical biomarkers that can predict treatment evaluation.

Other ongoing clinical trials are BEATcc (ENGOT-Cx10//9), which evaluated the efficacy of atezolizumab, an anti-PD-L1 antibody, on top of paclitaxel and platinum-based therapy with bevacizumab in chemotherapy-naïve patients with recurrent, residual, or metastatic cervical cancer, and BEATcc (ENGOT-Cx10/GEICO 68-C/GOG3030/JGOG1084) study, which investigated the efficacy of atezolizumab in combination with paclitaxel and platinum-based therapy [21]. In addition, the phase I/II CheckMate358 trial investigates the combination of nivolumab, an anti-PD-1 antibody, and ipilimumab, an anti-CTLA-4 antibody, for treating recurrent or metastatic cervical cancer. Anti-CTLA-4 antibodies, immune checkpoint inhibitors, can reactivate T cells by inhibiting the binding of CTLA4 on activated T cells and regulatory T cells (Treg) to B7 (CD80/CD86) on antigen-presenting cells. In this study, it was confirmed that the drug was very effective with an ORR of 46% in treatment-naïve patients regardless of PD-L1 expression in the tumor [22], and these may also be promising agents in the future. The phase II RaPIDS study (GOG-3028) showed the efficacy of the anti-PD-1 antibody Balstilimab in combination with the anti-CTLA-4 antibody zalifrelimab in patients with recurrent or metastatic cervical cancer [23]. In the SKYSCRAPER-04 study (NCT04300647), the anti-TIGIT antibody drug tiragolumab was combined with the PD-L1 antibody atezolizumab and is now accepting enrollment. In addition, a phase III clinical trial is underway to evaluate the add-on effect of immune checkpoint inhibitors to concurrent radiation chemotherapy for locally advanced cervical cancer; the efficacy of durvalumab, a human immunoglobulin G1κ monoclonal antibody that blocks the interaction between PD-L1 and PD-1, is also being investigated in the CALLA study [24] and ENGOTcx11/KEYNOTE-A18 study investigating the add-on effect of pembrolizumab is underway [25]. Although still in phase I trials, the efficacy of ipilimumab, an anti-CTLA-4 antibody, as monotherapy after concurrent radiation chemotherapy for advanced cervical cancer with positive lymph nodes has also been demonstrated. Thus, clinical trials are being conducted overseas to investigate the efficacy of immune checkpoint inhibitors in treatment-resistant or recurrent cervical cancer and in combination with concurrent radiation chemotherapy [26].

16.4 Development of PARP Inhibitors and Tisotumab Vedotin

As the efficacy of immune checkpoint inhibitors for advanced, recurrent, and metastatic cervical cancer is demonstrated, the potential for treatment with PARP inhibitors, which target DNA damage repair enzymes, is also being investigated. The phase I/II TOPACIO/KEYNOTE-162 study of the PARP inhibitor niraparib in combination with pembrolizumab in advanced or metastatic triple-negative breast cancer and recurrent platinum-resistant ovarian cancer suggested a synergistic effect of these agents [27, 28]. In cervical cancer, it has been shown that cervical cancer cell lines are highly sensitive to the PARP inhibitor olaparib, which is associated with high cellular poly ADP-ribosylation, although this is an in vitro study [29]. Enrollment is now underway for a trial to test the efficacy of veliparib, olaparib, and rucaparib in treatment-resistant or recurrent cervical cancer [30–32].The phase II innovaTV 204/GOG-3023/ENGOT-cx6 trial demonstrated the efficacy of tisotumab vedotin monotherapy in previously treated recurrent and metastatic cervical cancer with an ORR of 24% [33]. These are very noteworthy results indicating the potential of a new molecular-targeted therapy, and the U.S. FDA granted expedited approval of tisotumab vedotin in September 2021 for "recurrent or metastatic cervical cancer that has relapsed during or after treatment." A phase III trial is currently ongoing, with enrollment underway.

16.5 Development of Therapeutic Vaccines

Cervical cancer is caused by HPV infection, and as the disease progresses, Th1 cells and CD4+ and CD8+ T cell-derived cytotoxic T cells become strongly involved [34]. Cellular immunity is more critical than humoral immunity for the clearance of viral infection, and therapeutic vaccines that induce cellular immune responses in cervical precancerous lesions have been developed in many countries. The efficacy of these therapeutic vaccines has been confirmed in patients with cervical precancerous lesions, where induction of HPV-specific T cell responses has been shown to result in clinical regression. Clinical trials are ongoing for pembrolizumab in combination with the therapeutic vaccine GX-188E [35] for advanced cervical cancer as well as cervical precancerous lesions [36]. Reported at ASCO in 2021 as the KEYNOTE-567 trial, this trial is designed to evaluate pembrolizumab in HPV type 16 and 18 positives recurrent or metastatic cervical. The median PFS and OS were 4.1 and 16.7 months, respectively, in patients with HPV type 16 or 18 positive recurrent or metastatic cervical cancer treated with the combination of pembrolizumab and GX-188E. The median PFS and OS were shown to be improved over pembrolizumab monotherapy, as shown in KEYNOTE-158 above. In particular, patients with PD-L1-positive, HPV-16-positive, squamous cell carcinoma showed a high response rate of 48.0% with this combination, suggesting that pembrolizumab plus GX-188E may be a new treatment option for patients with advanced, recurrent cervical cancer.

16.6 Cancer Gene Panel Test for Molecular Target Therapy

The Comprehensive Cancer Genome Profiling (CGP) test can collectively detect mutations in target genes by analyzing them using next-generation sequencers (NGS). The test can be broadly classified into the amplicon method, which can screen for hot spots of specific gene mutations, and the hybrid capture method, which can comprehensively analyze base substitution/insertion/deletion mutations, copy number changes, and fusion genes. The CGP test is currently being carried out based on the guidelines for chemotherapy issued by relevant academic societies. The CGP tests can only be calculated if the attending physician judges, based on the patient's general condition and organ functions, that there is a high probability that chemotherapy will be indicated after the test is performed. However, as each CGP test usually takes at least three weeks to return results, it is necessary to explain the test and ensure that it is not missed in order to ensure therapeutic benefit. The evidence for the efficacy of the CGP test in lung cancer patients has been accumulated and is well known. In several clinical trials for other types of cancer, the detection of driver genes by the CGP test has increased survival rates [37]. In August 2020, the European Society of Clinical Oncology (ESMO) announced that it had approved the use of the CGP test for the treatment of advanced non-squamous, non-small cell lung, prostate, and ovarian cancers, as well as advanced non-squamous, non-small cell lung, prostate, and ovarian cancers [38]. Candidate driver genes for cervical cancer have been identified based on the results analyzed by The Cancer Genome Atlas (TCGA) [39], but those that can be used as companion diagnostics have not been determined. Recently, the results of a basket study [40] against representative driver genes have been shown, which may apply to cervical cancer patients in the future. In addition, the results of measuring TMB in 100,000 samples using the F1CDx, as mentioned above, showed that in cervical cancer (squamous cell carcinoma), the number of samples with a TMB-high (high tumor mutation burden) of 20 mutations/Mb or more was relatively high at 6.7% (4.3–10.2) [41]. Based on the results of the KEYNOTE-158 trial [42], an international, non-randomized, open-label, phase II trial in unresectable locally advanced or metastatic solid tumours with mismatch repair (MMR)-deficient or MSI-high, including cervical cancer patients, TMB-high is a biomarker that predicts treatment response [43–45]. Conversely, based on the results of the KEYNOTE-826 study [19], which showed the efficacy of chemotherapy ± pembrolizumab combination in treatment-resistant, recurrent, or metastatic cervical cancer with positive PD-L1 test, TMB-high could be useful as a biomarker for predicting treatment response. However, the tumor proportion score (TPS) could also be devised to score the evaluation of PD-1 expression in tumor cells. The determination TMB-high, together with MSI-high and PD-1/PD-L1 protein expression, is a potential biomarker for anti-PD-1 (pembrolizumab, nivolumab) and anti-PD-L1 (atezolizumab, avelumab, durvalumab) antibody drugs that have been introduced into clinical practice [44].

While the ESMO recommends the CGP testing for patients with metastatic cancer [38], and the prognosis is expected to improve after testing in the treatment of cervical cancer, there is insufficient research on cost-effectiveness, and there are concerns that continued inappropriate use of the CGP testing will put pressure on healthcare costs due to high drug prices for molecularly targeted drugs [45]. It should be noted that the effectiveness of testing is also not apparent. In general practice, the appropriate timing of the CGP testing for cervical cancer patients and the effectiveness of the test is not precise at present, as the likelihood of actually reaching treatment after testing is never high. However, cancer treatment guidelines based on gene panel testing using next-generation sequencing recommend that "the timing of cancer genomic profiling testing should not be limited to the treatment line alone, but the optimal timing should be considered in light of the subsequent treatment plan" [46]. It may be possible to improve post-test survival in cervical cancer by selecting an appropriate time for CGP testing during treatment and suggesting treatment based on genomic abnormalities, rather than limiting it to when the patient has completed standard treatment.

16.7 Conclusion and Future Direction

Advanced recurrent cervical cancer is refractory, and the development of novel, more personalized therapies and new treatment strategies is needed. In particular, developing immune checkpoint inhibitors and therapeutic vaccines holds promise. Ongoing clinical studies of phase I, II, and III are summarized in Tables 16.1, 16.2, and 16.3 [47–66]. Clearly, there is progress in drug discovery in the field of immune checkpoint inhibitors and therapeutic vaccines. In addition to these novel target drugs, research into the benefits of using radiotherapy and angiogenesis inhibitors in combination is ongoing [47–50, 58, 59, 63–65], Further researches on CTCs obtained from cervical cancer patients must be a future challenge. The ability to detect CTCs with greater accuracy and predict treatment response using minimally invasive methods will open new vistas in future cervical cancer treatment strategies. Although the onset of cervical cancer can be prevented by "cervical screening and HPV vaccination," at present, except for some countries where both screening and vaccination rates are high, many countries, especially developing countries, have not yet reached the stage where cervical cancer can be eradicated. Treatment strategies are needed for advanced, recurrent cervical cancer that is difficult to treat with existing protocols. Along with the development of genomic medicine, we strongly hope for the improvement of precision medicine for treatment-resistant cervical cancer and breakthroughs in new drug discovery.

Table 16.1 Ongoing clinical studies for advanced cervical cancer: phase I

National Clinical Trial (NCT)	Title	Phase	Primary end point	Reference URL
NCT03298893	Nivolumab in association with radiotherapy and cisplatin in locally advanced cervical cancers followed by adjuvant nivolumab for up to 6 months (NiCOL)	I	Dose-limiting toxicity	https://ascopubs.org/doi/abs/10.1200/JCO.2022.40.16_suppl.5534 (ref. [47])
NCT03738228	Atezolizumab before and/or with chemoradiotherapy in immune system activation in patients with node-positive stage IB2, II, IIIB, or IVA cervical cancer	I	T cell receptor beta (TCRB) clonal expansion in peripheral blood	https://ijgc.bmj.com/content/30/5/701.long (ref. [48])
NCT03277482	Durvalumab, tremelimumab + radiotherapy in gynecologic cancer	I	Maximum tolerated dose	https://jitc.bmj.com/content/10/Suppl_2/A590 (ref. [49])
NCT03452332	Stereotactic body radiation therapy, tremelimumab, and durvalumab in treating participants with recurrent or metastatic cervical, vaginal, or vulvar cancers	I	Adverse events	https://www.mdanderson.org/patients-family/diagnosis-treatment/clinical-trials/clinical-trials-index/clinical-trials-detail.ID2017-0548.html (ref. [50])
NCT02379520	HPV-16/18 E6/E7-specific T lymphocytes, relapsed HPV-associated cancers, HESTIA (HESTIA)	I	Dose-limiting toxicity	https://clinicaltrials.gov/ct2/show/NCT02379520 (ref. [51])
NCT03578406	HPV-E6-specific anti-PD1 TCR-T cells in the treatment of HPV-positive NHSCC or cervical cancer	I	Maximum tolerated dose	https://clinicaltrials.gov/ct2/show/NCT03578406 (ref. [52])
NCT02172911	A study of INO-3112 DNA vaccine with electroporation in participants with cervical cancer	I	Adverse effects	https://clinicaltrials.gov/ct2/show/NCT02172911 (ref. [53])

Table 16.2 Ongoing clinical studies for advanced cervical cancer: phase II

National Clinical Trial (NCT)	Title	Phase	Primary end point	Reference URL
NCT02635360	Pembrolizumab and chemoradiation treatment for advanced cervical cancer	II	Change in immunologic markers	https://clinicaltrials.gov/ct2/show/NCT02635360 (ref. [54])
NCT03612791	Trial assessing the inhibitor of programmed cell death ligand 1 (PD-L1) immune checkpoint atezolizumab (ATEZOLACC)	II	Progression-free survival	https://clinicaltrials.gov/ct2/history/NCT03612791 (ref. [55])
NCT03833479	TSR-042 as maintenance therapy for patients with high-risk locally advanced cervical cancer after chemoradiation (ATOMICC)	II	Progression-free survival	https://ijgc.bmj.com/content/32/9/1196.long (ref. [56])
NCT01693783	Ipilimumab in treating patients with metastatic or recurrent human papilloma virus-related cervical cancer	II	Number of adverse events Objective response rate	https://jamanetwork.com/journals/jamaoncology/fullarticle/2663280 (ref. [57])
NCT03614949	SBRT and atezolizumab in the management of recurrent, persistent, or metastatic cervical cancer	II	Overall response rate	https://www.sciencedirect.com/science/article/abs/pii/S0360301622012226 (ref. [58])
NCT03192059	Study of pembrolizumab, radiation and immune modulatory cocktail in cervical/uterine cancer (PRIMMO)	II	Objective response rate	https://link.springer.com/article/10.1007/s00262-022-03253-x (ref. [59])
NCT03444376	The combination of GX-188E vaccination and pembrolizumab in patients with HPV 16 and/or 18+ advanced cervical cancer	II	Overall response rate	https://ascopubs.org/doi/10.1200/JCO.2021.39.15_suppl.5511(ref. [36])
NCT03260023	Phase Ib/II of TG4001 and avelumab in HPV16 positive R/M cancers	Ib/II	Overall response rate Progression-free survival	https://www.annalsofoncology.org/article/S0923-7534(19)59422-4/fulltext (ref. [60])
NCT04405349	Investigating the combination of VB10.16 and atezolizumab in patients with HPV 16 positive cervical cancer	II	Adverse events Overall response rate	https://www.annalsofoncology.org/article/S0923-7534(20)41016-6/fulltext (ref. [61])

(continued)

Table 16.2 (continued)

National Clinical Trial (NCT)	Title	Phase	Primary end point	Reference URL
NCT04646005	Cemiplimab and ISA101b vaccine in adult participants with recurrent/ metastatic human papillomavirus (HPV)16 cervical cancer who have experienced disease progression after first-line chemotherapy	II	Objective response rate	https://clinicaltrials.gov/ct2/show/NCT04646005 (ref. [62])

Table 16.3 Ongoing clinical studies for advanced cervical cancer: phase III

National Clinical Trial (NCT)	Title	Phase	Primary end point	Reference URL
NCT03830866	Study of durvalumab with chemoradiotherapy for women with locally advanced cervical cancer (CALLA)	III	Progression-free survival	https://ijgc.bmj.com/content/30/7/1065.long (ref. [63])
NCT04221945	Study of chemoradiotherapy with or without pembrolizumab (MK-3475) for the treatment of locally advancedcervicalcancer(MK-3475-A18/KEYNOTE-A18/ ENGOT-cx11/GOG-3047)	III	Progression-free overall survival	https://ascopubs.org/doi/abs/10.1200/JCO.2020.38.15_suppl.TPS6096 (ref. [64])
NCT03556839	Platinum chemotherapy plus paclitaxel with bevacizumab and atezolizumab in metastatic carcinoma of the cervix (BEATcc)	III	Overall survival	https://ijgc.bmj.com/content/30/1/139.long (ref. [21])
NCT03912415	Efficacy and safety of BCD-100 (anti-PD-1) in combination with platinum-based chemotherapy with and without bevacizumab as first-line treatment of subjects with advanced cervical cancer (FERMATA)	III	Overall survival	https://clinicaltrials.gov/ct2/show/NCT03912415. (ref. [65])
NCT03257267	Study of cemiplimab in adults with cervical cancer	III	Overall survival	https://www.nejm.org/doi/full/10.1056/NEJMoa2112187 (ref. [20])
NCT04697628	Tisotumab vedotin vs chemotherapy in recurrent or metastatic cervical cancer (innovaTV 301)	III	Overall survival	https://ijgc.bmj.com/content/31/Suppl_3/A1.1 (ref. [66])

References

1. Kaufmann SH. Paul Ehrlich: founder of chemotherapy. Nat Rev Drug Discov. 2008;7(5):373.
2. Obermair A, et al. Tumor angiogenesis in stage IB cervical cancer: correlation of microvessel density with survival. Am J Obstet Gynecol. 1998;178(2):314–9.
3. Ferrara N. VEGF and the quest for tumour angiogenesis factors. Nat Rev Cancer. 2002;2:795–803.
4. Cheng WF, Chen CA, Lee CN, et al. Vascular endothelial growth factor and prognosis of cervical carcinoma. Obstet Gynecol. 2000;96:721–6.
5. Bremer GL, Tiebosch AT, van der Putten HW, et al. Tumor angiogenesis: an independent prognostic parameter in cervical cancer. Am J Obstet Gynecol. 1996;174:126–31.
6. López-Ocejo O, et al. Oncogenes and tumor angiogenesis: the HPV-16 E6 oncoprotein activates the vascular endothelial growth factor (VEGF) gene promoter in a p53 independent manner. Oncogene. 2000;19(40):4611–20.
7. Tewari KS, et al. Improved survival with bevacizumab in advanced cervical cancer. N Engl J Med. 2014;370(8):734–43.
8. Schefter TE, et al. A phase II study of bevacizumab in combination with definitive radiotherapy and cisplatin chemotherapy in untreated patients with locally advanced cervical carcinoma: preliminary results of RTOG 0417. Int J Radiat Oncol Biol Phys. 2012;83(4):1179–84.
9. Chuai Y, et al. Vascular endothelial growth factor (VEGF) targeting therapy for persistent, recurrent, or metastatic cervical cancer. Cochrane Database Syst Rev. 2021;3(3):CD013348.
10. Tewari KS, et al. Circulating tumor cells in advanced cervical cancer: NRG oncology-gynecologic oncology group study 240 (NCT 00803062). Mol Cancer Ther. 2020;19(11):2363–70.
11. Krishnamurthy S, et al. Targeting the mutant PIK3CA gene by DNA-alkylating pyrrole-imidazole polyamide in cervical cancer. Cancer Sci. 2021;112(3):1141–9.
12. Ji J, et al. Activation of mTOR signaling pathway contributes to survival of cervical cancer cells. Gynecol Oncol. 2010;117(1):103–8.
13. Bahrami A, et al. The potential value of the PI3K/Akt/mTOR signaling pathway for assessing prognosis in cervical cancer and as a target for therapy. J Cell Biochem. 2017;118(12):4163–9.
14. Enwere EK, et al. Expression of PD-L1 and presence of CD8-positive T cells in pre-treatment specimens of locally advanced cervical cancer. Mod Pathol. 2017;30(4):577–86.
15. Mezache L, et al. Enhanced expression of PD L1 in cervical intraepithelial neoplasia and cervical cancers. Mod Pathol. 2015;28(12):1594–602.
16. Qin S, et al. Novel immune checkpoint targets: moving beyond PD-1 and CTLA-4. Mol Cancer. 2019;18(1):155.
17. Yang W, et al. Increased expression of programmed death (PD)-1 and its ligand PD-L1 correlates with impaired cell-mediated immunity in high-risk human papillomavirus-related cervical intraepithelial neoplasia. Immunology. 2013;139(4):513–22.
18. Chung HC, et al. Efficacy and safety of Pembrolizumab in previously treated advanced cervical cancer: results from the phase II KEYNOTE-158 study. J Clin Oncol. 2019;37(17):1470–8.
19. Colombo N, et al. Pembrolizumab for persistent, recurrent, or metastatic cervical cancer. N Engl J Med. 2021;385(20):1856–67.
20. Tewari KS, et al. Survival with Cemiplimab in recurrent cervical cancer. N Engl J Med. 2022;386(6):544–55.
21. Grau JF, et al. A randomized phase III trial of platinum chemotherapy plus paclitaxel with bevacizumab and atezolizumab versus platinum chemotherapy plus paclitaxel and bevacizumab in metastatic (stage IVB), persistent, or recurrent carcinoma of the cervix: the BEATcc study (ENGOT-Cx10/GEICO 68-C/JGOG1084/GOG-3030). Int J Gynecol Cancer. 2020;30(1):139–43.
22. Hollebecque A, et al. An open-label, multicohort, phase I/II study of nivolumab in patients with virus-associated tumors (CheckMate 358): efficacy and safety in recurrent or metastatic (R/M) cervical, vaginal, and vulvar cancers. J Clin Oncol. 2017;35:5504.

23. O'Malley DM, et al. Phase II study of the safety and efficacy of the anti-PD-1 antibody balstilimab in patients with recurrent and/or metastatic cervical cancer. Gynecol Oncol. 2021;163(2):274–80.
24. Mayadev J, et al. CALLA: efficacy and safety of concurrent and adjuvant durvalumab with chemoradiotherapy versus chemoradiotherapy alone in women with locally advanced cervical cancer: a phase III, randomized, double-blind, multicenter study. Int J Gynecol Cancer. 2020;30(7):1065–70.
25. Lorusso D, et al. 164 ENGOT-cx11/GOG 3047/KEYNOTE-A18: a phase 3, randomized, double-blind study of pembrolizumab with chemoradiotherapy in patients with high-risk locally advanced cervical cancer. Int J Gynecol Cancer. 2020;30:A71 LP–A71.
26. Mayadev JS, et al. Sequential Ipilimumab after Chemoradiotherapy in curative-intent treatment of patients with node-positive cervical cancer. JAMA Oncol. 2020;6(1):92–9.
27. Vinayak S, et al. Open-label clinical trial of Niraparib combined with Pembrolizumab for treatment of advanced or metastatic triple-negative breast cancer. JAMA Oncol. 2019;5(8):1132–40.
28. Konstantinopoulos PA, et al. Single-arm phases 1 and 2 trial of Niraparib in combination with Pembrolizumab in patients with recurrent platinum-resistant ovarian carcinoma. JAMA Oncol. 2019;5(8):1141–9.
29. Bianchi A, et al. PARP-1 activity (PAR) determines the sensitivity of cervical cancer to olaparib. Gynecol Oncol. 2019;155(1):144–50.
30. Thaker PH, et al. A phase I trial of paclitaxel, cisplatin, and veliparib in the treatment of persistent or recurrent carcinoma of the cervix: an NRG oncology study (NCT#01281852). Ann Oncol. 2017;28(3):505–11.
31. Kunos C, et al. A phase I-II evaluation of veliparib (NSC #737664), topotecan, and filgrastim or pegfilgrastim in the treatment of persistent or recurrent carcinoma of the uterine cervix: an NRG oncology/gynecologic oncology group study. Int J Gynecol Cancer. 2015;25(3):484–92.
32. Jackson CC, et al. A phase II trial of bevacizumab and rucaparib in recurrent carcinoma of the cervix or endometrium. J Clin Oncol. 2021;39:5527.
33. Coleman RL, et al. Efficacy and safety of tisotumab vedotin in previously treated recurrent or metastatic cervical cancer (innovaTV 204/GOG-3023/ENGOT-cx6): a multicentre, open-label, single-arm, phase 2 study. Lancet Oncol. 2021;22(5):609–19.
34. van der Burg SH, et al. Therapeutic vaccination against human papillomavirus induced malignancies. Curr Opin Immunol. 2011;23(2):252–7.
35. Kim TJ, et al. Clearance of persistent HPV infection and cervical lesion by therapeutic DNA vaccine in CIN3 patients. Nat Commun. 2014;5:5317.
36. Park JS, et al. Efficacy and safety results of GX-188E, a therapeutic DNA vaccine, combined with pembrolizumab administration in patients with HPV 16- and/or 18- positive advanced cervical cancer: phase II interim analysis results (KEYNOTE-567). J Clin Oncol. 2021;39:5511.
37. Kris MG, Johnson BE, Berry LD, Kwiatkowski DJ, Iafrate AJ, Wistuba II, et al. Using multiplexed assays of oncogenic drivers in lung cancers to select targeted drugs. JAMA. 2014;311:1998–2006.
38. Mosele F, Remon J, Mateo J, Westphalen CB, Barlesi F, Lolkema MP, et al. Recommendations for the use of next-generation sequencing (NGS) for patients with metastatic cancers: a report from the ESMO precision medicine working group. Ann Oncol. 2020;31:1491–505.
39. Ojesina AI, Lichtenstein L, Freeman SS, Pedamallu CS, Imaz-Rosshandler I, et al. Landscape of genomic alterations in cervical carcinomas. Nature. 2014;506:371–5.
40. Jhaveri K, Chang MT, Juric D, Saura C, Gambardella V, Melnyk A, et al. Phase I basket study of Taselisib, an isoform-selective PI3K inhibitor, in patients with *PIK3CA*-mutant cancers. Clin Cancer Res. 2021;27:447–59.
41. Chalmers ZR, Connelly CF, Fabrizio D, Gay L, Ali SM, Ennis R, et al. Analysis of 100,000 human cancer genomes reveals the landscape of tumor mutational burden. Genome Med. 2017;9:34.
42. Marabelle A, Fakih M, Lopez J, Shah M, Shapira-Frommer R, Nakagawa K, et al. Association of tumour mutational burden with outcomes in patients with advanced solid tumours treated

with pembrolizumab: prospective biomarker analysis of the multicohort, open-label, phase 2 KEYNOTE-158 study. Lancet Oncol. 2020;21:1353–65.
43. Luchini C, Bibeau F, Ligtenberg MJL, Singh N, Nottegar A, Bosse T, et al. ESMO recommendations on microsatellite instability testing for immunotherapy in cancer, and its relationship with PD-1/PD-L1 expression and tumour mutational burden: a systematic review-based approach. Ann Oncol. 2019;30:1232–43.
44. Vanderwalde A, Spetzler D, Xiao N, Gatalica Z, Marshall J. Microsatellite instability status determined by next-generation sequencing and compared with PD-L1 and tumor mutational burden in 11,348 patients. Cancer Med. 2018;7:746–56.
45. Haslem DS, Van Norman SB, Fulde G, Knighton AJ, Belnap T, Butler AM, et al. A retrospective analysis of precision medicine outcomes in patients with advanced cancer reveals improved progression-free survival without increased health care costs. J Oncol Pract. 2017;13:e108–19.
46. Sunami K, Ichikawa H, Kubo T, Kato M, Fujiwara Y, Shimomura A, et al. Feasibility and utility of a panel testing for 114 cancer-associated genes in a clinical setting: a hospital-based study. Cancer Sci. 2019;110:1480–90.
47. Rodrigues M, et al. Combination of nivolumab with chemoradiotherapy for locally advanced cervical cancer: NiCOL phase I trial. J Clin Oncol. 2022;40:5534.
48. Mayadev J, Zamarin D, Deng W, Lankes H, O'Cearbhaill R, Aghajanian CA, et al. Anti-PD-L1 (atezolizumab) as an immune primer and concurrently with extended-field chemoradiotherapy for node-positive locally advanced cervical cancer. Int J Gynecol Cancer. 2020;30(5):701–4.
49. Lee L, Konstantinopoulos P, Matulonis U, Liu J, Horowitz N, Lee E, et al. 563 a phase I clinical trial of radiation therapy, durvalumab and tremelimumab in recurrent gynecologic cancer. J Immunother Cancer. 2022;10:A590 LP-A590.
50. Stereotactic body radiation therapy, tremelimumab and durvalumab in treating participants with recurrent or metastatic cervical, vaginal, or vulvar cancers. https://www.mdanderson.org/patients-family/diagnosis-treatment/clinical-trials/clinical-trials-index/clinical-trials-detail.ID2017-0548.html
51. HPV-16/18 E6/E7-specific T lymphocytes, relapsed HPV-associated cancers, HESTIA (HESTIA). https://clinicaltrials.gov/ct2/show/NCT02379520
52. HPV-E6-specific anti-PD1 TCR-T cells in the treatment of HPV-positive NHSCC or cervical cancer. https://clinicaltrials.gov/ct2/show/NCT03578406
53. A study of INO-3112 DNA vaccine with electroporation in participants with cervical cancer. https://clinicaltrials.gov/ct2/show/NCT02172911
54. Pembrolizumab and chemoradiation treatment for advanced cervical cancer. https://clinicaltrials.gov/ct2/show/NCT02635360
55. Trial assessing the inhibitor of programmed cell death ligand 1 (PD-L1) immune checkpoint atezolizumab (ATEZOLACC). https://clinicaltrials.gov/ct2/history/NCT03612791
56. Garcia-Duran C, Grau F, Villacampa G, Oaknin A. ATOMICC trial: a randomized, open-label, phase II trial of anti-PD1, dostarlimab, as maintenance therapy for patients with high-risk locally advanced cervical cancer after chemoradiation. Int J Gynecol Cancer. 2022;32:1196.
57. Lheureux S, Butler MO, Clarke B, Cristea MC, Martin LP, Tonkin K, et al. Association of ipilimumab with safety and antitumor activity in women with metastatic or recurrent human papillomavirus-related cervical carcinoma. JAMA Oncol. 2018;4(7):e173776.
58. Ahmed KA, Quick AM, Bixel K, Kim Y, Lemerond E, Chon HS, et al. Atezolizumab and stereotactic body radiation therapy in metastatic, recurrent or persistent cervical cancer: interim results from a non-randomized, open-label phase II multi-institutional study. Int J Radiat Oncol. 2022;114:S89–90.
59. De Jaeghere EA, Tuyaerts S, Van Nuffel AMT, Belmans A, Bogaerts K, Baiden-Amissah R, et al. Pembrolizumab, radiotherapy, and an immunomodulatory five-drug cocktail in pretreated patients with persistent, recurrent, or metastatic cervical or endometrial carcinoma: results of the phase II PRIMMO study. Cancer Immunol Immunother. 2023;72(2):475–91.
60. Le Tourneau C, Delord J-P, Cassier P, Loirat D, Tavernaro A, Bastien B, et al. Phase Ib/II trial of TG4001 (Tipapkinogene sovacivec), a therapeutic HPV-vaccine, and Avelumab in patients with recurrent/metastatic (R/M) HPV-16+ cancers. Ann Oncol. 2019;30:v494–5.

61. Hillemanns P, Baurain J-F, Blecharz P, Lindemann K, Nicolaisen B, Schetne K, et al. 881TiP a multi-centre, open-label phase II trial of the combination of VB10.16 and atezolizumab in patients with advanced or recurrent, non-resectable HPV16 positive cervical cancer. Ann Oncol. 2020;31:S645–6.
62. Cemiplimab and ISA101b vaccine in adult participants with recurrent/metastatic human. https://clinicaltrials.gov/ct2/show/NCT04646005.
63. Mayadev J, Nunes AT, Li M, Marcovitz M, Lanasa MC, Monk BJ. CALLA: efficacy and safety of concurrent and adjuvant durvalumab with chemoradiotherapy versus chemoradiotherapy alone in women with locally advanced cervical cancer: a phase III, randomized, double-blind, multicenter study. Int J Gynecol Cancer. 2020;30(7):1065–70.
64. Lorusso D, Colombo N, Coleman R, Randall L, Duska L, Xiang Y, et al. 164 ENGOT-cx11/GOG 3047/KEYNOTE-A18: a phase 3, randomized, double-blind study of pembrolizumab with chemoradiotherapy in patients with high-risk locally advanced cervical cancer. Int J Gynecol Cancer. 2020;30:A71 LP-A71.
65. Efficacy and safety of BCD-100 (Anti-PD-1) in combination with platinum-based chemotherapy with and without bevacizumab as first-line treatment of subjects with advanced cervical cancer (FERMATA). https://clinicaltrials.gov/ct2/show/NCT03912415.
66. Vergote IB, Randall L, Kalbacher E, Madsen K, Van Nieuwenhuysen E, Gonzalez-Martin A, et al. 40 InnovaTV 301/ENGOT-cx12/GOG-3057: tisotumab vedotin vs investigator{\textquoteright}s choice chemo in second- or third-line recurrent or metastatic cervical cancer. Int J Gynecol Cancer. 2021;31:A1.

MIX
Papier aus verantwortungsvollen Quellen
Paper from responsible sources
FSC® C105338

If you have any concerns about our products,
you can contact us on
ProductSafety@springernature.com

In case Publisher is established outside the EU,
the EU authorized representative is:
Springer Nature Customer Service Center GmbH
Europaplatz 3, 69115 Heidelberg, Germany

Printed by Libri Plureos GmbH
in Hamburg, Germany